SAVE DOGS FROM DISTEMPER

The 'Impossible' Cure of Dr. Alson Sears

Ed Bond

> "Those who say, 'It can't be done,'
> are usually interrupted by others doing it."
> – *Joel Arthur Barker*

Foreword

Dr. Alson Sears,
D.V.M. U.C. Davis '63

Perhaps one individual, primed by education and inclination, will find this material and put it to good use. Eventually, I hope these procedures can be appreciated by as many professionals as possible in the alleviation of pain in canines and other species suffering from the ravishes of morbillivirus.

What I discovered in the late 1960s/early 1970s was a variation on the method to make interferon. I made a mistake, but it was serendipitous. Instead of interferon, we made a material that to this day I have not been able to identify. But the 12-hour Newcastle's Disease Vaccine-induced serum [NDV-induced serum] was able to cure rather than ameliorate previously untreatable diseases, including distemper.

If you Google "distemper virus," you will find page after page on the Internet telling you that acute systemic distemper virus has no cure, and the only treatment possible is supportive. Don't believe this. Within this book, you will find the protocol for an effective treatment for acute infectious distemper. However, the dog must be treated early to get the full effect.

Unfortunately, my attempts to get this out into the world failed. So, after reaching advanced age and having retired some years ago, I decided it was time to record what I discovered. The question of why it worked is the great unknown. In the 1960s and 70s, I had no idea nor could I find out what I had discovered. Today, I have more of an idea from reading scientific journals about new discoveries in the immune system. I am indebted to the library of the University of Utah for access to their library stacks and the journals they had. Information vital to what I was doing was and is critical. The librarians of the LDS Medical Hospital were also instrumental in helping. Thanks to these people for access to the literature.

I am indebted to Ed Bond and J.D. Ward for their interest in keeping this protocol alive after rejection by the guardians of veterinary literature.

This book will cover diagnosis and treatment of canine distemper (CDV): a member of the Paramyxoviridae family, in the morbillivirus genus, as well as the diagnosis and treatment of Old Dog Encephalitis (ODE), which includes chorea, paralysis, seizures, blindness. Notes are available only through kindheartsinaction.com on how the 12-hour NDV induced serum was used to treat a variety of other diseases including herpes, canine influenza and interstitial cystitis. Respiratory herpes virus may mimic distemper, but the serum can also control this disease.

It is my hope that these treatments can further eradicate more diseases from more species. I see no reason that this protocol could not be used in other species infected with morbillivirus diseases. NDV-induced serum from individual species should have the same effect as this serum does in canines. I would suggest that it be tried in humans with measles, Hendra virus and Nipah virus.

A key principle behind the success of these treatments is the need for quick and reliable diagnosis. Diagnosis is extremely important, mainly because you cannot treat what you do not know. There are many lookalike viruses to contend with. Not all respond to NDV-induced serum as distemper does. Vets need to take samples and send them to a lab, but immediately institute treatment to stop acute distemper. To wait is to lose your patient. Reports from the lab may confirm distemper. By the time you get the report, if you had distemper and treated it, the dog will be cured. If not distemper, then you have done no damage. The fastest way to test for distemper without sending off to a lab would be a bladder cell study, which will be explained in Chapter Three.

Websites run by Kind Hearts In Action and Project Hope have been instrumental in not only keeping these protocols alive but in finding veterinarians willing to use them. It seems that the halls of academia are slow to accept techniques developed in the field of clinical practice. For those individuals needing help, please contact one of the named websites for help. God bless and good luck.

– February 2011

> **"Do what you can, with what you have, where you are."**
> – motto made famous by Theodore Roosevelt

Introduction

I don't like dogs dying when they don't have to.

I also don't like giving up if I still have cards to play.

Those are the reasons behind everything I did and why I wrote this book.

This book won't prove Dr. Sears' treatments can save dogs from canine distemper. But it will show that many dogs are dying needlessly.

Rather than proof, I offer a prediction. If his NDV-serum treatment for dogs in the pre-neurologic stage of canine distemper could be put to the test by approved scientific methods, they would dramatically outperform the survival rates of traditional veterinary medicine. The result would be faster recoveries, fewer cases reaching the neurologic stage, a decrease in long-term symptoms and more distemper dogs surviving.

Unfortunately, neither Dr. Sears nor myself have the means to test this hypothesis. He is a retired veterinary clinician who did not get the guidance he needed to present this properly during his career, and I am just an average guy with a computer. You may also learn something about the challenges the veterinary community must overcome to defeat this disease. The first challenge is to realize that distemper has not been defeated.

The title of this book "Save Dogs From Distemper" is not a statement. It is a request, a plea, and an ongoing cause. Somehow the system has broken down, and it needs to be fixed. Dogs are dying all over the world, veterinarians are losing their patients, humans are losing beloved members of their families, and more needs to be done about it. We can save the lives of many of these dogs.

We don't even know how many die because canine distemper is not a reportable disease in most regions. No one is keeping an overall tally of the stats.

The term, canine distemper, strikes terror into the heart of any loving dog owner, and not enough is done to address this terror. More research, education and communication would give dog owners a way to cope with their fears. It would be helpful for dog owners to know how many dogs get distemper, how many survive, and why.

In the accepted literature, the main tools still seem to be vaccination, supportive therapy and euthanasia. Vaccination is absolutely the best first line of defense against this completely preventable – but completely possible and persistent – disease. It is far, far better for dog and owner to avoid this nightmare.

When dogs do get sick, the response from some vets is not always useful, sympathetic or accurate. Too often, I have heard from dog owners who said their vet's first response had been: "We don't know if it's distemper." Or worse, "We won't know until the seizures begin." Or even worse, "It's just kennel cough." If the dog recovers, they may say, "Well, it wasn't distemper." If the dog began neurologic trouble: "Well, nothing to do but euthanize."

If nothing else, I hope this book will demonstrate that dogs in the neurologic stage of distemper do not need to be immediately euthanized. As I often tell the dog owners who write me, distemper is a terrible, nasty, cruel disease that does not play fair. It is not easy to defeat and not every dog can be saved from distemper. But more dogs are saved when their owners and vets are willing to give them a chance to live. Dogs can survive distemper and often enjoy a decent quality of life for years after. For many of the survivors discussed in this book, euthanasia would have usually been the only option available to them.

But I also will never quarrel with an owner who chooses to spare their dog further pain. Sometimes the disease does strike too quickly and with devastating power. Euthanasia is a blessing in those cases. However, we are dangerously ignoring to our need to learn. Researchers still need to help clarify when vets have an active case of distemper on their hands. Some dogs may survive because of their age, genetics or the particular strain of the virus. These factors need to be studied further to determine which treatments increase the chances of survival.

Tragically, today in 2020, the human world has been brought to its knees by the power of a different disease, the novel coronavirus (COVID-19). This virus is unrelated to distemper, and I need to be clear that we do not claim that any of the methods in this book would help against COVID-19. But there are lessons to be learned from the human crisis.

For instance, panic and bad information are the allies of the virus and the tools of the con artist. Someone watching a loved one – human or dog – suffer from a fatal disease is vulnerable. They can become desperate to try any option, pay any price to save that life. It has been distressing to watch the rich and powerful exploit the panic by promoting unproven cures as treatments for COVID-19. Not only does this not save the life of the patient, but the false hope allows the virus to spread. Similarly, I have heard over the years about quick and easy "cures" for canine distemper. But their proponents may not offer any track record or supporting information. In these cases, the strategy seems to bypass or ignore the scientific method. That is not our goal. Our goal is to participate in the scientific method and see the NDV treatments put to the test. When someone writes to me, I try to be honest and realistic. I have no interest in peddling false hope to anyone desperate or vulnerable.

My previous career as a journalist gave me a skeptical approach. As a reporter, I learned that science needs to be done by scientists. So, there is a part of me that understands I should not be involved in this. I am not a veterinarian, a doctor, a scientist or a researcher. I have no standing in the scientific world. I am not an expert. So, no one should listen to what I have to say about canine distemper.

Having said that, however, I have participated in a story, witnessed events and collected information that has overcome my natural skepticism and compelled me to act. I have pragmatic reasons to believe that in the right hands this information could save lives. I do believe there is hope for distemper dogs, and I wrote this book to explain why.

Getting attention for a dog disease that many experts already believe to be solved by vaccination has been difficult. Now that so much of the world's resources are focused on fighting COVID-19, the challenge of finishing the battle against canine distemper becomes that much steeper. So, the timing of the release of this book may not be the best, but during this world crisis, the motto "now or never" motivates me more than before. As Dr. Sears has often said, it may be years before someone picks up these theories and carries them across the finish line, but publishing this book at least puts them on the record in a format that cannot be lost and may be used by some future researcher.

In recent years, I have noticed a shift in approach among shelter vets and rescue groups. More are willing to try to save dogs from this disease and find options to "depopulating" – killing – an entire shelter when an outbreak occurs. This is a welcome change even though many remain skeptical of the NDV treatments.

Even if you do not believe in the "impossible" treatments discovered by Dr. Alson Sears but are at least willing to try anything to give these dogs a chance to live – either as a scientific researcher, veterinary clinician, rescue group or an advocate for dogs – I am grateful. We have something in common. We don't like dogs dying, and we don't give up.

– **Ed Bond**
May 2020

Table of Contents

Finding Galen

The red dog swaggered with the machismo needed to survive on the streets of Los Angeles. If you dared get close enough to look, his tongue hinted at his half-psycho nature. Genetics had stained the back half of the tongue dark blue, like the Chow Chow. The front half showed typical dog-tongue pink. From the length and texture of his fur, plus the flop-over ears, he appeared at least part Labrador. But he had the stocky, muscular build of the Chow Chow, the aggressive breed the ancient Chinese employed in guarding temples.

My sister, Karen Bond, spotted him from the back seat of her friend's SUV as they drove through the intersection of Pico and Alvarado late one afternoon in January 1997. Karen and her friends Steven Schwartz and Casey Hale quickly agreed on a plan of action. Karen and Casey stepped out of the car to stalk the stray while Steven drove to a nearby 7-11 to buy food.

Karen fashioned a rope from the car into a lasso. When Steven returned with a can of cat food, she set the trap.

As Steven and Casey stayed back, Karen pulled the top off the can and set it on the sidewalk, encircled by the lasso. She retreated back to her friends, took hold of the other end of the rope and waited. The smell of wet cat food drew the dog to the bait. When his snout fully engaged, she flipped the rope up and lassoed the red dog around the neck.

They pulled the Chow-Lab into the SUV and slammed the doors shut. Success! But a switch flipped in the dog's head, and he snapped into full Chow Chow mode. He growled and barked and lunged, defending the car as his new territory. "THIS IS MY TEMPLE! STAY AWAY!"

When Steven tried to open his door, the red dog leaped. Quickly, he shut the door to save himself. Same thing happened when Karen tried another door, same again with Casey. The frantic humans ran in circles around the car, each trying a door and each time the dog lunged and barked, teeth snapping. Steven had lost ownership of his SUV to a psycho dog.

Amidst the chaos, Casey tripped on a parking block and face planted onto the pavement. Karen and Steven had no idea where he'd gone until it was over.

As an account executive with AT&T, Karen had experience diving into tough negotiations. She would be the one to leap into the danger zone and end the standoff. As Steven opened a front door, the dog lunged to the front seat, and Karen slid in the back seat with the can of cat food.

"Here! Yumblies!" she called, holding out the can.

He lunged again, but for the cat food. Hunger had won out over fear and aggression. As he sucked up the remainder of the juicy, smelly meat, the anger subsided. His belly appeased, he dropped his head into my sister's lap and ceded ownership of the car.

Capturing the dog had been step one. Step two: find the sweet little psycho a home.

Meeting Amy

On an evening a few days later, my wife, Amy, and I walked through a cobbled courtyard and opened the wooden gate to Karen's patio. This set the canines in her living room on alert. They leapt to their feet before we reached the door. Any knock on the front door of Karen's two-story unit triggered a tornado of barking and twirling fur. We knew this well because we had lived with Karen for a couple of years after moving to Los Angeles from Upstate New York. This evening, the usual three-dog dog tornado at our knock had increased by a fourth dog – the Chow-Lab mix. Karen had mentioned the red dog in passing when I told her we would needed to stop by to borrow money needed to get Amy's car fixed. She also casually mentioned the dog needed a home. After we made our way through the chaos, Amy sat down on the couch where the red dog also settled.

Vaccination – The administration of a dead, weakened or altered version of a microorganism (vaccine) with the intent to trigger the immune system. After a vaccination, the body's immune system should be able to recognize and destroy the full-strength version.

Perhaps dogs have a sense about people. Perhaps he sensed Amy had a place in her heart for another dog. Perhaps he sensed the pain and loss we had been through in the previous year.

Or maybe he just saw an easy mark.

Either way, he knew what to do. First, he placed one paw on Amy's lap, then the other. Then he laid his chin on his paws and gazed up into her eyes. He may have survived on the streets with swagger and aggression, but he'd also picked up a substantial amount of charm. I don't know how Karen had changed him, but this dog was determined to only show us his sweet, gentle side. Amy petted his head and looked up at me with hope and worry in her eyes. Once again, she was falling in love with a stray Karen had found, and she had damn good reason to be wary. Lately, almost every dog Amy had fallen in love with had died.

"Nah," I thought. "It couldn't possibly happen again."

We told Karen we needed time to think. She did not tell us about his psycho side until later.

"You don't have any reservations about him, do you?" Amy asked on the drive home.

"None," I said defiantly.

We were newlyweds – only six months earlier we'd returned to Upstate New York to get married – now living in a Los Angeles rental house with two cats and one very exuberant puppy named Shadow. Perhaps this stray red dog could be a good companion for our puppy?

But we had also just gone through a year of hell with canine distemper, a disease I had not even heard about before moving to California. Where I grew up in New Jersey, and elsewhere in the Northeast, the disease is rare and well controlled by **vaccination**. Most people I have met don't know anything about it and few want to.

"You guys are on restriction," our vet had told us after our second puppy in a row died of distemper. "The next dog you get, I have to approve it."

The next dog was Shadow, who we found at a pet store adoption event. A rescue group had pulled her from a South-Central animal shelter in August and held on to her for a month to make sure she was healthy. Because of her dark, brindled color and pointy ears, they told us she was an Australian Cattle Dog/German shepherd mix. But I wondered whether she had some pit bull in her too.

She was playful and quick to lick Amy. Shadow's tongue snaked out of her mouth like an anteater. You could hold her at arms length and somehow she could twist and stretch enough to smack your face with slobber. If her tongue didn't get you, her tail would. She wagged with the entire back half of her body, thumping anything in range. We called her the half-tongue, half-tail puppy.

Most importantly she met with approval from our vet, who wanted to spare us from any more heartbreak. The weeks it took to get her fully vaccinated were nerve wracking. Until Shadow was fully vaccinated, I didn't let her off our property. And, when I found a foreign deposit on the front lawn from a strange dog, I not only picked it up, but I wrapped the newspaper I picked it up with in a plastic bag. Then I wrapped that bag in another plastic bag. I guess I would have wrapped Shadow in plastic bags if it would have helped.

In December, she got her final vaccination shots, which included the shot for rabies. I clasped the rabies tag in my hand. "Now we have a real dog," I said.

However, our worries had made her the most paranoid animal. Since we had kept her away from other dogs, she didn't know how to play with them. She was high strung and exuberant, and we were getting tired from her constant need for play. We took her to a dog park, but Shadow's social skills were awkward and undeveloped.

"Maybe Shadow needs a friend," Amy caught herself saying on the way home from the park. She slapped her hand over her mouth. Did she just say that? "No, I never said that," she said, laughing. "Never tell me I said that."

Amy had always suspected my secret plan was to flood our home with dogs. After all, she had first-hand experience of Karen and her dog tornado. She knew of our older sister, Jane in western New Jersey, who also had three dogs and multiple cats. She also knew that we had grown up in a house on the Jersey Shore with a constant menagerie of dogs, cats, hamsters, etc.

Amy's family also had dogs and cats, but not as fanatically as mine. Amy grew up as the youngest of eight kids in Horseheads, N.Y. Her father worked for the phone company as a lineman, and her mother was a nurse. They raised their kids to be practical and to love each other. I met Amy in the newsroom of the Star-Gazette in Elmira, N.Y., where I had been a reporter. Amy was the newsroom assistant, and the first time I saw her she stormed out of the editor's office. Tall, with short-cropped, brunette hair, she strode quickly and with determination. I came to an immediate conclusion. "Boy, she's pissed."

But along with her determination came a sense of humor and pragmatism that would carry us through many adventures. Breaking down in the middle of Nebraska the first time we drove to Los Angeles, finding work in a new city and living through the Northridge Earthquake gave our relationship a resiliency we would need in our next challenges. We made accommodations for each other. Because she knew I'd like it, Amy grew out her hair. I resolved not to bring home strays without her approval.

By now, Amy worked at a company in Sherman Oaks called WITI that advocated for stronger roles for women in technology. At night, she bartended at an upscale restaurant near the intersection of La Brea and Third. Meanwhile, I was a full-time, freelance reporter for the Los Angeles Times-Valley Edition and taught journalism classes at two community colleges.

Sometimes I would tease her about my love for dogs. We'd be driving around Los Angeles, when I would announce, "Oh look! A dog! I think it needs a home!" To which Amy would reply, "Uh, no. It's on a leash ... with its owner."

Still, we agreed Shadow needed a friend. So, Karen's rescue of the red dog seemed serendipitous. The red dog also already had our vet's approval. Karen went to the same vet we did, and she'd already checked over this Chow-Lab and given him a clean bill of health. The red dog had survived into adulthood and was not a young, unvaccinated puppy with a developing immune system. The risks seemed minimal. We trusted our vet because we knew how protective she was of us. Maybe this could be the canine friend Shadow needed?

Karen brought the red dog to visit Shadow at our house on the next Saturday afternoon. We took the dogs out to the small yard out back bordered by a cinderblock wall and punctuated with a lemon tree. Shadow, a 6-month-old puppy, was already even in height with the new dog. She was boisterous and playful. He was older, just as strong and just as willing to get into a tumble. They played a constant game of wrestling with their mouths and teeth. They reached a balance, an instant friendship.

That satisfied everyone. Karen left the red dog with us.

"How do you keep doing this to me?" Amy asked.

"What did I do?" I asked innocently.

"Look, now we have two cats and two dogs. How did that happen?"

Only through mutual agreement, I reminded her.

A load of bad memories

We decided "red dog," as Karen had named him, needed a better moniker. So far, the dog had only shown us a sweet, gentle side, so we named him Galen, which means calm in Gaelic. But as he settled into the house, Galen taught Shadow his view of the world. He didn't like the cats, and Galen showed Shadow how to chase them. We put up a baby gate in the bedroom doorway to create "Cat Switzerland" in the back half of the one-story house where Stevenson and Seneca could find safe refuge.

One night, I heard Galen coughing.

It was familiar.

Too familiar.

In the next couple of days, we watched him carefully. His eyelids became heavy. The nose dried up and filled with snot. We had him tested for canine distemper, our old enemy. "If anything happens to Shadow," Amy said. "I'll never forgive myself."

We hadn't recognized the early symptoms of distemper with our first puppy, Tug. Neither did our vet. Tug McDog had been a throwaway dog, an eight-week old shepherd-mix pup with fur ravaged by mange. Karen had found her in the women's restroom at the Farmer's Market, a popular tourist destination at the corner of Third and Fairfax.

"I just don't know about this," Amy said as we watched an exhausted puppy walk in circles around Karen's courtyard that evening. This had been about six months before we got married and moved into the rental house. We were then living in a one-bedroom apartment near Los Angeles International Airport.

"We'll try it for a week and see what happens," I said. We kept her for her lifetime. As she rested, ate and adjusted to life with us, the real puppy emerged. We treated her mange and gave her oatmeal baths to restore her coat. With her pointed ears, she was clearly a shepherd-mix, mostly black, with tan legs. Her face was black with tan on either side of her snout and tan eyebrows above her eyes. As we walked, I would spin the leash in front of her. She would catch it and tug back. That's how she got the name Tug.

Then one day, Amy surprised me. "You really picked a great dog," she said. That morning, she brought Tug back to the apartment after a walk, but before they could get inside, the puppy plopped on the concrete patio in protest, refusing to budge.

"It was as if she was saying, 'You know you are forgetting something, aren't you?' " Amy said. Then she remembered the squeaky toy in her pocket. The two of them played for about 15 minutes. Tug chased the toy in and around Amy's legs. "I love this dog," she declared.

Tug had a sniffle, but it didn't worry us. The vet diagnosed it as kennel cough, a harmless bacterial infection. We didn't realize it was canine distemper until the seizures began. We fought to save her life for three weeks, giving her 24-hour nursing care, bottle-feeding, diapering, and administering seizure-control medications. Finally, she died at the vet clinic. We went to bed exhausted and defeated that night. "I'll never give my heart to another animal like that," Amy said.

Within minutes of adopting our second puppy – this time from a rescue group – I was in an examining room presenting her to our vet. Our vet checked over Selkie, an all-black Lab-shepherd mix with flop-over ears. She gave her the usual shots and tests, then shrugged. "Feed her and love her," she said. A few days later the coughing began. She developed a fever. We had her tested again for distemper. She'd been tested before and was declared healthy. A second test may have been pointless, since the earlier vaccination may have thrown off the results.

Antibodies – Proteins in the blood that can attach themselves to attacking foreign bodies such as bacteria, viruses and other pathogens.

Distemper tests check the blood for levels of **antibodies** to the virus, not the virus itself. After vaccination, it becomes difficult for vets to tell whether the distemper antibodies are from the vaccine or from the contagious "hot" version of the virus. But a dog already exposed to the "hot" version before the vaccination could still get sick.

All we could do was wait. We put aside the fear for the worst and did what we could to boost her immune system. At least that might help her with the kennel cough — or whatever that constant coughing was. We called her "The amazing coughing dog." A local animal group recommended a diet of vegetables and raw lamb. I chopped vegetables for hours, but Selkie wouldn't eat the special food.

Then, as Amy drove to work with Selkie, the puppy's mouth snarled, smacked and drooled with foam. Vets call this a chewing gum seizure because the dog looks like it is munching on a stick of gum. Amy immediately turned the car around and headed to the vet's office. When I got to the exam room, our vet was very direct. She told us we should consider putting her to sleep. "I can't do that," Amy said, crying. "Not while she's still with us."

We didn't get much of a choice. Two nights later, we put her in the tub to clean the mucous and saliva from her fur. The cool water triggered an unstoppable seizure. Her teeth clenched, the gums flared, and her head thrashed back and forth, spraying saliva. We pulled her out. It didn't stop after we got her out of the bath. It didn't stop after we dried her off. It didn't stop to let us get her evening medication into her. We could only drip a drop or two into her mouth as her head jerked side to side, throwing spit.

Our friend Margaret Owens happened to stop by that night. A local singer and songwriter, she waited tables at the same restaurant where Amy bartended. She helped us see the truth. "It's not fair to her anymore," she told us.

Our vet had already closed for the night. We could not wait until morning, so we flipped through the phone book. Just before midnight, we climbed into the back of Margaret's four-wheel drive and she drove us to an emergency veterinary hospital on Sepulveda near Westwood. The vet on duty euthanized Selkie early on the morning of my 31st birthday.

So, Galen's coughing set off alarm bells for us. When Amy called from the vet's office to tell me Galen had been confirmed with distemper, we both knew what it meant. No federal agency tracks distemper cases so there was no way to know whether our misfortune was unique among dog owners. The possible odds of one couple dealing with three unrelated distemper cases within a year still left us numb.

Numb like a tractor-trailer hitting you with a load of bad memories. They jumble together in my mind … Tug in a cage at the vet clinic, drawing herself up on her front paws – despite the heavy load of drugs – to try to say hello, to say that she still loved us … Carrying Tug unconscious in a basket everywhere we went, including a viewing party for an episode of "Star Trek: Voyager" I'd co-written with my best friend, Jeff Schnaufer … Sitting in the waiting room at the emergency vet, watching a terrible episode of classic "Star Trek," while Selkie sprayed spit back and forth during that last unstoppable seizure … The odd experience of watching our calm puppy return as the euthanol stopped Selkie's heart … Seeing how much Tug had grown during her three-week illness as she lay dead on the cold, metal exam table. She looked more like an adult dog than I realized.

I remembered early on in Tug's illness – before the seizures – wrapping little pills of antibiotics in pieces of bread for her. She learned to sit quickly, as if to tell us, "I will sit because I love you." With Selkie, we had to force her mouth open and toss them down her gullet. But antibiotics have no effect against distemper. **Antibiotics** fight bacteria and do nothing against viruses.

Still in the early stage of the disease, Galen's cough progressed. The pads of his feet cracked like a dry lakebed. His nose dried up too. His eyelids bunched up and weighed heavily. Overall, he looked haggard and uncomfortable. Beyond those symptoms we could easily see, the virus most likely could have been attacking any of Galen's organs, causing damage we didn't even know about. But we knew what the next terrible stage would be. We'd seen it twice before.

Expecting the neurologic stage

Tug's first seizure happened at WITI, where she had become the office puppy. Tug had to be taken to a nearby vet we didn't know in Studio City. He diagnosed her with distemper the next day. But we could not bear to euthanize her.

Antibiotic – A material that can destroy or inhibit bacteria.

So, that afternoon, he handed us three prescription bottles: Phenobarbital, to controls seizures; Valium, to also ease seizures and reduce anxiety; **Antibiotics**, which also had to be taken every 12 hours to hopefully block those bacterial infections. This is the standard supportive therapy prescribed by veterinarians, based on the prevailing doctrine that nothing can be done against the distemper virus. There is no cure for canine distemper; at least that was the commonly held belief of the veterinary community. However, we were told a few rare dogs somehow survive it. This was the slim ledge of hope to which we clung.

"In about a week, she'll either get better," the vet said as we left. "Or the seizures will get worse."

A blonde-haired young man handed Tug to us through a back door. The muscles in Tug's head bulged stiffly. Saliva drained from her mouth, and snot and mucous coated the fur on her chest. I wrapped Tug in a blue towel as he put her into my arms. Then I placed her on Amy's lap after she got into the passenger seat of my Honda Civic hatchback. Throughout the long rush hour drive home in the sunset traffic on the 405 – over the hills separating the San Fernando Valley from the rest of Los Angeles – we took turns talking to her. "Good girl, Tug. You're going to be OK, Tug." But I couldn't get a good look at her as I drove. "How's she doing?" I asked. Amy shook her head grimly.

The struggle to save Tug had moments of false hope. One night, I dozed on our couch while Amy worked late at her bartending job. Tug lay in a basket on the floor, unconscious from a combination of seizures, Phenobarbital, and Valium. She had been like this for days. At about 12:30 a.m., something jarred my arm. I woke up. Tug jumped at my arm again. Then she cried. She was awake and had to go outside. Quickly, I grabbed her leash, hooked her up and took her to the front of the apartment building. Our puppy was back!

She staggered to one side or the other as she walked. Her legs wobbled when she stopped to pee. Back in the apartment, she kept walking. Making use of my best chance to feed her, I squirted a highly blended mixture of dog food and Pedialyte into her mouth with a syringe. Then I would follow that with a squirt of water. Tug and I kept that up for another hour, until Amy got home from her bartending job. "You're going to get better," I told Tug. "You're going to be playing on the beach with us real soon."

But in the following days, she returned to being mostly unconscious. The seizures did not get worse, just persistent, a gentle throbbing of the muscles in the top of her head as she slept. We learned that seizures are not painful. The puppy is just unconscious and unaware of her surroundings. Since she didn't seem to be in pain, we felt comfortable continuing the nursing care, but we lost a lot of sleep. The next couple of weeks were a blur of medications, checking to see whether she was seizing or just breathing heavily. Sometimes we weren't sure she was still breathing. Eventually, we could no longer keep her going. Neither could our vet after we had her hospitalized. But the vet and her clinic staff kept trying right up until Tug died.

Searching for options

Tug and Selkie were cremated. In separate ceremonies about three months apart, we scattered their ashes on the beach in Playa del Rey, a favorite spot to take them to play. Our fight to save their lives might have been futile, except it was because we fought so hard to save their lives we found the way to save Galen.

Our regular vet had been supportive of our fight to save Tug from the very beginning. She was willing to try any treatments such as acupuncture and vitamin C. These didn't help, but as Tug's battle went into the later stages, she kept looking for other options. Then, she remembered there was a vet who had some sort of unconventional treatment to save dogs from distemper. She didn't have the details but understood it had something to do with a blood transfusion. With our permission, she tried a transfusion of a distemper survivor's blood into Tug. This transfusion didn't help, but that was the first time I heard about Dr. Alson Sears of Lancaster, California.

The second time I heard about Dr. Sears was when Selkie started having seizures, when our vet told us we should consider euthanasia. Just then, another seizure hit Selkie, and her mouth locked into a twisted snarl. The vet picked up her front paw and pressed her thumb to its side, an acupressure technique that relieved the seizure. That's when I remembered Dr. Sears. "Who was this vet you told us about?" I asked. "The one up in Lancaster?"

They gave me the number for his clinic, and I called after we got Selkie home. A male voice answered, not Dr. Sears, but an assistant. I explained we had a distemper puppy with seizures. They had a serum treatment for distemper, he told me, but it would not help a distemper dog once the seizures started. I thanked him and hung up. We were too late to save Selkie.

> **Serum** – What remains when blood cells are removed from blood. The liquid usually has a yellowish tint from the fats present.

But maybe we weren't too late to save Galen? He hadn't had any seizures yet. I didn't know how Dr. Sears' **serum** – just blood without blood cells – could save a distemper dog, but there was one way to find out more. Amy asked our vet if we should take Galen to this Dr. Sears. "She said that wouldn't be a bad idea," Amy told me. But Lancaster is an hour north of Los Angeles, and with our work schedules, we couldn't get him there.

Taking a chance

Lancaster, California, could be described as the exact opposite of its namesake, Lancaster, Pennsylvania, famous for its lush, green Amish farmland. Getting to the California Lancaster – the bedroom community for Edwards Air Force Base – requires a long, hot drive into the desert of the Antelope Valley. The temperatures readily climb above 100 degrees. When Lancaster gets the rare brief rain shower, you can still kick the thin layer of wet dirt on the surface and find plenty of dusty, dry sand underneath. So, bring along extra water for the trip.

Karen volunteered to drive Galen up to Dr. Sears' clinic.

That night before Galen left, Amy and I sat with him in the home office in the back of the house where we kept him away from Shadow. This had been part of "Cat Switzerland." It was now a slap-dash isolation ward. If Shadow had not been fully vaccinated, she probably could have been in danger of infection. We petted Galen, scratched his head and took a few pictures. We had not had a chance yet to take any photos of him. We were saying good-bye.

The next day, Karen drove Galen to Lancaster. He threw up on the backseat. "I was so upset," Karen told me later. "I thought I was going to take him up there and he was going to die there."

That weekend, Shadow sulked. Galen was missing, and she knew something was terribly wrong.

Two days later, on a Sunday, I had to work but Amy went with Karen to pick up Galen from Dr. Sears' clinic. I was home when they pulled into the driveway at the side of the house and brought Galen through the gate into the backyard. He was breathing, walking, tail wagging. Strong. He wasn't cremated and scattered on a beach, not comatose or seizing, all qualities I prefer in dogs.

Shadow launched herself through the dog door into the backyard and gleefully welcomed her friend. In the ensuing chaos, Karen and Amy explained the virus had been turned off, according to Dr. Sears. However, the distemper had probably already done damage, possibly to the stomach, the lungs, most definitely the eyes, the skin on the pads of the feet and the nose.

Distemper attacks the tear ducts, shutting them down, making it difficult for the eyes to naturally rewet themselves. Along with treatments of liquid vitamin A on the pads of the feet and on Galen's nose, we also had to put ointment directly onto Galen's dry eyeballs.

Amy held Galen still, as Karen – who possesses a notable talent for these things, and a special relationship with Galen as his original rescuer – started to apply the ointment. My job was just to hold Shadow. But she broke free from me, and with front legs outstretched, she threw herself bodily against Galen. About the closest a dog could come to giving a bear hug, as if to say, "HOORAYYY!! Welcome home!"

We kept up the treatments for a couple of weeks. He hated the eye ointments and nose creams, so we had to put a muzzle on his snout. As we approached with the ointments, he would growl in protest, a low, threatening GRRRRRRR!

We watched him carefully, wondering whether a smacking of chops was a preliminary chewing gum seizure. But no, we finally realized, he was just smacking his chops.

As the fears subsided and our lives settled down into a happy home with two dogs and two cats, my journalistic curiosity rose up. I asked myself some questions.

If canine distemper is fatal, why is Galen alive?

If this Dr. Sears has a cure for this fatal disease, why aren't other vets using his treatment?

The story of an unknown veterinarian with a dramatic cure for a terrible, fatal dog disease intrigued me. I wanted to know more about him and where he came from. This could be a good story for the newspaper. However, I had two problems. Much as I enjoyed working as a full-time freelancer at the L.A. Times, my four-year career there was coming to an end. I was very close to being hired by L.A. Valley College in Van Nuys to teach journalism full time.

The other problem? Dr. Alson Sears was not returning my phone calls.

Meeting Dr. Sears

"Get me out of this," Dr. Sears told his wife, Ruth, when he heard the *L.A. Times* reporter was on the line again. "I just don't want to go out there again."

Newspaper reporters expect to have some phone calls dodged by potential sources. But since I'd taken over the "Personal Best" column at the *Times'-San Fernando Valley Edition* about the unsung heroes of the community, I'd become accustomed to having people call back quickly. Piles of letters, press packets, and notes on leads cluttered my desk. I kept track of tips and lists of people to track down, crossing them off as they either came through for a column or didn't pan out. These were mostly feel-good stories about people making the world a better place. Firefighters, police officers, addiction counselors, literacy volunteers, teachers, kids raising money for a cause, advocates for the homeless and many more had made their way into my columns.

I had no doubt Dr. Alson Sears had made our lives better by saving Galen. However, by now we had learned Galen's name – "calm" in Gaelic – had been an ironic choice. Distemper had dampened his aggressive side when he joined our family. After he recovered, the Chow Chow inside the sweet little psycho emerged.

He attacked the cats; Stevenson stood his ground and Seneca kept her distance in "Cat Switzerland." He barked and lunged at the front bay window whenever anyone walked by the house. When we took him to his first and last obedience class, he bit the trainer as she leaned over to pet him. He also once bit me on the hand. Another trainer came to the house and helped us unravel the problems. She taught us his time on the streets forced him to use a different kind of language, and we'd been misunderstanding his signals. We learned when he wagged his tail, it didn't signal happiness. It meant confident, as in "macho" or "I know I can kick your ass." Eventually, we learned his triggers, and he learned our rules. The sweet little psycho dog found a home.

Now, months after he was saved from distemper, I still wanted to know how it happened. The name Dr. Al Sears had reached the top of my list of column prospects a couple of times. But each time, my call went unanswered. I didn't see why a vet with a treatment for a terrible disease hadn't called back. So, I called again, and this time Ruth got on the phone to get him out of it.

Ruth Sears, who was also the clinic office manager, was very resistant to letting her husband talk to a reporter. She didn't want to see facts twisted, didn't want to see her husband turned into something he wasn't. Nearly 20 years earlier, the clinic had survived a lawsuit over a parvovirus case. They won the case, but at a lot of expense. The stinging memory was still fresh in her mind. Someone calling back about a case they had treated might mean bad news.

I claim no skill for manipulation. My approach in gathering information has simply been genuine curiosity. When I let the potential source know I honestly wanted to know their side of the story, I often succeeded. "Be an empty bucket and let them fill you with information," was the lesson I remembered about successful interviews. When someone resisted an interview, I'd usually point out that this was his or her opportunity to get on the record. Why not take advantage of it? Usually it worked.

But Ruth didn't want to see him hurt. She worried I might try to play him up as something he was not. I told her I didn't want that. "I just want to write this story about how he saved my dog," I said. Ruth put me on the phone with her husband. We set up the interview for the following week, late June.

Origins

The day of the interview, I drove up to Lancaster in time for lunch. The Sears Veterinary Clinic was a one-story building with a clean white lobby then overseen by Mitchell, a grey and white cat. He'd been dropped off by a client who never came back. He became the office cat and an unofficial greeter.

A big, friendly man in his early 60s with a full head of white hair came out to the lobby. He held out his hand. "Call me Al," he said as we shook hands. He employs a direct, country-wisdom when he talks, often punctuated with humor and a deep belly laugh.

This began an association with Dr. Sears that would outlast my relationship with the *Los Angeles Times*, my career in journalism, our residency in California, and even Galen's lifespan. Meeting Dr. Sears changed my life in ways neither of us would have expected. Either out of an abundance of politeness or a desire to give him respect, I still call him "Dr. Sears."

As he drove Ruth and I to their country club for lunch, I told him about Tug and her early symptoms. "There must have been something I missed," I said.

"You can't tell the difference between a real bad case of kennel cough and a mild case of distemper," Dr. Sears said. During distemper outbreaks in the 1960s, "we were losing ten dogs a week," he said. But now that vaccination had become common, Galen was the first distemper case he had seen in at least six years.

"The key to the whole thing is to turn the virus off," he said.

As we waited to order lunch at the country club, I told him more about the three cases of distemper Amy and I had gone through, and how rattled it left us. Dr. Sears listened to my story of worry and paranoia politely, and then he snorted.

"Try having kids," he said.

Al and Ruth Sears have three children, two sons and a daughter. They were all born while Al studied at veterinary school at U.C. Davis in Northern California from 1958 to 1963. Their first boy – Alson Jr. or "Skip" – had been born during his first year. Their daughter Patricia was born the following year, and their youngest son, Michael, was born in Al's last year at school. When Ruth went into labor with Michael, she had to call the school three times to get Al to come home. "I think I was in a very interesting small animal class," Al said. "It's very important that you don't miss very much in the way of clinical experience."

A bad cut to the hand brought them together. In 1957, the fall of his senior year at the University of Pennsylvania, Al sliced his palm as he pulled the top off a canned ham. He knew nurses lived in the building adjoining his apartment. So, he went over and knocked on a door and found Ruth, an RN going for her bachelor's degree.

"I looked at the cut and I was sort of smirking because it wasn't very big," Ruth said. "And then I looked at him. He was this great big tall, skinny kid. And I realized, 'Oh my gosh, he's going to faint!' So, I pulled him in, sat him down on the toilet and had him put his head between his legs, and that was our meeting."

Al kept a rabbit that ran loose in his apartment. "I thought if he ever looked at me the way he looked at that rabbit, it would be great," Ruth said. At 6 foot 1, his height made it a challenge for her to see him all at once.

"My mother wanted to know what color his hair was and I had only looked at his eyes and his eyebrows, which were white," Ruth said. The top of her head goes to about as high as Al's eyes. "And I said he was blonde. But he really wasn't. He had dark hair. My mother, when she saw him said, 'He's not blond.' But I'd only looked at his eyes. ... Oh, he had a red beard. And when it was time for me to take him home to meet my parents, I begged him to shave the beard off, which of course he did not."

He finally did, the day after he met her parents.

By March, Al gave Ruth his old fraternity pin. "It's a promise to be promised," Ruth says. "My father wanted to make sure I knew the difference between a proposal and a proposition."

The "pinning" meant that there was someone significant in her life, so she could turn down dates from anyone else.

"I thought she was pretty neat," Al says with a laugh. "Especially the fact that she was a nurse who could take care of me when I was wounded."

Al still faints at the sight of human blood even though he had been able to handle the ugliest of animal wounds as a teenager growing up in the Panama Canal Zone. In high school, he volunteered at veterinary clinics in the afternoons or on weekends. "It was my dream to do exactly what they were doing," Al said. "Of course, they would give me the nasty jobs like cleaning out rotten infected feet, which I did. In the tropics, if you get a cut, chances are you're going to get gangrene. It's a rotten infection of tissue that smells to high heaven and is full of pus and putrefying flesh. And the job is to clean all that out. You hold your nose while you're doing it and hope you don't throw up. But that was the jobs they gave to me. I think they were testing my mettle, to see if I really wanted to be a veterinarian, and I did it. I did what had to be done."

His family moved to New York City as he graduated from high school, and the University of Pennsylvania readily accepted him as an undergraduate. But he had always dreamed of going to school in California, which is where his parents had met. They had grown up on separate sides of the Panama Canal and met during college. His mother went to Stanford, and his father attended Berkeley.

After graduating from Penn, Al married Ruth in New York City in 1958. They drove cross-country to Berkeley, where they put a deposit down on an apartment before Al went to register as a student. But when they showed up at Berkeley's admissions office, they found out they had no veterinary school. The Sears had to cancel the apartment in Berkeley and head to U.C. Davis, about an hour and half north.

After graduating and passing the veterinary boards in 1963, an interest in cats drew the freshly minted Dr. Alson Sears down to Southern California.

"I really thought they were a great species, and there were a few specialists out there who were doing work, research type, clinical work," Al says. "And I thought that would be a great place to be."

But as it turned out the vet he had joined in Pasadena was not so much a cat expert but just a dairy practitioner who didn't like working with cows, who then switched to small animals and found out he was afraid of dogs. "So, he opened a cat practice and he really didn't know a hell of a lot about them," Al says. "It didn't take me long to figure that out."

When Ruth arrived in Pasadena with the kids, after spending the summer on the beach with her family in New Jersey, they discovered another problem. "What's wrong with the children?" she asked. "They're all crying and their eyes look terrible." The Pasadena smog had affected them.

The other vet had Al perform all the surgeries, but they didn't get along. Al knew he was either going to quit or be fired. He searched for other options, and visited three other vets in Southern California, including one in Lancaster who he liked named Dr. Bill Zontine. But he also considered moving back to Panama to work with cattle. Panama had been a paradise for Al in his childhood. "The Canal Zone was a garden with flowers and fruit and green grass and beautiful boulevards and royal palms and government buildings," he says. "It was a little piece of heaven." But when he returned to visit the hospitals where he volunteered as a teen, he was told there was no reason to come back because the United States would eventually be handing the Canal Zone over to Panama. He called Ruth. "I guess we're going to go to Lancaster. Don't go without me."

"Which translated to, he was worried if I saw it I would say, 'Not a chance.'" Ruth says. "Of course I packed the kids up in the car and went up there. Tumbleweeds were rolling across the road, and it was a dustbowl as far as I was concerned. But wherever he went, I was going."

They moved to Lancaster in November 1963, the same week as the John F. Kennedy assassination. Bill Zontine told Al, "I've got a large animal practice you can have. You can understudy me and take care of my emergency calls and my weekend calls and you can have the large animal part."

Taking over the large animal part of Bill Zontine's practice meant caring for about five horse herds and about six dairy and beef herds. A lot of wealthy people had ranches in the area: racehorse, quarter horse and draft horse ranches. At that time, Lancaster was also known for alfalfa and poultry farms. Electricity and pumps delivered water from the aquifer 300 feet below the Antelope Valley to the alfalfa fields, which fed the local herds and also dairy farms in Los Angeles.

Al Sears enjoyed working with the herds. "To go out and look at cases and try to help them, that was what it was all about," Al says. "I was a young vet full of enthusiasm and was more than willing to use the training I had."

They put together broken bones for animals injured in auto accidents, sutured wounds, treated scrapes, scratches and ulcers. "As I look back on it, Bill Zontine was probably one of the finest practitioners that I ever, ever had an association with or got a chance to see at work," Al says.

In the 60s, veterinarians didn't have access to the lab tests they have today. Bill Zontine gave Al Sears indispensible diagnosis training using "touch, feel, smell and see what you can do."

"He could look at an animal and within seconds have an idea where to go to get the diagnosis," Al says. "That is what he was able to teach, and I have been forever grateful. Because even though you know everything in the books and you know every disease that exists at that time, putting it together with an animal that walks in and gets plopped on the table in front of you is pretty tough to do. But there's an instinct that goes with it that you develop after a bunch of years in practice."

The best advice Bill Zontine gave was to "work hard, learn as much as you can, practice, and remember it ... See as many cases as you can and learn what the outcomes of what you do are. That's what medicine is all about. The idea of medicine is to reduce pain and suffering and try to save lives as best you can."

But they had few tools to combat disease, especially viral diseases, which were difficult to diagnose and impossible to treat. When Al started in Lancaster, they would often discover which disease had attacked the animal only after the patient died. "We could vaccinate and prevent," Al says. "But we couldn't treat."

Even though vaccinations were available against rabies and distemper, about half the animals in the Antelope Valley were not vaccinated. About 1 in 5 of the cases that walked in door were viral diseases. "So we had a large pool of susceptible animals that were constantly getting ill, and these were ones that we were frustrated with," Al says.

Many of the farming clients didn't vaccinate and didn't even spay their animals. "We don't believe in spaying dogs," they would tell Al. How about vaccinating? " 'Oh no, we don't vaccinate. When I was a kid, we used to shoot 'em if they got sick, and we'll do the same with this one.' Welcome to the desert. We ran into that attitude all the time."

By 1969, Al had his own small, cramped storefront practice, and the Antelope Valley had become a dramatically different region. Within his first couple of years in Lancaster, the price of electricity had jumped. So, pumps could not draw water from the aquifer to irrigate the alfalfa. Without alfalfa to feed the horses and cows and sheep, the herds disappeared. The agricultural clients withdrew into the minority, replaced by a very different clientele.

Lancaster also served as the bedroom community for Edwards Air Force Base and Plant 42, an Air Force manufacturing site. In the 60s, the race for the moon was on, and more and more pilots, astronauts, scientists, and engineers moved into town. Rockets from the moon program – and later the space shuttle program – would light up the entire valley at night. "The whole place went from primitive backyard farming to suburban within a year," Al says. "It was really a glorious thing to live through."

The discovery

With the new clients – and their kids who were all "little geniuses" – Al Sears had switched from large animals, such as cows and horses, to small companion animals like dogs and cats. The major dog disease he faced in his storefront clinic was distemper. At first, Al followed the officially sanctioned treatment for distemper – fluids, antibiotics, and watching them die.

"Most of the dogs that came in with distemper died." Al says. "We're talking many, many, many boxes of dead dogs. Those that did survive went on to see horrible secondary neurologic problems from which many lingered and eventually died. Once sick, there did not seem to be much that could be done to help them."

Al Sears voraciously read everything he could on treating the disease. Although as a student he had no interest in joining the research side of the profession, he still had an endless curiosity about the advancements reported in medical and veterinary journals. One of his major sources of information was the *Journal of the American Animal Hospital Association*.

"His office wasn't big," remembers Chuck Whitt, Al Sears' longtime assistant. "But it was totally full of journals and veterinary books and whenever the new veterinary books would come out and therapies would come out, he would buy them and he would read constantly, just all the time."

When Chuck would visit Al at home, he would notice the journals stacked around his reading chair and all over the house. "He read at night, at home, before he went to bed," Chuck says. "He wasn't a typical TV watcher. He would read journals."

His collection of veterinary and medical journals only got bigger throughout the years and filled any available space. Chuck remembers that when they built shelves in the X-ray room, Al said, "That would be a good place for my journals." His collection later expanded into an outside storage shed.

Al's memory and mental sharpness impressed Chuck. He knew where each article was. Whenever he needed one, he'd call on Chuck to go get it.

"That was always fun to go back and dig out different journals and different articles for him," Chuck said. "He would use them in different cases. A case would come up, and he would remember something about reading something, and he would remember the date and the year of the journal."

And he would remember where it had been stored.

Al Sears tried every procedure he could find against distemper, ranging from simple to complex to bizarre: large and small amounts of vitamin C, Chinese herbs, acupuncture, aromatherapy, skim milk injections, plus Ribavirin, Acyclovir, Vidarabine and Levamisole. One technique called for having the dog breathe ether for 24 hours while unconscious.

None worked.

He guesses at least 90 percent of the distemper dogs he treated in those early days died. A small number lived. This had been the small ledge of hope that Amy and I clung to while fighting to save Tug and Selkie. Most dogs die from distemper, a few live. Dr. Sears attributes their survival to genetics and the strength of a particular dog's immune system. "But we were rather frustrated with this disease because we were seeing a lot of death and a lot of unhappy owners," Al says.

Interferon – A protein made by immune cells that inhibits the replication of viruses and some cancers.

Inducer – A microbe such as a virus or bacteria that prompts a cell to create interferon or other desired effect.

NDV – Newcastle's Disease Vaccine.

Meanwhile, a friend had a yacht who invited Al to join him on excursions to the islands off the California coast. Al learned to scuba dive. "I always took reading material because there was a lot of laying around time."

One weekend in late 1960s/early 1970s, they took the boat to Santa Barbara, and Al ended up sitting on the seawall near the Pacific Coast Highway. He took out a pamphlet from the *Journal of the American Animal Hospital Association* and read an article that gave him a flash of insight.

The article described an experiment in which cats were given injections of Newcastle's Disease Vaccine (NDV), which is used to inoculate chickens against this disease, but also was known to prompt interferon production in mammals. NDV in cats had not been studied before, and the article reported the cats showed significant increase in interferon levels after an NDV injection. "It clicked in my head that this might work against distemper," Al Sears says. "I thought, 'Damn, if it works in cats, here's a viral technique we haven't tried.'"

Interferons are proteins made by immune cells to inhibit the replication of some viruses. Al Sears had been an undergraduate at Penn when the first paper on interferon was published in 1957. Sitting there on that seawall in Santa Barbara, Al Sears decided to make canine interferon using Newcastle's Disease Vaccine, a bird-disease virus.

When he got back to his storefront clinic, Al needed two things: a healthy dog and NDV. They borrowed the healthy dog from the local shelter. This was before rules were changed to prevent using shelter dogs for such a procedure.

Fortunately, of the half-dozen materials used to make interferon, NDV is also the cheapest and readily available. He just went down to the local agricultural store – which supplied chicken ranches – and bought a box off the shelf. A box of six bottles of the La Sota strain of NDV cost $10.

After injecting about 2 to 3ccs of NDV into a vein of the healthy shelter dog, Al waited until the next day to collect serum from the dog. The dog was anesthetized and placed on a splint designed to hold it on its back on a surgical table. An IV was set up to keep fluids going into the dog's body. They shaved the neck and inserted a catheter into the jugular vein to withdraw blood into vials.

Serum is blood without the blood cells. To separate the blood serum from the blood cells, the vials of blood are placed in a centrifuge that spins them like a mini-carnival ride. Physics sends the heavier red blood cells to the bottom of the tube, leaving the serum at the top where it can be easily collected. Blood serum can be transferred from one animal to another without problems, so long as they are the same species and the serum contains no red blood cells. In theory, whatever disease-fighting material Al had created with the NDV injection was now floating in the serum of the donor dog.

"But there was a hitch, which at the time we didn't recognize," Al says. "Time."

He had done all of this without realizing the journal article on interferon he was trying to follow had called for the serum to be withdrawn 6 to 8 hours after the injection. Dr. Al Sears had waited 11½ to 12 hours.

"I pulled it off at the time I thought was appropriate," Al says. "What did I know? We'd never done this before."

Looking back, he calls the change in timing serendipity. Perhaps, it was a happy accident of science. "Some mistakes are beneficial and some mistakes are not," Al says. "In this case, the mistake was hugely beneficial."

Acute phase – When the symptoms of the disease last for a short period of time, as opposed to the chronic phase, where symptoms persist long-term. In distemper, the respiratory symptoms are acute. The neurologic symptoms can often be chronic.

Subcutaneous injection – An injection made just below the skin, as opposed to a vein. Frequently referred to as "sub-Q."

They returned the blood-serum donor dog to the shelter, unharmed, and stored the vials of serum in the clinic's refrigerator. Al sent a sample to Cornell University and asked them to check whether it contained interferon. Now, he had to wait.

Four days later, a client brought in a canine distemper case, a 6- to 8-month-old shepherd-lab mix that had never been vaccinated.

"He came in with a real nice **acute** case," Al says. "One of the classics, you know. You get a high fever. He had a little diarrhea and vomiting and a runny nose, gooped up eyes, and a cracked nose. He was just a classic."

Without time to get the response from Cornell, Al didn't know whether the serum in his refrigerator had interferon. But he had a patient likely to die without treatment, and he needed to know whether this material worked.

Late that afternoon, he injected the serum into his patient "sub-Q," shorthand for **subcutaneous**, meaning the needle slid just under the skin to make its delivery. "There was no reason to give interferon in any other way," Al says. "It was just a matter of getting it into the body is all. As long as you got it in the body, it would absorb."

They put their patient back into its cage for the night. "I figured, 'We'll see,' " Al says.

When Chuck and Al returned in the morning, the dog bounced around happily. "The dog was jumping up and down in the cage, and its nose was cleared up, and its eyes were cleared up," Al says. "His fever was gone. I put him down on the floor and he ran around. We put some food out and he jumped into the food like he hadn't eaten for three or five days, which he probably hadn't. I'm looking at the dog and thinking, 'Geez, this dog's not sick.' "

In vitro – Outside a living body, usually in a test tube or petri dish. From the Latin for "in glass."

In vivo – Inside a living body.

After years of watching distemper dogs die, Al could not believe his eyes. "We made a mistake," he thought. "That couldn't have possibly have been distemper."

Nothing he had learned in veterinary school, in his training and his experience would allow him to believe what he saw. "I'm a veterinarian," says Al, who at first sounded just like the skeptics who would later besiege him for his entire career and beyond. "I'm rational. You can't cure viruses like that."

He was sure he must have misdiagnosed the distemper, "I'm lucky I didn't take the serum and throw it away and say, 'Well, yeah, it didn't work.'"

But he didn't.

Within a week, they treated another case and saw the same recovery. After five cases, Al felt confident these were distemper cases and they were being cured. "I kept saying, 'That's not possible.' But I'm looking at it, I'm looking at it, I'm looking at it. These dogs are cured. And so we said, 'Jesus, we've got something really great here.'"

In the meantime, Cornell's report on the serum sample finally came back.

"They wrote back and said 'It has a very small antiviral activity. We do not suggest using it,'" Al says. He wrote back to Cornell to report that the serum cleared a dog of distemper within 24 hours. Cornell didn't respond.

Later, he'd realize one possible explanation for Cornell's result. The test for interferon is performed in glass tubes – **in vitro**.

"They tested it in vitro, which means they grow cells in a glass [dish]," he says. "They infect the cells with a virus. They then instill the serum against that virus and wait to see how many of the cells remain alive and how much of the virus is killed. They wrote back and said the interferon level is very low."

Since his serum did not have interferon, what was saving these dogs? Why couldn't Cornell see the potential in his discovery? As Al puzzled through these questions over the years, he concluded that if he did not make interferon, he must have made something else. He also guessed that most likely happened because of the mistake in the timing for the withdrawal of the serum from the donor dog.

The other reason is whatever material was created by the NDV injection could not be tested in vitro. He suspects that this material works only **in vivo** – inside a living body, not in a glass tube. Dr. Sears believes the material created by the NDV injection sparks further reactions inside a living dog's body that work together to stop the distemper virus.

"This material was killing the distemper virus and killing it quickly," he says. "These animals were recovering almost absolutely in front of our eyes, to the point where we almost couldn't believe what we were doing."

In the years since my first interview with Dr. Sears, I've learned a few things from reading journal articles and talking to people who know more than I. One flaw pointed out to me here is that viruses are not living organisms, so it is problematic to claim that a treatment has killed the virus. Viruses are inert packets of genetic material wrapped in an envelope, often made of protein. They don't move on their own. When they get picked up by a living being, they can attach themselves to cells if possible, pass through the cell membrane and then use the energy and material of the cell to replicate thousands of copies of themselves.

Even so, Dr. Sears watched his patients making speedy recovery from a dangerous and often fatal disease. What to do with this discovery?

Rejected by the big guns

"Here we were, a little tiny practice up in the desert area of California and we had a way to treat a disease for which there was no answer," Al says.

So, he drove to a veterinary convention in Las Vegas to share his discovery with one of the biggest experts in the field.

Thousands of veterinarians had descended on Vegas for a conference with lectures on a wide range of topics. Dr. Richard L. Ott, one of the primary experts on veterinary virology would be lecturing on canine distemper.

Taxonomy – How organisms are classified.

When Al got to Ott's distemper lecture, he found himself in an auditorium with about 300 other vets. One he recognized as a colleague from Palmdale, about 10 miles away from Lancaster. Al Sears was in his mid-30s with reddish brown hair and a clean-shaven face.

Ott strode back and forth onstage, explaining the latest research about distemper. He explained basics, such as the **taxonomy** and categorization of the distemper virus. He explained which animals get infected and what the virus looked like. But when it came to treating patients, the options were simply vaccination to prevent the disease or treat them with antibiotics, fluids, and tender loving care before eventually euthanizing them.

Attendees are allowed to interrupt lectures of this kind because they were talking professional to professional. Al saw his opportunity. Nervous, he raised his hand.

"Dr. Ott was a giant in the field," Al says. "He's like the Numero Uno virologist in veterinary medicine. He's the specialist. He's the god."

When Ott acknowledged Al Sears in the audience, the young vet stood up and said, "Dr. Ott, we have a way to treat distemper."

Al then explained his procedure, the NDV injection, the serum withdrawal, the subcutaneous injection, the dramatic recovery. Ott took this in and paced back and forth on the stage for about a minute and a half. Al expected to maybe get at least a pat on the back.

Instead, he stopped pacing and turned to face him.

"Son, that's impossible. Sit down."

Al fell back into his seat, shattered and dejected. At the end of the lecture, he got up to leave. As he exited the room, his colleague from Palmdale caught up with him at the door. "Jesus, Sears," he said. "Where did you come up with that?"

The god of virology had shot him down. For the more than 3-hour drive home, "I was so mad I was spitting nails," Al says.

"It is frustrating when you deal with people who won't listen and just look at you like you're nuts," Al says. "I know exactly what was going through Ott's head. All of these guys are well versed in interferon, and my procedure was very similar. So, he looked at me thinking, 'Interferon. It doesn't work against distemper. Sit down, son, you're just giving us the wrong information.' I can see it going through his head. I understand it, but it doesn't change the fact that he was wrong."

It didn't help matters when Al went back to U.C. Davis for his 10-year reunion in 1973. He walked into another room full of veterinarians – his classmates – and announced, "I discovered how to cure distemper." They looked at him doubtfully and said, "Yeah, yeah. Have another drink and sit down."

Al nursed his wounds for months, then years. But even though he could not get anyone to listen, he still took comfort in his discovery. "I'm a clinical veterinarian," he says. "My job is to relieve suffering and prevent death. The fact that I could do that was more than a thrill. So, we continued to treat cases successfully, but I wasn't interested in talking to anybody about it."

Now I knew why he didn't want to get on the phone with a newspaper reporter. When he finished the story, I asked him what was in the serum and how it worked.

"I don't know," Dr. Sears said. "What we don't know to this day is what the material is."

Sending more samples to a university would be pointless, he said. They wouldn't know what to look for.

"If you send it to the lab and say 'find it for me' they'd just laugh at you," Dr. Sears said. "They're set up to look for things specifically. So, if you don't know the specific thing you're looking for, how are you going to tell them what to look for? You can't. So, we didn't."

This is yet another example of the limitations Dr. Sears had been saddled with as a clinical veterinarian in an isolated community and far away from the resources of a university. From his point of view, the only analysis available was from clinical diagnostic lab which is set up to identify known pathogens such as the distemper virus, rabies, parvovirus, etc. I would learn years later that a research lab equipped to perform a mass spectrum analysis of the NDV-induced serum compared with serum that had not been treated with NDV could possibly identify the unique compounds responsible for the recovery of the distemper patients. Mass spectrometry may not have been common in the 1970s, but the comparison could be done today.

Still, the money, resources and knowledge to do this were far out of reach for a small-town vet struggling to pay salaries and stay ahead of monthly bills. We finished lunch, and he drove us back to the clinic.

I asked him to tell me more about Galen's case.

Galen had a fever when Karen brought him in. They treated him with fluids and antibiotics. The old methods may not cure the disease, but they have a role in saving the animal, such as preventing opportunistic infections like pneumonia. Distemper had sapped all energy from Galen. "He wasn't fighting anyone," Dr. Sears said. He took me to the refrigerator in the back of his clinic where he kept the serum, the color of weak honey beer. Serum often has a yellowish tinge from the fats present. He had not yet settled on a name so he called it "Goofy serum." But Ruth told me she preferred the more respectable name of "Serum X." Later, we would realize a poorly worded name hurts its credibility.

He kept the serum in vials, sealed in plastic bags. To begin treatment on Galen, he used a syringe to draw 5ccs of serum and injected it just under the skin in his rump. Galen got another injection 12 hours later, and a third injection 12 hours after that. The repeated injections are a result of Dr. Sears tinkering with his protocol over the years as he found out what method saved the most dogs. The answer was three shots over 24 hours, each given 12 hours after the previous one.[1] Galen's fever was under control only 18 hours after the first injection.

"But why don't you get this published?" I asked.

"I've been burned a couple of times by the big guns before," he said. "I finally said, 'I don't care.'"

Getting published in a veterinary journal is the path to acceptance and availability of a treatment. Otherwise, few veterinary clinics will consider using an unknown treatment. Without publication in a journal, it was only a matter of luck that our vet in Los Angeles had even heard of Dr. Sears.

"I'll probably publish, but it will be when I'm ready to get out of the firing line," he said as he put the serum back in the clinic refrigerator. He planned to wait until he retired because of the examples of Copernicus and Galileo. Even though Copernicus knew the Earth revolved around the sun, he feared the wrath of religious critics and did not publish until the year of his death. Even Galileo, who proved Copernicus right by looking through one of the first telescopes, had to recant under threat of excommunication from the Catholic Church.

Dr. Sears feared that declaring an effective treatment for canine distemper would prompt a similar response in the veterinary community as Galileo's supposed heresy against the church. When he publishes, "Everybody will yell and scream, but then, I'll be saying, 'Fine, yell and scream, but this is what I found.'"

I thanked Dr. Sears and drove back to Los Angeles. Although we would stay in contact, I would not see him again until 12 years later. For now, I saw his story had much more potential than just a 400-word column. This was possibly a good feature article, and I worked on drafts when I had spare moments from my regular beat. Finally, I had a version of more than 6,000 words I felt was ready to show my editor. It needed a lot of work, but it could at least enter the shepherding process from *Times* editors that might eventually get it into print. My expectation for a feature of this kind was that it would need multiple drafts as various editors weighed in. It needed perspective, more reporting on the science, and more sources. I turned in the draft on my last day of work at the *Times* before starting at Los Angeles Valley College. My editor and I agreed we would keep working on it as a freelance feature.

The story had a critical flaw. A vet saving the life of one dog – mine – was not enough to prove he had found the cure to canine distemper. As I had said to Ruth, I had just wanted to write about how he had saved my dog. I didn't ask about all the other dogs he had treated over the years. I also found myself overwhelmed with the responsibilities of teaching a full schedule, advising a student newspaper, and supervising a journalism department and photography lab. Meanwhile, my editor moved on to a job at another *Times* section. We both let Dr. Alson Sears' cure for canine distemper fall into the cracks between us.

So much for that opportunity to tell the world, but there would be others. Besides, Dr. Alson Sears had not even told me the full story yet.

The NDV Spinal Tap

For most of their time in Lancaster in the 1960s, Al and Ruth Sears worked in different spheres. Ruth focused on raising the kids while working as a director of nursing at Antelope Valley Convalescent Hospital. Al worked six days a week, striving through a handful of attempts to get his own clinic. Had veterinary school taught him about financial management and legal contracts, it might have gone smoother. Although he'd enjoyed a good relationship with Bill Zontine, when he struck out on his own he ran into problems with a lease-to-buy contract that fell through and then a series of bad partnerships.

Finally, in 1969 Al opened a clinic by himself in a cramped storefront. That summer, Chuck Whitt walked into the new business fresh out of high school. When he was 14, Chuck's parents had moved from San Antonio to Lancaster to work in civil service for the Air Force. As a high school student, Chuck worked as a kennel man at another clinic where Al had practiced. Al quickly hired Chuck and they began a working relationship and friendship that would last decades.

"Both of us just worked together every day and just came in and worked as hard as we could work," Chuck says. "I never thought he would retire, honestly, up until the time it came. We would come in probably around 8 o'clock and we would start seeing clients at nine. We were a non-appointment hospital. So, we handled whatever came through the door and whatever surgeries were scheduled. We would leave at 8 p.m., sometimes 9."

But Al also maintained a playful attitude. "He was about the animals," says Chuck. "That's one thing I can say. He was always about the animals. Not about the business end of it."

Cats were his real passion, and he and Chuck sometimes joked about opening a cat-only practice someday.

"He never turned anybody down," Chuck says. "Anybody could come in, and they would say, 'Well, I don't have this much money.' And he would say, 'Don't worry about it, we'll take care of it.' And figure out a fair price and bring it in and he would just treat the animal."

Sometimes people would take advantage of him that way. They might offer to pay a little bit each month, then only pay one month and never come back. "It happens," says Chuck. "But you move on and go to the next one."

Al Sears would serve as Chuck's best man, twice. "You've got to love him for that," Chuck says.

Sundays were the only days Al could connect with his family. On those days, the whole family would ride bikes into town for breakfast. Al would take the kids ice-skating at a local rink. Or when they had more time off, they'd go on family trips together.

Then, an ectopic pregnancy almost killed Ruth.

"And when I was in the hospital and came to, I realized I had worked all of my life with three kids at home and it was time to stop," Ruth says. "So, I quit work as a director of nursing, but as I recovered I was bored."

So, Ruth stopped in to visit the storefront clinic and found out how much Al needed her.

"Chuck was so grateful when I started wandering in because I was bored at home," Ruth says. "And I'd see all these bills stacked up. And Chuck would say, 'He hasn't paid them.' So, little by little, I began to do things. In the beginning, I had to only write the checks and then Al would sign them."

But Ruth also saw that the storefront wasn't a good place for an animal hospital, cramped and poorly designed for the purpose. She bought herself a briefcase and went around to banks saying, "We want to build our own clinic." Al ignored what she was doing and focused on treating animals, but that gave her free reign to do what she wanted. An empty piece of property across the street from the storefront had caught her eye.

She found a bank willing to give them a small business loan. "You know," Ruth told Al. "I think this is going to work."

"I'll believe it when I'm signing on the dotted line," he replied. It took almost 8 or 9 months to get final approval, but as Al was signing for the loan, Ruth asked, "Do you believe it now?" And he said, "Well, no. Not really."

So in the early 1970s, Al and Ruth were busy planning the new clinic when Al made the first batch of what he now calls 12-hour NDV-induced serum. They found a builder but couldn't afford an architect. Instead, they hired a draftsman, who came and sat in Al's office and watched how he worked. Al didn't want hallways. Al didn't want wasted space. It would take a few years before the new clinic was ready, but this would be their chance to have an independent clinic, tailor-made for their needs.

Testing the limits

Meanwhile, Al and Chuck kept treating distemper dogs, tweaking the protocol to find a way to save the most dogs, learning the boundaries of the cure. The major obstacle became the neurologic stage of the disease, when the dogs suffered from seizures, twitching, blindness and paralysis.

"So there was a lot of jockeying with the material and the dogs that we treated to figure out what worked best and why it worked and how much it took and what the timing was," Al says. One shot of serum eventually evolved into 3 shots, each 12 hours apart.

"As it turned out, the timing was simply a priori," Al says. "It was a matter of trying it out to see what worked best and the idea of giving the shot every twelve hours for three times came out because that was what worked best for us."

Six days became the limit. If a dog could be treated with the serum before going through the sixth day of showing symptoms, it had a very good chance of survival. Beyond the sixth day, the neurologic stage would begin and in most cases, the dog would die. This stage was also called Old Dog Encephalitis – ODE – a swelling of the brain. Al describes four main problems in this stage:

- **Optic neuritis**, damage to the optic nerve, which blinds the dog.
- **Encephalitis,** when dogs begin to exhibit the neurological symptoms of disease, such as seizures.
- **Chorea**, a type of twitching, which may be just in one muscle or throughout the entire dog.
- Ascending paralysis, meaning the dog loses the ability to move the back legs and this keeps climbing up the spine until the dog loses control of the lungs, can't breathe and then dies.

Saving dogs came down to a race for Al's serum to stop the distemper virus from reaching the nervous system. If the distemper virus crossed the **blood-brain barrier** protecting the nervous system and brain, the dog usually died. If the serum stopped the distemper virus before it breeched the blood-brain barrier, the dog usually lived.

"Once we got it down to where we were curing most of the dogs, then we kind of stopped experimenting with it and just ran with it from there," Al says. "How old the dogs had to be, we knew. How long they had to be sick, we knew. Basically how much serum to give them we knew."

Encephalitis – A swelling of the brain, often caused by trauma or infection, as with Old Dog Encephalitis (ODE).

Optic neuritis – A swelling of the optic nerve, which connects the eye to the brain. An infection could be a cause.

Chorea – Also called myoclonus, it is a spasmodic twitching of the muscles.

Blood-brain barrier – A semi-permeable barrier that separates the brain and spinal cord from the rest of the body. It allows some materials to pass, but blocks others.

To win the race against distemper, Al needed to get the jump on the disease by getting a diagnosis as early as possible.

"If you send the sample to the lab, it takes 2 to 3 to 5 days to get the answer back," Al says. "Now, you're into day six-seven already. Too late to treat. So, what have you done in the meantime? You gave him antibiotics. You gave him fluids. Is he still sick? Yeah, he's still sick. Or you get a **conjunctiva** smear and you send it in. How long does that take? Three to four days. The dog's still sick. Now, you're up to day four, five or six again. So, again, you are pushing the limits of what your stuff can do."

What he needed was a way to know if a dog had distemper without having to send a sample to a lab. He needed to diagnose in his clinic. Al says:

"So we looked at this and tried to figure how we can handle this. What we decided was one, you pull the blood from the dog to send to the lab. Then you immediately treat the dog. Treat the dog immediately. Because if you're wrong, it doesn't make any difference. If you're right, by tomorrow the dog's well. That makes sense. It doesn't cause any harm, and yet it clears the dog. If it's one of the other viruses and it doesn't do anything, so what? Now you need to know whether you have distemper not. What we realized was, there are several areas where the distemper virus is always found. It's usually found in the **conjunctiva.** It's almost always found in the **macrophages** in the lung, but you've got to get that out and that's

Conjunctiva – Mucous membrane of the eye and eyelids.

Macrophages – White blood cells, which capture and destroy foreign materials, such as viruses and damaged tissues. They also prepare antigens for the B and T cells to process

Trachea – The windpipe.

Inclusions – Foreign granules, particles or droplets caused by infection, such as viruses in stained nuclei.

hard to do. [By either a needle in the chest or a tube down the **trachea**, AKA the windpipe.] But there's an easy place to look, and that's in the bladder. The transitional cells of the bladder are highly sensitive and highly reactive to the virus. They always have the virus. So if you have distemper in the **acute phase**, pull some cells out of the bladder, which is as easy as passing a catheter, drain the urine out, run it back and forth against the bladder wall, get some cells loose, suck them up into the catheter, bring them out, put them on a slide."

By staining the slide[2] and looking at it under a microscope, Al could look for the signs of the distemper virus – red spots alongside the nucleus of the cell called **inclusions**. Within 15 minutes, he'd know he had a dog with distemper and should start his serum injections.

This was called the Brush Border Smear. The "brush border" is the surface area of accessible cells, which a vet could gather up and "smear" on a slide.

"We began to run that in all the cases that came in, and it was positive in all those acute cases," Al says. "So, it became a definitive test for us. We stopped running stuff off to the lab. We just did it ourselves."

But the later into the disease the dog went, the number of cells that showed **inclusions** decreased. "Those cells that are infected are sloughed off the bladder surface and they're gone," Al says. So, the Brush Border Smear was a more accurate diagnosis within the first 10 days of symptoms. [As of June 2020, I had learned the distemper tests are much faster. One dog owner wrote to tell me a veterinary hospital was able to confirm distemper via lab test within 10 minutes.]

In my series of interviews with Dr. Sears, most of which happened years after his retirement in 2006, I would often ask what year he began a particular procedure such as the Brush Border Smear. Very often, I wouldn't get a specific answer because the years of running a business had tended to blend together.[3]

Dogs kept dying if they were brought to Al already in the neurologic stage. Al kept reading journal articles, trying to understand why his serum worked, why it didn't and to find ways to improve his success rate. He often drove to the library at the University of California Los Angeles on the weekends to read up on the latest journals.

In 1973, he read an article in *The California Veterinarian* (Adams and Snow 1973)[4] co-authored by John Adams, UCLA's retired professor of pediatric virology. Adams had been the founding chair of the Department of Pediatrics at the UCLA School of Medicine. A specialist in immunology, **multiple sclerosis**, and sudden infant death syndrome, Adams had retired in 1972 at the age of 67 but was energetically continuing his research.

The article asked for veterinarians to bring him dogs with ODE. Adams had a theory that dogs with ODE were equivalent to people with multiple sclerosis. He believed distemper and measles were equivalent diseases. (Adams et al. 1958) In the 1930s, he'd written one of the first papers on the similarity of distemper and measles. The connection between measles, also known as rubeola, and distemper was later confirmed through genetic comparisons of the viruses.

A paper published in the International Journal of Paleopathology in March 2019 used modern methods to determine canine distemper evolved as a mutation of the measles virus in South America during the period of European colonization.[5] The Spanish explorers brought diseases like measles and small pox to the New World, and these viruses became unwitting allies in the conquest of the Americas.

The modern researchers point to an outbreak of canine distemper around Quito in 1746. Native populations of dogs almost completely disappeared during the period of European colonization in an epidemic similar to that ones that devastated the native human population.

But long before that determination, Adams had made microscopic photos comparing the brain cells of humans with MS and dogs with distemper. When the slides were placed side-by-side, the similarities were striking to him.

> **Multiple sclerosis** – A disease that destroys the oligodentrocytes that generate the protective myelin of nervous system and causes a range of neurologic problems. Suspected causes are genetics, environment or an attack from a virus.
>
> **Myelin** – Fatty white material that insulates the nerve cell, the neuron. Loss of myelin causes a disruption in nerve function.

He thought it possible that in the way the distemper virus eventually caused ODE in dogs, measles was what eventually caused MS in people. The neurologic problems suffered by MS patients were similar to dogs with latter-stage distemper. For example, in both diseases, there was a loss of **myelin** – the fatty white protein that provides insulation to the nerves – as well as lesions on the brain. So, Adams saw dogs in the neurologic stage of distemper as an animal model for the study of measles and MS.

Adams occupied an office two doors from the library entrance Al used. So, Al stopped in to introduce himself to the grey-haired professor with horn-rimmed glasses. "We are in a hotbed of distemper, and I have plenty of cases," Al said. "Would you be interested?"

"Absolutely, we want as many as we can get," Adams replied.

Ethics and experimentation

Dogs have been used in scientific experiments going back to the 19th Century. Scientists used dogs to make breakthroughs in diabetes research in 1889. Louis Pasteur used dogs to understand and prevent rabies, and Ivan Pavlov famously used dogs to understand the connections between the digestive and nervous systems.[6]

However, because dogs have become a favorite companion to people, the public has often expressed outrage when some experiments using dogs become known. In the early 1960s, a group of veterinarians formed the Animal Care Panel and published "The Guide for the Care and Use of Laboratory Animals." In 1966, media reports on the treatment of laboratory animals – including the story of a stolen dog dying in experimental surgery – helped to galvanize Congress to pass the Animal Welfare Act. Under this act, the USDA would establish regulations for the acquisition and transport of animals used in experiments as well as required licensing and inspection of dealers and research facilities.

In 1971, amendments to the act allowed institutions to comply with the act by establishing animal care committees, which in 1986 evolved into the "Institutional Animal Care and Use Committee" or IACUC to oversee and approve animal experiments. Critics and animal welfare advocates complain this system is plagued with loopholes that leave animals with little to no protection. Since the head of the facility selects the members, the committees become self-regulating. According to the website of the New England Anti-Vivisection Society, a Boston-based, national animal advocacy organization dedicated to ending the use of animals in research:

"Recent incidents at several major research institutions point to profound inadequacies within the federal enforcement program, and to AWA regulations that are so limited that physical and psychological cruelty and suffering continue. For example, while the AWA stipulates that researchers '... avoid or minimize discomfort, distress, and pain to the animals,' procedures that cause pain and distress merely require that the 'principal investigator has considered alternatives to procedures that may cause more than momentary or slight pain or distress to the animals, and has provided a written narrative description of the methods and sources...used to determine that alternatives were not available.' While the AWA 'requires researchers to provide anesthesia or pain-relieving medication [to regulated animals] to minimize the pain or distress caused by the experiment...' they can withhold anesthetics, painkillers, and tranquilizers if deemed 'scientifically necessary.' This same vacuous 'protection' applies to conducting multiple survival surgeries on an animal, where the animal will recover from one major experimental surgery and then be subjected later to more surgery. The AWA prohibits this, yet it is allowed if called for by an IACUC-approved experiment."[7]

The first edition of "Animal Liberation" by Peter Singer in 1975 addressed many of the ethical problems in using animals for experimentation. With today's heightened awareness of the treatment of animals in scientific experiments, it may be useful to compare the ethics in cases cited by Singer with Adams' canine distemper study.

In Chapter 2 of Singer's book, "Tools for Research,"[8] he runs through a series of examples of animal experimentation that "appear to be trivial or misconceived, and some were not even designed to yield important benefits."

These experiments included:

- A 1927 U.S. Naval Medical School study that showed dogs placed in a hot humid chamber would develop heat stroke and die.
- A U.S. Army study that showed feeding TNT to Beagles would make the dogs sick and die.
- A 1953 Harvard University study that shocked dogs through an electrified floor to induce a state of hopelessness and despair.
- A 1969 University of Rochester study of microwaves that killed dogs and rabbits.
- A 1971 study by the United States Public Health Service that showed running dogs on a treadmill in 113 degrees would induce heat stroke. Many died.
- A plan in 1973 by U.S Air Force plan to test poisonous gases on Beagle puppies. (The Air Force switched to other experimental animals because of a public outcry.)

Many of these studies came to obvious conclusions that were already well established in human medicine, Singer pointed out.

Singer concludes it does not seem likely that any major Western democracy will abolish all animal experimentation, but he contrasted the looser regulations of U.S. animal testing with those in Britain. To perform an experiment on an animal, Britain requires a license issued only after the Secretary of State "weighs the adverse effects on the animals concerned against the benefit likely to accrue." [9]

In the 2002 edition of his book, Singer writes:

"In the United States, where the present lack of control over experimentation allows the kinds of experiments described in the preceding pages, a minimal first step would be a requirement that no experiment be conducted without prior approval from an ethics committee that includes animal welfare representatives and is authorized to refuse approval to experiments when it does not consider that the potential benefits outweigh the harm to the animals."[10]

In 2013, approximately 74,000 dogs were used in scientific research, according to the Humane Society of the United States' tabulation of data provided by the U.S. Department of Agriculture.[11] More than 25 million animals are used in scientific research in the U.S. each year, most often mice.[12] Throughout this book are references to breakthroughs and research made possible because of laboratory animals.

In the context of these broad ethical concerns, a few points are needed to be understood about Adams' plan to euthanize dogs and remove their brains and other tissues for a scientific study:

- Rather than starting with healthy dogs, these dogs would be in the advanced, neurologic stage of canine distemper and were likely to be dying soon, either from the disease or from euthanasia.
- Rather than prolong the dog's pain and suffering, Adams would humanely release them from their misery as part of his study.
- Adams had a reasonable scientific goal – to understand the similarities and possible connections between distemper, measles and MS.
- Adams' research had the potential to help humans with Multiple Sclerosis.

"Let's give it a try"

While other vets were bringing one or two dogs to Adams, Al brought dozens to UCLA. Adams finally asked Al, "Why are you getting so many of these cases?" Al Sears told him about the widespread cases of distemper in the Antelope Valley but also about the success he had in treating it.

Adams listened.

Following the stinging rebuke of Dr. Ott in Las Vegas and the dismissive response from his own classmates at U.C. Davis, Al Sears had found someone open to a new idea.

"He was a gentlemanly scholar educator is what he was," Al says. "He was willing to listen and he was willing to expound on the ideas and if an idea that I presented came across something that he was involved in or had literature on he would dig into his desk, and pull out the information and copy it and give it to me."

Al Sears describes Adams as dynamic, with a brain working "a mile a minute." He wanted to get his work done before the end of his life. He was "a very smart man, and the smarter they are, the more willing they are to listen, apparently," Al says.

When Adams eventually published his comparison of old dog encephalitis with demyelinating diseases in humans, such as MS, he listed Alson Sears as one of the nine authors of the paper. (Adams et al. 1975)[13]

In their long conversations, Adams realized they didn't just have a chance to understand MS and distemper. If Dr. Al Sears had found a cure for distemper, then perhaps Dr. Adams might find a treatment for people with MS.

The two men faced a similar problem from different sides. Al Sears could not save dogs in the neurologic stage of distemper, and if the two diseases are equivalent, people with MS are already in the neurologic stage. So, an NDV treatment would be too late for those with MS. Their common problem lay with the blood-brain barrier.

When talking about the immune system, there are two environments within the body. There is the neurologic environment – the brain and spinal cord – and there is the rest of the body. The blood-brain barrier keeps them separate. The barrier is semi-permeable. It allows some materials to cross, but stops others. To cross the barrier, a molecule would have to be small enough. For example, vaccine-induced antibodies are too big. They can't make the trip. But an infectious viral particle, which is hundred or thousands of times smaller than a human cell, can easily cross the barrier. Dr. Sears believed that whatever component of the Newcastle Disease Vaccine serum that was saving dogs in the early stages of distemper was not able to cross the blood-brain barrier. It needed extra human intervention.

"So I said it might be worth a try on one of these dogs to put this stuff into the spinal canal to see what we can do," Al says. Adams agreed to perform the first NDV spinal tap, an injection of the Newcastle Disease Vaccine directly into the spinal canal.

In the desert, the city of Lancaster formed a triangle with the towns of Mojave and Boron, where Al Sears saw a special form of distemper. As puppies, the only symptoms they showed were mild symptoms for a couple of days – just some sniffling or sneezing – from which they quickly recovered. The owners of these dogs often didn't even bring them into a hospital, and the dogs showed no other symptoms for years. Then, six to eight years after the sniffles as a puppy, Old Dog Encephalitis showed up. It was one of these dogs, a 7-year-old Pointer named "Joe" from Rosamond north of Lancaster, that Al Sears took to Dr. Adams for the first NDV spinal tap on Nov. 14, 1974.

About two months earlier, Joe had begun staggering and leaning to the right as he walked. His front leg also jerked. Joe's owner had told Al, "I donate him." By the time he was brought to UCLA, Joe could not walk or see.

"He was a big dog, but I'm a big guy, so I just picked him up," Al says. He carried him into the Rigler Research Center in the basement at UCLA along with a bottle of NDV.

Adams looked at the dog and said, "Let's give it a try." As with other cases of neurologic distemper, Joe was not expected to survive, and Dr. Adams would euthanize him as planned within a couple of months.

Dr. Adams wrote in his notes: "When admitted, the dog was unable to walk, pupils were wildly dilated, and the animal appeared to be in acute distress."

They prepped the dog for surgery and put it under anesthesia. Al inserted the needle in the back of **foramen magnum**, an opening at the base of the skull, which allows access to the spinal canal. It is a procedure that requires precision. If the needle is pushed in too far, it can hit the spinal cord, damaging or severing it – pithing – and cause permanent paralysis. From that needle, Al withdrew 10 milliliters of **cerebrospinal fluid** from the spinal canal. Then, 2 milliliters of Newcastle's Disease Vaccine in solution was injected into the spinal canal.

The injection sent the dog into immediate shock with spasms.

"Well, we all stood there looking at this dog in shock," Al says. "Since I was clinical veterinarian, I yelled for an IV catheter. I put an IV catheter in him and got this dog on fluids, and of course it recovered in a matter of minutes."

Al left Joe in Dr. Adams care from then on.

While Dr. Adams proceeded with his study on Joe and neurologic distemper, the date for breaking ground on the new Sears clinic approached. But when the builder met with Al and Ruth, he told them, "Well, we hit a snafu."

"I went to the snafu place and cried," Ruth says. The water department wouldn't turn the water on. Al and Ruth had to give answers to a long list of questions such as how much animal feces would go down the drain. Finally, the service was approved, and the builder broke ground.

Foramen magnum – An opening at the base of the skull, through which the spinal cord passes to connect with the brain.

Cerebrospinal fluid (CSF) – A clear protective fluid found in the brain and spinal canal.

In January 1975, Dr. Adams compiled his notes on Joe into a rough draft of a case report. The results of the NDV spinal tap were apparently dramatic, considering this was a dog that had been blind, paralyzed and twitching in his front leg.

"In 24 hours, the patient was responding to voice and vocal stimulation," Dr. Adams wrote. "In 48 hours, the forelegs moved in an attempt to rise, rear legs appeared to be useless and paralyzed."

In his notes, Dr. Adams reported drawing a new sample of spinal fluid a week after the tap. He sent that off to Cornell for testing. Then, he continued:

> "The dog continued to eat and drink well and gradually showed increased muscular activity, forelegs permitted moving to food and water, and the dog made an effort to use his hind limbs, rising partially and collapsing into a lying position. This type of activity has continued, and it is the impression of the examiners that 'Joe' is improving very gradually, but still weak and partially paralyzed, particularly in the pelvic limbs. Tail wagging has been noticed by some observers."

Dr. Adams wrote that as of Dec. 12, nearly a month after the spinal tap, "the patient is continuing to eat and drink lustily and makes a real effort to rise on all fours and to walk, but fails to accomplish this act completely."

On Dec. 15, he noted, "the dog rose on all fours and 'walked' out of his cage for a brief period, but then returned to a prone position. Tail wagging in response to voice." However, the pupils of his eyes were widely dilated, an indication that he was still having trouble seeing. Then Dr. Adams wrote:

> "During the final 2 weeks of December, the dog continued to make slow progress in standing on all four legs and rather vigorous tail wagging when spoken to. He responds to commands and tries very hard to rise on all four legs and manages to walk out of cage area and into the room, which has a tile floor and is slippery, offering very little resistance or help to the animal in his efforts to walk. Vision also appears to be improved, but pupils remain widely dilated except when a bright light is shown into the eye, the pupils responded sluggishly to light."

On Jan. 2, 1975, and according to plan, Dr. Adams euthanized Joe so that the final spinal, blood and tissue samples could be drawn for the study. The brain, along with a piece of the spinal cord, was removed for Dr. Adams' research. "Grossly, no distinct lesions could be seen," he wrote.

How Joe's recovery happened has been a matter of debate. In Dr. Sears' interpretation, this unknown factor created by NDV crossed the blood-brain barrier to stop the virus and allow the nervous system to repair itself. Others might argue it was somehow a modulation of the immune system. Or it could have been because Joe's nervous system had been given enough time to experience neurologic retraining, where healthy neurons are used to take over the tasks performed by the damaged neurons.

When I tell this story to dog lovers, the euthanasia of Joe draws a reaction. Many would second guess putting a dog to sleep when he seemed on the path to recovery. But despite his improvement, Joe was still a part of the study, and the purpose of the study was to help humans, not dogs. But even though studies such as these are conducted for the benefit of humans, the case of Joe would have an unusual twist. Because of Dr. Sears' involvement, this scientific study of a dog helped other dogs more than 30 years later.

Construction on the clinic went forward. At Christmas, the builder had given Ruth a hard hat so she could supervise. By now, Al was taking his lunch breaks across the street to watch the construction. But the building project was Ruth's baby. She oversaw every detail. Al didn't believe in getting a decorator, but Ruth hired one anyway to design the waiting room. She needed help deciding all the details, such as the type of benches or what kind of handles to have on the drawers.

"Anyway, little-by-little, it all came together," Ruth says. "And one day it was ready for occupancy. And I was still lining shelves in the surgery, and Al came in and said, 'Get out of my way.' And literally, it was his place. And I backed off."

When they opened for business in 1975, they called the phone company and said, "OK, we'll initiate that phone that we contracted with you." And they were told, "You canceled it."

Al said, "I did what?"

"You canceled it."

A rival vet had canceled their phone. There are dirty tricks in veterinary medicine, just like politics, Al says. So, the new clinic was not in the phone book for the first year. This was scary because at this time, vets were not allowed to advertise. A number in the phone book was the only advertisement allowed.

"Well, if I can't get in the phone book and nobody knows I'm here, I've got to let somebody know I'm out here," Al says. So, he ran a small newspaper ad, "and it got me in all kinds of trouble with the state of California."

"But you know what? When people like you, they find you," says Ruth.

CDV – Canine Distemper Virus

Dr. Adams never published the report on Joe's treatment and recovery. But he updated Al as he continued to explore the possibilities of NDV against distemper. In one unpublished experiment, he tested two groups of ferrets with distemper. "Ferrets are also highly susceptible to **CDV** and the disease is virtually 100% fatal." (Kapil and Yeary 2011)[14] One group was treated with NDV; the other wasn't. All the ferrets in the untreated group died. The group treated with NDV lived but some died four months after treatment. He also wrote up a proposal to study NDV on puppies.

"And unfortunately he did something that sort of brought everything to a halt," Al says. "He died."

Dr. Adams died on June 30, 1980, at age 75. Al received the news via a phone call and then a letter from the university. Al and Ruth sent flowers and condolences to his family. He got a letter from one of his colleagues, and from his wife. But he could not attend the funeral. "To walk away from my practice was to leave 20 or 30 or 40 people without treatment and I still had to pay my payrolls," Al says.

Dr. Adams papers were archived in a box at the UCLA library.

After he died, Al tried to get medical researchers interested in Dr. Adams' work. He contacted the National Institutes of Health and told them what had been done. He was told, "Look you're a veterinarian. We will put you in touch with Cornell, and you can talk to somebody at Cornell."

So, Al talked to someone at Cornell Vet School, and he says he was told, "Well, send us $500,000, and we'll initiate a study. We'll put it in your name." And Al said, "Look, I'm a clinical vet in California. I can barely make my payroll. You've got to be kidding me." He called his alma mater, U.C. Davis Veterinary School, and they gave the same answer.

"So, it kind of died," Al says. "And no one else seemed to be interested."

Skeptics

As a schoolboy in England, Edward Jenner and a group of fellow students were starved, bled, deliberately scratched with small pox and locked into a stable.

They were kept there until either the disease ran its course or they died.

This method of **variolation** came to Britain in the early 18th Century and had been the best idea medical science had on how to stop the spread of small pox. The death rate for those treated with variolation was 10 times lower than from naturally occurring small pox, but still 2 percent to 3 percent of those inoculated died.[15]

Jenner survived but would never forget the ordeal.

Later, as a country doctor, Jenner learned from farmers that anyone who caught cowpox from their cows would not come down with small pox. In 1796, when a dairymaid showed Jenner a cowpox rash on her hand, Jenner saw an opportunity.

Variolation – Scratching material taken from a smallpox victim into the skin of a healthy person. This would result in sickness, but if the person survived they should have immunity to small pox. Used before the development of vaccination.

Fauces – Part of the pharynx at the back of the mouth and nasal cavity.

He needed someone who had not previously been exposed to small pox for an experiment. So, he borrowed the 8-year-old son of his gardener. He took material from the dairymaid's rash and scratched it into the boy's arm. The boy became mildly ill from cowpox but recovered a week later. About six weeks later, Jenner variolated the boy with small pox, and to his great relief the boy did not get sick. He had found a way to safely protect a person from disease: the first vaccination. [16]

But his discovery met with immediate resistance.

He submitted the technique in a paper to the *Royal Society Journal*. They rejected him with the message, "he was in variance with established knowledge" and that "he had better not promulgate such a wild idea if he valued his reputation."[17] Jenner would have to self-publish the discovery and it would take decades until variolation was banned and cowpox vaccination became compulsory in England.

However, his discovery would eventually eradicate smallpox from the world in the 1970s.

As an English doctor of the Age of Enlightenment, Jenner had a wide range of interests beyond human medicine. He experimented with balloons, wrote poetry, studied bird migration, fossils and geology as well as played the flute and violin. In 1809, he also took great interest in a disease suffered by the foxhounds of the Earl of Berkeley.

His interest may have been triggered by another memory of his youth. When he was a teenager – and an apprentice surgeon – a gentleman Jenner knew had "destroyed the greater part of his hounds, from supposing them mad, when the distemper first broke out among them; so little was it then known by those the most conversant with dogs."

The horror of rabies – also known as hydrophobia – had been known since ancient times. The name hydrophobia comes from the overpowering fear of water victims of rabies suffer from. This is one of the devastating symptoms of the disease, which also causes convulsions, hallucinations and fits before death.

In the 18th Century, wiping out a pack of dogs to stop the spread of rabies made sense, not only to save other dogs but also to save humans from a horrible fate. But an assumption of rabies was not enough to satisfy Jenner. When the hounds of the Earl of Berkeley fell ill, he studied them carefully.

He described the disease as beginning with an inflammation of the lungs, vomiting and diarrhea. A dark mucous covered the teeth. The eyes were inflamed and also covered with mucous. In his paper, "Distemper in Dogs," he goes on to write:

> "The brain is often affected as early as the second day after the attack. The animal becomes stupid, and his general habits are changed. In this state, if not prevented by loss of strength, he sometimes wanders from home. He is frequently endeavoring to expel, by forcible expirations, the mucus from the trachea and **fauces**, with a peculiar rattling noise. His jaws are generally smeared with it, and it sometimes flows out in a frothy state, from his frequent champing. During the progress of the disease, especially in its advanced stages, he is disposed to bite and gnaw any thing within his reach. He has sometimes epileptic fits, or quick succession of general, though slight convulsive spasms of the muscles. If the dog survives, this

affection of the muscles continues through life. He is often attacked with fits of a different description. He first staggers, then tumbles, rolls, cries as if whipped, and tears up the ground with his teeth and forefeet." (Jenner 1809)[18]

To any other English gentleman, these symptoms might have been enough to justify a conclusion of rabies and slaughter these dogs. Instead, Jenner looked closer. His careful observations established a separate disease in the first scientific paper on canine distemper. Most importantly, he noted:

- The dogs were not afraid of water. He said of one: "his thirst seems insatiable, and nothing seems to cheer him like the sight of water."
- This disease was not communicable to humans.

The name of the disease had been born out of ignorance and superstition.

The word distemper came from Old French meaning "to disturb." In the Middle Ages, any illness was thought to be caused by a disturbance of the four bodily humors – Yellow Bile, Black Bile, Phlegm and Blood. So, distemper – disturbance of the humors – at first described any illness in a human or animal.

Over the years, as other diseases – such as measles or small pox – were identified and named, distemper ended up with its name by default.

Figuring out the cause of canine distemper would take another century. It would take a lot of guesswork and overcoming the wrong assumptions. Even though Jenner could successfully use one disease to stop another and establish the distinction between rabies and distemper, he never knew they were viruses.

Searching for cause and cure

It was not until the mid-1800s that **bacteria** were recognized as the source of some maladies. These are single-cell life forms that could be observed under the microscopes of the 19th Century. The German physician, Robert Koch, refined his "Koch's postulates" between 1884 and 1890 to establish how to determine which bacteria caused which disease. Koch would be hailed as the founder of modern bacteriology for his work identifying the causes of tuberculosis, cholera and anthrax.

Scientists of the time used porcelain filters to establish the size of a bacterium. They would pass infectious material through the filter, and if the resulting material were no longer infectious, they'd know the bacteria had been stopped by the filter and were therefore bigger than its holes. Bacteria were relatively easy to recognize because they could also be grown in cultures outside of a host body.

At the end of the 19th Century, scientists found the sap from a diseased tobacco plant could pass through any bacterial filter and still be infectious to healthy tobacco plants. In 1898, this unseen agent became the first recognized plant **virus**. [19]

Viruses were a difficult concept for 19th Century scientists because they could not be seen under a microscope and they could not be grown in culture. Compared with a bacterium, a virus is miniscule. Bacteria are complete cells. Viruses are merely small packets of genetic material that invade living cells to replicate themselves. They would not be seen directly until the first electron microscopes in the 1930s.

Bacterium – (bacteria is the plural form) A single-celled organism. Some bacteria are responsible for disease.

Virus – A small packet of genetic information, usually covered in an envelope of protein. It causes disease by invading a living host cell and using the cell's energy to replicate itself and spread.

The first scientists searching for the cause of canine distemper encountered plenty of bacteria. Beginning in 1875, researchers reported finding various microscopic candidates they thought were responsible for canine distemper. Between 1875 and 1910, nearly two-dozen theories had been proposed. Most of these were bacteria.[20]

Among the din of claims was a report by a 35-year-old French scientist named Henri Carré, director of the Research Laboratory of Maisons-Alfort outside of Paris. Through experimentation, he concluded in 1905:

- Distemper was a filterable virus.
- It could be found in the watery nasal discharge (and some other fluids) of the sick dog.
- Two or three drops were enough to induce the disease and often death.
- There was no organism that could be cultivated.
- Survivors would be immune to further attacks.

However, Carré could not actually show the world his distemper virus. And for years later, most veterinarians assumed distemper was some form of bacteria. In 1910, American researcher Newell S. Ferry and British researcher J.P. M'Gowan reported that the agent responsible was *Bacillus bronchisepticus*, which was at the time one of the smallest known organisms. (Ferry 1911; M'Gowan 1911)[21] Work by other researchers supported this conclusion. For someone in the 21st Century, the reason for the confusion is obvious. Anyone who has tried to save a distemper dog knows the virus knocks down the immune system and this allows bacterial diseases to attack. These early researchers were finding the bacteria taking advantage of the distemper attack, not the attack itself. In fact, *Bacillus bronchisepticus* is a known cause of pneumonia, which shows up in distemper dogs.

Throughout this period, researchers made several attempts to either prevent the spread of the disease or to find a cure. These included:

- Cow-pox vaccination, which failed.
- Inoculating the healthy dog with the nasal discharge of a sick dog – or having the dogs make nose-to-nose contact – as a form of variolation. This usually killed the dog they were trying to protect.
- Copeman's Vaccine, which in 1900 was derived from a broth culture of bacteria from a distemper dog. Dr. Monckton Copeman's product was sometimes called an "anti-distemper serum."[22]

In 1922, the veterinary and scientific communities were still grasping at straws over the problem of canine distemper when British veterinarian Hamilton Kirk wrote a book summarizing what was then known about the disease. At the time, the cause was still very much in debate. He wrote:

> "In the discovery of a prophylactic or curative vaccine or serum lies the only hope of salvation for the canine race against the dread scourge of distemper, and the bacteriologist who can accomplish this will deservedly become famous in the annals of veterinary science." [23]

Despite his expressed hope for either a preventative or a cure, Kirk had strong words for "quack remedies.":

> "It is really surprising what faith some members of the community place in these quack nostrums, and withal rather pathetic to think of the poor sick dog being regularly dosed with them, irrespective of whether they are suited to his particular case or harmful. He is lucky in the possession of the power of voluntary emesis. In view of the diversity of this disease, it must be obvious to all how impossible it is to expect to derive benefit from any one prescription. Each case must be treated on its merits, and since no specific therapeutic agent exists, one must necessarily treat the symptoms as they arise." [24]

Kirk then goes on in detail to describe the supportive nursing care for distemper dogs, including the need for hygienic conditions, keeping the animal warm, using steam kettles, proper diet and medications to treat symptoms as they occur.

The resistance to "any one prescription" curing this disease invokes a battle that the emerging sciences of the 20th Century had been having with the patent medicines popular in the 19th Century. In 1905, Collier's magazine published a series of articles by Samuel Hopkins Adams exposing the fraud of the patent medicine industry.[25] Patent medicines were the creations of advertising companies and con men who would sell concoctions as cure-alls for a wide range of diseases or conditions without any proof that they worked. These "miracle cures" were often peddled from town to town by traveling medicine shows in which crowds of people would be tricked into buying worthless product. These con artists were often called snake oil salesmen.

The Collier's series led to the U.S. Congress passing the Pure Food and Drug Act of 1906. In Britain, doctors and scientists had to overcome an ethical struggle because medical journals had accepted advertising from producers of patent medicines. Action on the issue had to wait until after the conclusion of World War I. The first legislation against patent medicines in Britain would not be adopted until the 1920s. So, Kirk writes at a time when the scientific method battled with quackery for the public's trust.

This battle created a powerful – and reasonable – skepticism in the scientific community against anyone who claimed a cure-all for disease.

"Saving the lives of our dogs"

The turning point in fighting canine distemper would happen – as it did with Jenner – because of the much-loved dogs of the British aristocracy.

Throughout the 19th Century, the British love of dogs had deepened. They celebrated new breeds of dogs at dog shows. They hunted foxes with their dogs, and they mourned the loss of these dogs when they died of distemper.

In 1923, *The Field,* a weekly country journal for sportsmen, landowners and farmers published an appeal for a distemper fund to support a massive research project to save dogs from canine distemper. This appeal was made out of a love of dogs as much as for a need to advance medical science. Members of the landed aristocracy and others donated £55,000 – £8.8 million in today's economy – which was spent on distemper research between 1923 and 1932. [26]

The research happened through a collaboration between veterinary professionals, the Medical Research Council and Burroughs-Wellcome, a pharmaceutical company. At the center of the effort were two pathologists named Patrick Laidlaw and G.W. Dunkin. Their first job was to settle the argument about the cause of canine distemper. Dogs were bred specifically to be free of diseases on a farm at Mill Hill in North London to ensure no other **pathogen** was affecting the results.

Through experiments in which healthy puppies were exposed to dogs infected with distemper, they were able to rule out *Bacillus bronchisepticus* as the cause of canine distemper. By early 1926, they concluded 'the infecting agent of dog-distemper belongs to the class of filter-passing viruses.'

So after more than 20 years, Carré's theory had been validated, and later academic papers would refer to distemper as the "Virus of Carré" until viruses were reclassified in the latter part of the 20th Century.[27]

But Laidlaw and Dunkin now had to develop an effective vaccine, and they decided dogs were not suitable as long-term laboratory animals. They did not endure the isolation well.

Ferrets, another **canid** susceptible to distemper, proved to be more useful because they thrived in small spaces and bred quickly. In their research, they found the spleen of the ferret collected the most virus and was the most useful to create a vaccine for other ferrets.

The ferret vaccine did not translate well over to dogs. So, they created a dog version by grinding up the spleen, liver and glands of infected distemper dogs. This created an extract with live virus that would then be chemically treated with **formalin**. The killed virus would then become the vaccine that would trigger the immune system of healthy dogs to recognize the distemper virus and stop them from getting the disease.

Pathogen – A microorganism that causes disease.

Canid – A mammal related to the dog.

Formalin – An antiseptic, which also acts as a fixative so tissue can be preserved.

They found the best way to vaccinate would be to first use the killed version of the virus, followed two weeks later with the full-strength live version. Early trials in estates, homes and kennels were encouraging. Distemper cases were cut to 1 out of 100 vaccinated dogs. But problems arose in ensuring the consistency of how the double dose of vaccine was used, and the first commercial version of the vaccine was pulled from the market after only 16 months.

But this was enough for *The Field* to declare victory. On Feb. 4, 1933, *The Field* published a twelve-page special supplement celebrating the conquest of canine distemper: 'Saving the lives of our dogs.' However, the first reliable commercial version of the vaccine would not be developed until 1950.

The scientific search to save dogs from distemper apparently ended with the development of the canine distemper vaccine. Dogs could be saved from the disease if vaccinated in time. But if already sickened, vets had to rely on supportive methods, treat each symptom as it arose and hope for the best. A cure for distemper became seen as unnecessary, impossible and likely quackery.

But unlike the small pox vaccine, the development of a canine distemper vaccine would not end the virus. When the World Health Organization launched its final assault on small pox in 1967, they had a key strategic advantage: Small pox only infected humans. Teams of vaccinators could travel the world and vaccinate every human in areas at risk. They could track the disease, and in 1977 when the last scab fell off the last victim of the disease – a Somali hospital worker – they knew they were close to finishing off their foe. WHO declared complete victory over small pox in 1980.

Distemper does not sicken humans, but it can infect a wide range of canid animals (dog, fox, coyote, wolf) as well as large wild cats, river otters, bears and even Rhesus monkeys. The distemper virus exists wherever there are carnivores. Domestic dogs – the most numerous of carnivores on the planet at more than 500 million – are the main reservoir for canine distemper. This means they are the animal population where the virus is naturally found, from where it grows and spreads to other susceptible species. "In the United States, spillover of infection from domestic dogs with spillback from raccoons, which may serve as intermediate hosts, and other susceptible wildlife is well documented." (Kapil and Yeary 2011)[28] Raccoons are considered to be a secondary reservoir for the disease.

From an expert overview about the disease:

"Vaccine coverage of 95% of domesticated dogs is needed to control canine distemper in these pets. Currently the best means for breaking the circulation of CDV between susceptible wildlife populations and domestic dogs is through regular vaccination of pet dogs and preventing them from roaming freely and interacting with unvaccinated dogs and wildlife that may harbor the virus." (Kapil and Yeary 2011)[29]

So, even with perfect vigilance and nearly complete vaccination of domestic dogs, the virus would most likely still be waiting to attack from the surrounding wildlife. And I would wager that even today the 95 percent mark is not being reached in many regions. The virus transfers from one animal to another in a variety of ways:

CNS – Central nervous system

"Transmission of CDV between animals is via aerosol or respiratory secretions (coughing, sneezing, barking, licking) and bodily excretions (urine and feces) or through direct contact with shared, virus-contaminated food and water bowls, garbage, compost piles, and other organic materials. Other disease-causing contacts include chasing, mating, fights, simultaneous and sequential feeding events at carcasses, and grooming. Wild animals with distemper have similar symptoms as infected dogs. They are often mistaken as rabid because they display unusual behavior, disorientation, aimless wandering, and/or aggression and walk with an unusual gait due to **CNS** involvement. The majority of cases in wildlife are most often observed in spring and summer since juveniles are more susceptible to infection, but cases occur year round." (Kapil and Yeary 2011)[30]

In June 2011, I asked Dr. Sears about whether a treatment for distemper would always be needed. His answer:

"The answer to your question is yes, and there's several reasons for it. One is, even vaccinated dogs especially young puppies that are taken into facilities and are exposed, some of them are going to break. And the only way you are going to stop that is to use the serum to stop it after they become infected. The problem is at the present time they're not doing that. What they are doing is destroying the animals. Well, if destroying the animals is the answer to the problem, they wouldn't be seeing it anymore. Yet, you know and I know that it is occurring in large quantities across the United States, especially in California, Florida and Texas because they're willing to admit it. Some of the other pounds in the rest of the country are not willing to admit it. They just are being very quiet about it. So, the disease is out there in large numbers. Here's your problem: The veterinary profession has said vaccine has controlled the disease. OK? So, if a dog is vaccinated, it's not supposed to get sick. Well, that's just not true. You know that from the information I've given you and the stuff that I've seen. That's a fallacy to begin with. So, the numbers of the cases have been reduced. Veterinarians that are in the field are seeing less and less of it because of the vaccine. Veterinarians at the university level where the research goes on see hardly anyat all. Because the ones that are seen in the field are basically destroyed and the ones in the pounds are destroyed. So, they don't even get the cases. So, as far as they are concerned, it's gone. Well, you and I both know it isn't gone. It's just in hiding. We have reduced it by 75 or 80 percent. There's no question about that. The vaccine has worked, but it doesn't work in all cases and in all facilities."

"Voodoo medicine"

In the same year that WHO declared victory over small pox, Dr. Alson Sears found himself with few allies. In 1980, his major supporter and friend in the academic community had died. His colleagues had dismissed him, and universities offered a path seemingly impossible for a country vet with a small clinic to follow. But he could still use his serum to treat his distemper patients.

In the early 1980s he found a new ally with the emerging Internet. Using Tandy computers and the Internet billboard system, Al could let other veterinarians know about his serum.

"I had Tandy computers with the great big floppy disks," Al says. "Remember those things? In fact, we ran those out of the front office, we ran them in the back office. We did all sorts of cross checking on the practice with that sort of thing. I got really good at rewriting those floppy disks because they got hair and debris and dust from the clinic in them and they'd shut down. So, at least once a week I had to go in and resurrect floppy disks. So, you could imagine what that was like. I had four computers running in the clinic."

Because of a gap in enforcement on federal laws, he could send his serum to those who were willing to use it.

In 1913, Congress had passed the Virus-Serum-Toxin Act, which had been written in response to the unregulated manufacture and distribution of anti-hog cholera serum. A government official testified that the bill was necessary to protect the farmer and stock raiser of hogs. The act banned the shipment of "any worthless, contaminated, dangerous, or harmful virus, serum, toxin, or analogous product intended for use in the treatment of domestic animals."

Enforcement of the act fell to the U.S. Department of Agriculture. When the Food and Drug Administration was created in the 1940s, much of the food and drug regulatory power transferred there. However, Congress left meat inspection and veterinary biologics with the USDA. But for a practical matter, the federal government had a hands-off approach to veterinarians. "Regardless of where the authority lay, until relatively recently, the federal agencies regulating animal health products have taken the position that they do not regulate the practice of veterinary medicine. Until the 1970s, there were very few cases or regulatory initiatives by the agencies targeting veterinarians." [31]

The reason for this was pragmatic. While the interaction of drugs in humans could be reliably established in humans through trials, veterinarians treat several different species of animals and they knew which drugs were effective with which animals and in what combination. The federal agencies were more interested in human health and did not take an interest in the complexities of veterinary methods.

Also, the expense of running FDA approved trials becomes prohibitive if a drug's effectiveness must be tested in multiple animals and a variety of combinations. Veterinarians knew which combination of drugs worked for their patients, and "were left alone to produce biological products to use in their practices." [32]

To quote from a white paper on legal issues faced by veterinarians, when it discussed the hands-off policy:

> "For longer than any of us can remember, veterinarians have been skilled in the 'art' of producing vaccines, toxins, antiserums, etc., for treatment of a client's herd or flock. If the product worked well, the veterinarian might use it in a neighbor's herd, as well." [33]

So, in the beginning, the federal government took little interest in Dr. Sears and his serum. The clinic received requests for the serum through the Internet billboard. Among those who received the serum was a dog adoption agency run by an American in the Baja California Peninsula in Mexico who treated 14 street dogs infected with distemper. They wrote back to say the serum saved about half of the dogs treated early in the disease, but the rest – treated later in the disease – still died.

"In fact, I have a whole lot of reports, e-mails on the fact that we shipped the serum to people," Al says. "We shipped it to their veterinarians, is what we did. People would get to our e-mail, tell us what they had, and we would agree. They would give us the size of the dog and how long it was sick. We would determine the dose that they needed, we'd pack it up, take it over to FedEx and FedEx it overnight to their vets. They would give them the shot and respond as to how things came out …

"Initially, we did that for free just because we wanted to get as many cases as we could under our belts. Then we started charging. We realized we were putting a lot of money into this; let's see if we can get a return on it. So, we started charging $5 a cc. So, a 10cc bottle was costing $50, which to vets that were treating, was really nothing."

That caused some consternation among some customers who saw the earlier posts that the serum had been free. It took a while to untangle that problem.

Meanwhile, other vets in the Antelope Valley seemed to tolerate but privately grumble about Dr. Sears' serum.

"I had one veterinarian across the valley who called my techniques voodoo medicine," Al says. " 'Oh yeah Doctor Sears practices voodoo medicine.' And at one time I was going to call the damn stuff 'voodoo serum' just to piss him off. I didn't do it."

Throughout this period, Al got plenty of patients referred to him from around the Antelope Valley and Los Angeles, but the referrals were not made because the other vets had faith in his treatment.

"The joke in those days was 'Give all the bad cases to the new guy,' " Al says. "I was the new guy in town."

"So I ended up with tortoises and snakes and birds and rats and you name it," Al says. "And I also ended up with a lot of the distemper cases because they'd say, 'Well, I can't treat that. I can put it to sleep, but you can send it down to Dr. Sears. He thinks he's got a way to treat it.' So they would send a lot of the cases to me, not because they thought I had a cure but because they knew they couldn't treat it and why not give it to the guy down the street and let him have a problem with it. So that was the attitude that we ran into."

At least he had the ability to make plenty of NDV serum because of his good relationship with local dog breeders. Dog breeding had become big business in the Antelope Valley because of the wide open spaces free of city regulations. Al Sears became a favorite of theirs.

"One time I had a veterinarian ask me, 'How come Dr. Sears got along with all the breeders?'" says Chuck Whitt. The answer was that he listened to them. "They know everything they need to know about their breed of dog," Chuck says.

For example, Dr. Sears says a big issue with some breeds of dogs is whether they can handle particular combinations of vaccines. The wrong combination in the wrong breed could kill the dog, he says. But some vets would not listen to the advice of the breeders and didn't want to work with them. Al did.

"So, if you listen to them, they will tell you their problems," Al says. "Because the problem with one breed is not going to be the problem with another. So, if you listen to the breeders and treat their dogs according to the way they feel they should be treated, you become very popular with them."

Because of the massive numbers of distemper cases, Antelope Valley dog breeders often volunteered their dogs to be donors of the serum.

"I really liked my breeders," Al says. "I've had many many different kinds of breeds. They would adopt dogs and raise them out to make serum. We could make serum with them at 9 to 10 months of age and we would of course run all the lab work on them for free, and we would make serum and share it with them."

Because of this cooperation, Al not only could produce plenty of serum, he would also learn which breeds and kinds of dogs were best at creating a potent NDV serum. Over the years, Al would find mixed breeds were the best source of NDV serum.

A leap of faith must have been necessary for these breeders, who no doubt heard the grumbling and worries from other vets that Dr. Sears' methods were dangerous. Each animal could be worth hundreds or thousands of dollars, and Al was asking them to trust him by letting him inject them with a virus and then draw off their blood.

"They were doing this because they believed in what we were doing and what they saw," Al says. It was also worth it because they believed the NDV serum could save their dogs from distemper as well as from respiratory herpes, another disease Al Sears realized his serum could treat.

During his entire veterinary career, no harm came to any of the dogs used as serum donors, Dr. Sears says.

Federal handcuffs

The hands-off approach from the federal government would not last. In the 1970s, "the scientific community became concerned about the effects of residues of animal drugs in the human food supply. Toxicologists were quantifying the effects of low doses of these chemicals, and, equally importantly, test methods made it possible to find minute levels of residues in meat, milk, and eggs." [34]

The FDA would eventually conclude veterinary prescriptions used in food animals were the source of these trace amounts of illegal drugs in human food. This brought about a series of changes to the law beginning in 1985:

- Amendments to the Virus-Serum-Toxin Act extending USDA jurisdiction to all veterinary biologic products in the U.S. The statute covered any veterinary biologic product handled by any person in any place in the country.

- USDA is granted the authority to make "such rules and regulations as may be necessary."

The relationship between the government and veterinarians changed dramatically. "In a span of less than 10 years, USDA's jurisdiction went from a position of keeping its hands off the so-called 'intrastate' veterinary biologics industry to declaring that all veterinary biologics are governed by federal standards and any conflicting state laws are pre-empted." [35]

For Dr. Sears, the finality of the changes to the law were clear enough when an editorial in the Journal of the American Veterinary Medical Association arrived at his clinic in January 1987. After summarizing the current laws, the editorial concluded, "What must veterinarians do to practice effectively and responsibly under the conditions just mentioned? The first priority should be to protect themselves and their practices. When called upon to do favors for clients, practitioners should ask themselves, "Will this put me or my practice in jeopardy?"

JAVMA went on to write:

> "Employees and practice colleagues should be carefully instructed that such drugs are to be sold only when a **veterinarian-client-patient relationship** has been established. A veterinarian-client-patient relationship means that a veterinarian in the practice has seen the animals to be treated, is familiar with the premises and management system, and has established a tentative diagnosis for the condition to be treated. Records should be kept of all Rx drugs dispensed, who received the drugs, and for what purposes, and who ordered the drugs to be dispensed." [36]

Dr. Sears realized his use of emails, Internet billboards and FedEx could put his clinic and his license in danger. Heavy fines and jail time were possible, and he had only one safe way to proceed. "So, we pulled the website and we stopped shipping serum," he says. "If you came into our practice, we would treat you. But we're not shipping it to anybody, OK? It just stopped."

However, the new regulations handcuffed veterinarians. The American Veterinary Medical Association lobbied for some flexibility. In explaining the reasoning for what would become the Animal Medicinal Drug Use Clarification Act, the AVMA writes on its website:

> "A new animal drug was deemed unsafe unless it was subject to the FDA's stringent approval process – for exactly what was on the label – specific species, disease indication, dose, duration, frequency, and route of administration. **One of the main reasons why fewer drugs exist in veterinary medicine is that FDA's new drug approval process is very costly and time consuming for pharmaceutical companies, with little return on investment for animal drug products when compared to the return on investment associated with human drug products**, creating a relative disincentive for companies to put resources toward creating new veterinary drugs. Given the relatively few numbers of drugs available to veterinarians, AMDUCA created the professional flexibility that veterinarians need in order to adequately treat animals when their health is threatened. Additionally, many of the minor species have few to no drugs approved for various indications, making it very difficult for a veterinarian to

provide the best care for their minor species patient. With ELDU [Extra-Label Drug Use] regulation, many of these issues can be resolved and animals may be more readily relieved of suffering." [37]

The lobbying efforts resulted in exemptions for serums and "extra-label" use of prescription medications solely for animals under a veterinarian-client-patient relationship "when no FDA-approved product is available or when approved drugs are clinically ineffective." [38] Extra-label refers to the use of medications "not in accordance with the approved labeling." The Animal Medicinal Drug Use Clarification Act allowing extra-label use passed in 1994.

Options after rejection

When the Royal Society Journal had summarily rebuffed Edward Jenner for his "wild idea" about using cowpox against smallpox, he didn't give up. Two years later, he published a pamphlet on his methods at his own expense. The pamphlet described 20 patients who displayed lasting immunity to small pox after getting the cow pox vaccination. But he still faced popular opposition. Some leaders called it an outrage to infect a healthy person with repugnant material from an animal. Political cartoonists published drawings of people growing cow heads from their bodies. Religious leaders declared vaccination as against God's will. [39]

However, as Jenner's pamphlet circulated the method described was tried over and over again and succeeded. The success of vaccination silenced the critics and fear mongers, and Jenner later enjoyed accolades from all over the world.

Dr. Sears' 1980s Internet billboard and emailing were, in a way, an attempt to self-publish and get his methods out into the world when the standard path to acceptance was not open to him. However, he encountered a very different environment than Jenner. His obstacles included:

- The modern-day expense of scientific trials and studies, which make getting the approval of a new animal drug prohibitive for pharmaceuticals.
- A lack of interest in the treatment of distemper dogs since the disease was seemingly controlled by vaccination and euthanasia.
- A persistent worry of veterinary clinics about legal action. Malpractice insurance would not cover the use of any experimental or unproven techniques.

"You can't turn the ship of medicine that quickly," Al says. "You just can't do it. It refuses to change direction, and people are stuck in the way it's treated and professors teach it the way it's done and by God you better use that technique or you're in trouble. And it's getting in trouble that scares the bejesus out of people. Because the courts will clean you out and you will never recover, and it's not funny. You don't spend 16 years in school to have some lawyer take it all away from you. And it happens. If they don't have something from a specialist to put in the file, it doesn't count."

Oddly, the inexpensive cost of NDV creates another obstacle. Even today, NDV can be bought online at under $20 for a 5,000 dose bottle (free shipping if you get three or more). There would be little profit for a pharmaceutical company willing to navigate the costly and time-consuming drug approval process.

"We went to a party once," Ruth says. "And there was this physician who was very well thought of, and of course Al bends everybody's ear on this subject. And the man was so straight to the point, he said, 'How much money could the drug companies make?' And Al said, 'Oh, I don't know.' The guy said, 'There's your answer. Why should they put millions and millions of study and money into something that may not give them money back? And I said to Al, 'Are you listening? Are you listening to him?' Because he gets pretty frustrated, but that's the way it goes."

Leaving California

At the turn of the 21st Century, Amy and I lived a life completely untroubled by canine distemper. We had a baby boy, and I wanted to get a jump start on a healthier life for his sake. So I trained for and ran in the Los Angeles Marathon in March of 2000. The marathon wrecked my left foot, but I finished. This injury would bother me for years.

We had three dogs now, to my everlasting surprise. In 1998, I'd come home from work at L.A. Valley College one afternoon to find a 3-month old shepherd-mix puppy sitting under my desk in the home office.

Amy brought home a stray!

A drunk driver had smashed into her car as it sat unoccupied on the street one night. So, she needed a rental. The employees of the rental agency had caught a stray puppy and tied it to a fence hoping the owner would find it, but by the end of the day no one had come forward. When she arrived to pick up her rental car, Amy volunteered to take the puppy. "How hard could it be to find a home for a puppy?" she thought.

Actually, pretty hard. A couple of prospects fell through, and very quickly Wanda attached herself to me. She followed me wherever I went through the house. Although lighter in color, she was similar in breed and close to the age of Tug had been when she died. As Wanda grew, I could see what kind of dog Tug might have been. Giving her away became impossible.

So, in the spring of 2000, our lives revolved around our months-old baby boy – Jack – our three dogs, two cats and our jobs. One day, I searched through my desk for writing examples for my journalism students when I found a box of 3.5 inch computer disks. Curious, I popped one into the drive slot for my Mac and discovered my notes and rough draft of the Dr. Sears story.

Oh, that.

Amy and I remained grateful to have Galen. He was sometimes psycho, but also sweet and loyal. Three years had passed since Dr. Sears saved his life, and I continued to be amazed at how well he was doing. Out in the backyard, walled in with cement blocks so he couldn't see what was going on, he'd often bark wildly at any noise deemed a threat. (THIS IS MY TEMPLE!)

But despite his thuggish ways, he'd also play the sweet Labrador by napping with me on the couch. When we sat at the dinner table, he'd rest his snout on Amy's thigh or sometimes on mine. He never played fetch. As I threw the tennis ball for Shadow in the backyard, he would lie in the sun and contentedly chew on a stick. He and Shadow played a constant tug-of-war with a rope toy.

No traces of canine distemper troubled him. He never had any seizures. Galen lived the full life of a strong, healthy dog.

Too bad that story never got published, I thought, but too late. A shame that others won't find out about Dr. Sears and his treatment for canine distemper ...

As I mulled over this unpublished story, our local TV cable provider rolled out a new service: support and hosting for customers to create their own websites. I tried my hand at it, but my efforts did not impress Amy.

After all, Amy worked on the website at WITI. She had become quite the coding and web guru since we had moved to California. With her help and some space borrowed from a friend's server, we launched **http://www.edbond.com**.

This gave me an idea. I printed off a copy of the distemper story and mailed it to Dr. Sears. I asked for permission to publish it on edbond.com. A few days later, I came home to find a message from him on my answering machine. He said repeatedly that the story was "excellent" and enthusiastically agreed to have it posted.

In May of 2000, the canine distemper story went online in a series of primitive looking html pages. It opened with:

> *Let me tell you how we named our dogs.*
> *Tug was a throwaway dog, an eight-week old shepherd-mix pup with fur ravaged by mange. As Amy and I walked her around the block, I would spin the leash in front of her. She would catch it and, well, tug back. We got her a year ago in February. She left us that March.*
> *Selkie was a black lab, with some shepherd, a messy eater with a nose perpetually coated with her previous meal. She was named out of hope, from an ancient Gaelic mythical creature of the sea with an insecure relationship with man. The hope was that she would not leave us.*

We had rescued her in mid-May. She left in mid-June.
By the time we found Shadow, in October, we were
mentally exhausted, too drained for a creative name.
But she shadowed us around the house, so we applied
that verb to her. An Australian Cattle Dog - again with
some shepherd - she is muscular and high strung, taken
to barking at 1 a.m. Either Amy or I drag ourselves out
of bed, and if we have the patience, close our hands to
her head, make eye contact and as calmly as possible
say, 'No barking.'
Galen's first act with us - this February - was to put
his chin on Amy's thigh, followed by one front paw,
then another. His name means calm in Gaelic, but later
we would learn his demeanor was part fraud; he was
already weary from battling an old enemy of ours.
In a year, we fought that enemy four times, and became
too familiar with its attack, the silence, deception and
betrayal.
Thirty years ago, this enemy was as common as fleas.
Today, vets tell us how unlucky we were to have faced
it so often. Most vets never even see it.
The tally, so far: two dead, one survived and one never
attacked.
Now let me tell you how we fought canine distemper.[40]

By publishing this story on my website, I had no
intention of campaigning for Dr. Sears or proving the scientific
validity of his treatments. Saving one dog's life does not prove a
treatment. But I simply regretted missing a chance to put the
information out to the public. My hope was only that others in
Southern California – or anyone who could get their distemper
dog to Lancaster – could have their pets treated by Dr. Sears if
they wanted to.

Somehow, someday, Dr. Sears' treatments might get published in a journal and accepted by the veterinary community, but that was not going to be my job. I knew just enough about the world of science to understand I would be ill-equipped to fight that battle, and I had no interest. A colleague at the L.A. Times once put it to me this way: The purpose of the journalist was to illuminate the issues for others to act on. Posting a rough draft of a story to a website was intended to be minor act of journalism, not the declaration of an activist.

Only days after the story was posted, someone with a 6-month old puppy with distemper found the site and got her puppy Kassi to Dr. Sears right away. The puppy was still in the early stages of the disease and recovered quickly after the NDV serum treatment. In August, an Australian Shepherd/Corgi mix named Dot was saved. I began getting "thank you" emails every few months from owners of dogs Dr. Sears treated and saved.[41]

The call to home

Meanwhile, our world was about to be upended. Since our baby boy Jack had been born, we had a series of visits from Upstate New York family. Amy's mom and three of her sisters made treks to see the baby, and on one trip, her dad, Howard Clark, accompanied her sister, Mary Anne Bly.

Howie had always been a man of few words, but when he spoke they had impact. For example, we packed up Amy's car to drive to California in December 1992. In the driveway on Broad Street in Horseheads, I got behind the wheel for the first leg of the drive, when the driver's door opened and Howie loomed over me.

"You take good care of my daughter," he said. I gulped. Howie had a glint in his eye that reminded me of John Wayne. He made sure you knew his priorities. The safety and happiness of his children and grandchildren were paramount. I promised I would take care of Amy.

Then in July 1996, after our wedding ceremony at a winery on the eastern shore of Seneca Lake, Howie walked up to me. "Ten years of probation begins today," he said. Amy reassured me her dad had a very dry sense of humor, but I would never assume he was only kidding. After getting home from his California trip to visit the baby and us, Howie called Amy and asked, "So, when are you coming home?"

When Amy told me what he had asked, I knew our time in California had ended. In six words, Howie had not commanded us to return to Upstate New York, but he had shown us why we could not stay in California.

Amy was the youngest of eight. Most of her family either still lived in Horseheads or visited regularly. By living in California, we were 3,000 miles from the love and support of her family as we raised our son. By staying, Jack would miss out on the closeness of her family. His uncles and aunts and cousins would just be strangers who occasionally visited.

On the other hand, we also realized the dangers we lived with in Los Angeles. Before Jack was born, we had felt relatively safe in the niche we had created for ourselves in our Mar Vista neighborhood, which abuts Venice Beach. But after Jack came along, we saw the crime around us with new eyes. Drug dealers down the street from us. Our local bodega shot up in a drive by. At Valley College, one of my students showed up at the newspaper one morning and said he had nearly been shot the night before. He'd been saved only because the gun misfired. Another student missed class for a week and then called to say he'd been in jail. A former student at another college went to prison for murder.

When Amy and I visited Horseheads, our muscles relaxed once we were picked up from the Elmira-Corning Regional Airport. We hadn't realized how tight they had been in L.A. The release of tension surprised us and felt so good.

I'd come to Los Angeles to pursue a writing career, and I was happy with what I had achieved: writing for the Los Angeles Times, becoming a college professor, and – oh yeah – co-writing an episode of Star Trek: Voyager with my best friend, Jeff Schnaufer. Jeff and I met at the Times and teamed up on many adventures, including launching a newspaper in Santa Monica, teaching at community colleges and writing the Trek episode. Although we only sold the one episode, I pitched stories to the producers of Star Trek throughout the entire 7-year run of Voyager. Sci-Fi ideas now constantly flowed out of my head, a fire hose I could no longer shut off.

Amy had grown a lot in California. Not only could she now make margaritas and bloody marys, she learned web skills and trained in karate. We loved the excitement and culture of the city, the celebrity sightings, going to plays and concerts, visiting movie studios and museums. But we also knew we needed to return to Horseheads, to be close to her family and to have a better environment to raise our son. If it didn't happen right then when Jack was still little, it might never happen. I still had goals as a writer – including finishing a screenplay about time travel – but I realized I could achieve them from wherever we lived. The time had come to let go of Los Angeles.

I notified L.A. Valley College that Spring 2001 would be my last semester, giving them almost a full year to search for my replacement, a search that I helped get started. WITI agreed to allow Amy to work remotely from Horseheads after the big move.

But canine distemper had become part of my life now, and it would follow me wherever I went. During my last year at Valley College, I got emails like this:

Date: Wed, 7 Feb 2001
Subject: A Great Big Thank You

Hello Ed, I just wanted to write you a note to say thank you for taking the time and effort to post all of the information about Dr. Sears.

I live in Riverside, CA and have a 4 month old Aussie.

She came home from the humane society with Distemper and my vet told me there was really nothing they could do.

I did not accept this and went on a hunt for more information...that is when I found your site.

We took Cookie to Dr. Sears and now she is fine.

Dr. Sears is such a great guy...how do we get the word out to more dr's? I am e-mailing Oprah!!! and everyone else I can think of!

Well, Thanks again- you can go to bed tonight feeling like a hero because you literally saved my puppy's life!!!!!

Best Wishes to you and your family!

Dawn H.

In June 2001, I turned in my keys at the college. We began saying our goodbyes. Amy earned her black belt in karate. She had begun training in May 1998 and immediately fell in love with it. She had even kept up her training all through her pregnancy, until just shortly before Jack was delivered by C-section.

We celebrated Jack's 2nd birthday in July with a trip to the Santa Monica Pier, and at the end of July, Amy's friends from the karate school helped us sort our belongings and pack the moving truck I'd be driving cross-country with Jeff. The plan had been for Amy, Jack and all the pets to fly home to Horseheads, but the night before the flight our little black cat, Seneca, disappeared. So, Amy and Jack flew home one pet short.

The morning Jeff and I were to start driving the truck, Seneca showed up at the bedroom window. So, she got to fly to Horseheads all by herself. A week later, Jeff and I drove into Horseheads with the moving truck and my car in tow. I'd contacted my old newspaper, the Star-Gazette, to see if any jobs were available. My old boss told me there were two jobs: either reporting or copy editing.

Since I had already been a reporter at the Star-Gazette, I opted to be a copy editor this time around. They scheduled my first day at work for September 11, 2001.

Even though Elmira is about 5-hour drive from New York City and had a limited impact from the 9/11 attacks, the newsroom churned with activity that day. For the first time in decades, the little morning newspaper put out an afternoon edition. Even though I was supposed to be a copy editor that day, they pressed me into duty as a reporter.

Meanwhile, after staying with Amy's sister Kathy Wigsten and her family for a couple of weeks, then in a rental for a couple more weeks, we bought a house, something we would not have been able to do in Los Angeles. The closing had been delayed because of 9/11 when all aircraft were grounded and FedEx air deliveries were shut down. But in mid-September, we moved into a house just down the road from where Amy grew up, near a dairy farm and a string of horse farms.

Settling in

Our ranch house has a massive Norway maple in a large open back yard and two more maples in the front yard. The back property had no fencing, so the dogs could not run loose at first. The first night, I hooked up all the dogs on their leashes and took them out into the backyard in the rain. Just as we got past the maple tree, they spotted something in the dark.

All three dogs bolted at once, knocking me to the ground. I found them with their leashes tangled together, wrapped around branches, thorns and thin tree trunks in the brush on the far end of the property. They had trapped something amidst them.

A skunk!

My memory only recorded flashes of what happened next. Somehow, I extracted them from the brush and dragged them away. We made it back into the house in a muddy mess and a pervasive fog of skunk. Amy had already gone to bed and slept through the chaos. After years of living in the city, she could now sleep through cannon fire, apparently. I called my brother-in-law, Bill Clark, for advice. He laughed loudly and said, "Welcome to the country!"

Meanwhile, as he had said he would, Dr. Sears sent his protocols on treating canine distemper to nine veterinary journals. He received one reply, from the JAAHA on April 17, 2002. He sent me a copy of the editor's reply a few years later:

> Dear Dr. A.W. Sears,
> Thank you for your interest in publishing your protocol on treating canine distemper virus infection within the Journal of the American Animal Hospital Association. I have read your protocol summary titled Cellular Immunity Serum Protocol and cannot accept your article as currently submitted.
> For publication consideration, information must follow the guidelines for authors as detailed in various issues of JAAHA. It is also imperative that any suggested "new" treatment recommendations be validated through appropriately designed and carried out research protocols before it is disseminated as a valid clinical treatment option for readership consideration.

This includes ensuring that the research methodology used must meet recognized standards of animal care (usually through the review and acceptance by standing committees on animal care at the respective institutions where such investigative work is carried out). This latter point is especially relevant to your protocol because of the off-label use of Newcastle virus vaccine and the induction of shock in recipient dogs.

Unfortunately your article, as submitted, does not meet any of these requirements.

If I can be of any further assistance, please feel free to contact me either through the email address above or via AAHA at ....

Within a couple of years of our move, I'd found a gig as the part-time News Editing teacher at Ithaca College. I worked nights as a copy editor and days as a professor. This worked well for me because I could go into class teaching the print journalism skills I had been using the night before. My lessons were useful and practical because I focused on what the students would expect to do on a newspaper copy desk, editing stories, photos, writing headlines and laying out pages.

Amy's long-distance job at WITI did not last, and she ended up at her old job as the newsroom assistant. Eventually, she moved to the newspaper's online department. She worked days. I worked nights. So we only saw each other at home during a quick shift change where we only updated each other with key info about Jack and our youngest, Liam, who had been born in 2004.

After eating pancakes for Sunday breakfast in March 2006, a mild pain formed in my stomach. Just some gas, I thought. But it didn't go away for days, slowly getting worse each day. I finally went to the doctor on Thursday and ended up in the hospital. The hospital used a wide range of equipment on me: ultrasound, CT Scan, MRI, an endoscopic camera down my throat. For one scan, I had to lie in an awkward position while drinking barium, a chalky sludge that would show up on their imagers as it moved through my system.

They found a clot blocking a major vein that flowed through the liver, and the backlog shut off the flow of blood to my intestine. For a while, the doctors considered surgery to remove the damaged part of the intestine, but blood thinners began to relieve the clot and the intestine recovered. A hundred years ago, a clot like this could have killed me. I spent nearly two weeks in the hospital, but made it through thanks to the miracle of modern medicine and good health insurance. My doctor – Dr. Ed Foster – released me on Easter morning in 2006.

This experience gave me a unique perspective when Galen met his end.

Galen, the calm

Galen had become a different dog in Horseheads. With a large, open back yard and an invisible fence, he could see in all directions and feel less threatened. He calmed down. For the most part, he stayed inside the invisible fence, preferring to lie in a favorite sunny spot just beyond the maple tree. The only times he bolted was when spooked by loud noises.

During the replacement of our roof, I stood in the driveway as workmen chucked old shingles and debris into a dumpster. Someone tapped me on the shoulder, and I turned to find a man I had never met handing me a leash with Galen attached to the other end. The roofing work had spooked Galen, and he'd run from the back yard. This stranger had found him running loose in the neighborhood, tracked down his address through his tags and brought him back before I even knew he was gone. As far as he knew, Galen was simply a sweet, friendly dog.

If he only knew what trouble it had been to catch that dog back in the day.

Another time, I caught Galen jumping the invisible fence and when I brought him back, he knew I was mad at him. A little later that day, I took him with me on some errands. One stop happened to be at the Horseheads Animal Shelter. As soon as I pulled up to the shelter, Galen desperately put both paws on my thigh and lay his head across them, just as he did when he first met Amy. His claws dug into my leg. "Please, don't put me in there," he seemed to be saying. "I'll be a good dog."

It took several minutes of petting and talking to calm him down and reassure him I was not giving him up. But he knew what an animal shelter was, and what it could mean. His intelligence and ability to connect emotionally impressed me.

In July 2006, Howie and Amy's sister Mary Anne had come by to visit, when Mary Anne realized our recent wedding anniversary had been a landmark. She turned to her dad and me and said, "Shouldn't we have a ceremony to mark the end of Ed's probation?"

Howie and I looked at each other, and I realized how to spare him from wasting any words. I said, "I think we just had it."

We nodded to each other, and the ceremony was over without a word from him.

That October, I got up one morning to let the dogs outside. Galen took longer to get out the door than usual, so I scooted him through it because I was in a hurry. Later, I spotted him standing at the door waiting to come back in.

He looked like a distemper dog, haggard, drooling, eyes squinting. Clearly he was in a lot of pain and discomfort. This shocked me. As a distemper survivor, he should never have been attacked by that disease again.

He hadn't. From blood tests, the vet diagnosed the problem as being in the liver. The tests couldn't say whether it was cancer or some other liver disease, and the vet could only suggest some pills to try to correct the problem. The pills didn't help and each day Galen got worse. His only consolation seemed to be when he could lay down in his favorite sunny spot in the back yard.

My mind kept going back to my liver trouble only months earlier. As soon as I felt the belly pain, I could let someone know. When I realized it was getting worse, I could go to the doctor. I could cooperate with a series of expensive tests and give the doctors important clues to help them figure out what was wrong.

When Galen felt the beginnings of the same pain, he could tell no one. As it got worse, he could not let us know. We didn't realize he was sick until he looked so terrible. By then, the problem had gone on too long. He couldn't tell us exactly where and how it hurt. He couldn't participate in his own diagnosis. Even if we could run him through a battery of tests, he couldn't say what worked and what didn't. These are the limitations of animal medicine.

Every day, it became more difficult for him to reach his favorite sunny spot in the back yard. Every day, I knew we were getting closer to the end. "Ok," I thought. "If we're going to do this, I'm making a change."

I switched vets.

We had picked our vet randomly out of the phone book when we moved back to Horseheads. When our cat Stevenson got sick in 2004, I'd brought him to the clinic for tests. The vet barged into the exam room with: "Your cat has AIDS." He said it as directly as if he just told me my car needed brakes. The lack of bedside manner left a bitter taste when we euthanized Stevenson.

My in-laws had been saying good things about another veterinary clinic, so I ended up in their waiting room trying to explain the situation to the receptionist with tears in my eyes. How odd to ask to bring a dog in for its first visit just so it could be put to sleep.

They'd have to evaluate him first, of course, the receptionist said. "Yes, of course," I said. "That makes sense." They gave me an appointment for 9:30 the next morning. Amy had to work at the paper, so I would handle it. About an hour before the appointment, I put Galen in the passenger seat of my Toyota Camry. I wanted to spend some time with him before we got to the clinic. When I got into the driver's seat and closed the door – cut off from the rest of the world – I let loose with a good cry.

We stopped at a little park next to a fishing pond, and I sat there on a bench with Galen on my lap. I petted his head until it was time for the appointment and said goodbye, knowing it was for real this time.

The new vet evaluated Galen and agreed there was not much to be done for him. "Very often, dogs will just hang on because they don't want to leave us," she said. "They assume we don't want them to go. We have to help them."

We muzzled Galen. The vet approached with the injection.

"No more pain," she gently said to him.

Galen said, "GRRRRRRR!"

I buried him in some woods near a favorite creek. While I was at work that night, Amy noticed something odd. The boys had been playing with party balloons for a few days, and random balloons were still scattered around the house. One red balloon seemed to follow her as she went around the house. Half deflated, it scooted around the floor. It stopped when she stopped, stayed where she stayed, moved when she moved. This is how Galen sometimes followed Amy around. It only did this that one night. Had Galen come back to say goodbye?

Reaching Utah

Meanwhile, on the other side of the country, another ending approached. Dr. Al and Ruth Sears had maintained the two sides of their veterinary clinic for more than 30 years. Running a business together can stress a marriage and strengthen it. A sense of humor seems to be a key to survival.

"Credit to Al, he never brought problems home," Ruth says. "Credit to me, when he was wrong in a decision at the office – and I knew he was wrong – I would quietly give him the finger, but I left it at the office that day because there was no way you could not get into arguments over certain things."

This was from a phone interview I had with both of them in 2012. Throughout the interview, Al laughed as Ruth told her side of things.

"And in truth, we never brought it home, we always got over it and it was never a big deal," Ruth says. "But I knew one thing … the guy with the license is the most important guy there. And I knew that. And so it made it easy for both of us, for me to swallow when I knew he was wrong."

More laughter from Al.

"It's marriage," Ruth says. "But working together. Most people could not fathom how we managed to work together."

Ruth deeply admired what Al could do as a veterinarian.

"What Al did do was constantly try to find where the problem was," Ruth says. "And I told him one day, when we were in the office and he was doing something that was really quite clever, I said, 'If I wasn't already married to you, I would really make a pass.' "

But by the fall of 2006, Ruth came to a realization. Al had lost a step or two.

"My wife came to me and said, 'You're now 70. There's no reason for you to continue in practice," Al says. "You're deaf. You can't hear a damn thing and your memory is starting to fade. It's time for you to quit and put the practice up for sale.' I said, 'Ah, OK.' "

While not really deaf, he was having trouble hearing, and his powerful ability to recall information had been slipping. He got her point. They decided to retire to Utah.

"If it hadn't been for that I'd still be down there working," Al says. "I really love veterinary medicine. It's a wonderful thing to do as a profession."

When they put the Sears Veterinary Clinic up for sale in November 2006, the agent had told them to expect it to take two to three years to find a buyer. They found one within two weeks. The new vet paid in cash and asked for Al to stick around for a few weeks to help with the transition. "He bought it outright," Al says. "So I was out of the practice."

The rest of the clinic, including Chuck Whitt, would remain in place. However, the new vet had no interest in Al's distemper serum or in treating any distemper dogs. Even when Al successfully treated a dog with the serum during the transition, it did not change his mind. The new vet did not want infectious distemper dogs at his clinic. But as Al showed the new vet the animal treatment side of the clinic, Ruth helped his wife learn how to run the business side.

"But one day, I was home," Ruth says. "First day, I think, and I got a phone call from the wife. And she said, 'Mrs. So-and-so fell out in the parking lot.' As she said that, my stomach went bloop and then all of a sudden it dawned on me, 'Ah, not my worry.' That was the first realization. And I guided her to what she needed to do, but I realized the knots that were always there for all the little problems that occurred in the practice that went on all the time."

And now they were someone else's problem.

They still needed to put their house in order before they could make the move to their retirement in Utah. Years of pet ownership had taken a toll.

In their life in Lancaster, Al and Ruth had owned a lot of animals. On their property, they'd had a dozen chickens, two geese and usually no more than two dogs at a time, including two poodles and two Rhodesian Ridgebacks. They'd also had a rat who lived in a bowl at the clinic in the 1980s and 90s.

For a while, they also had a pet bobcat. "A beauty," Al says. "Would sleep in the bed with Ruth and I and purr the whole night long. Wonderful animal."

The bobcat had been brought to the clinic as a kitten to be vaccinated and neutered in the 1970s, but the owners returned with it a few months later, saying they could not take care of it any longer. The 38-pound animal fit in among Sears's pets after the mother cat of the house established her dominance.

"It used the doggy door to go out in the back field to hunt late a night," Al says. "He was generally a joy to have around. When we would go for a drive we would take the cat with us. He loved to relax on the shelf in the back window of the car, much to the amusement of drivers behind us. Got lots of honks."

But a neighbor became alarmed to see the bobcat on her back porch, looking through the door at her two Chihuahuas. That led to a visit from state officials and a letter informing them it was illegal to harbor wild animals in private homes. They had to send the bobcat to a friend in the mountains north of the valley where bobcats lived in the wild nearby. "To my knowledge he lived to a ripe old age able to play in the forest around his house," Al says.

Before they could sell the house, they needed to hire someone to clean the carpets, which had years of dirt ground in by the many pets.

When the man came to clean the carpets, he fell in love with their house.

"Oh this is lovely," he said. "What are you asking?"

The carpet cleaner bought their house.

"So, two months after we put all this up for sale, we were out of California," Al says. "We were gone. We put everything we owned into two big carriers and had people drive it up to Utah and moved into our home in Utah. But I was out of practice and gone in 3½ to four months. That amazed the hell out of me."

Al left most of his NDV serum at the clinic. Later, he would learn the NDV serum and the refrigerator he had stored it in had been thrown out. It had also been too difficult to separate out the files on the hundreds of distemper dogs he had treated.

"When I left the practice, it was pretty quick, so I did not collect all of that," he said. "I had over 5,000 records in my records file. To go through and pick out dogs that had been done 10 to 20 years before would have been impossible. So, I didn't collect any of that. When I left the office, I left everything behind. I just sort of walked away."

Reaching Utah brought Ruth joy. For years, Al had not been able to leave the clinic during the many crises and landmarks of their lives. That was over.

"I realized Al's all mine," she says. "I don't have to share him with anybody, except I have to share him with poker people four days a week."

They could do everything together now, including visit Panama to see Al's old schoolmates. They could ski together and get each other to doctor's appointments.

"He can't hear a damn thing," says Ruth as Al laughs. "But he's there. So, that is the big plus for me about being together. We do everything together except poker."

"And shooting," Al says, laughing. "She doesn't like to shoot."

Al shoots trap and skeet targets with a shotgun.

"The poker night is fine," she says. "It's a really good life. We can afford to eat."

They bought a farm in nearby Heber, and Al threw himself into new hobbies, gardening and growing citrus trees and experimenting with plant stem cells. Plant experiments or maybe a bagged stool sample from a neighbor's dog Al was helping for free often occupied the dining room table. Ruth's kitchen porcelain often got stained with dyes and the breakfast room filled up with plants.

"What was the movie where the captain has the tree that Roberts throws over the thing?" Ruth asks.

"Mr. Roberts," I answer. Al laughs.

"He has one of those trees that is quick growing and I think when it gets too big he'll put a hole through the roof. He's insane."

More laughter from Al.

"Do I mind?" Ruth says. "Does it keep life interesting? Yes, it does. So, it's never a dull moment, even though I have to club him frequently. "

Ruth laughs.

"He has brought a lot of his hobbies home because truthfully he doesn't like to be out at the farm by himself," she says. "He gets lonesome. He's very social. It's very hard for him to not have 50 to 80 people a day telling him how wonderful he is because he doesn't get that anymore."

They both laugh.

He did get a taste of his old life when he invited the neighbor of his property in Heber to have his cows graze on his land.

"So, one day I went out there, and one of the cows was down," Al says. "We call these downer cows. Basically I thought, 'Oh my God, the cow's got bloat. It's going to die.' "

But when Al went out to take a closer look, he found the real problem.

> **Dystocia** – A difficult birth, typically caused by the size and position of the fetus in relation to the mother's uterus, cervix or pelvis.

"She had two little hooves sticking out of her vagina," Al says. "I'm thinking, 'She's not down from bloat. She's in **dystocia**. She's having trouble delivering.' "

Al called the owner of the cow and told him to send for a vet. "You've got to bring some ropes, and you've got to bring some iodine, and you've got to bring somebody who knows what they're doing, and let's get this calf delivered,' " he told him.

But after finishing the call, Al stood there looking at the cow struggling in pain.

"She's straining and the calf's got little feet sticking out, and I'm thinking, 'That's stupid. I'm a vet. I can pull this damn calf,'" Al says. "So, I reached down and I pulled that calf. It was like one of those Christian pictures that you have with all the animals gathering around. All the other cows came around and gathered around, leaning over my shoulder and washing him. It was the strangest thing you'd ever want to see in your whole life. I'd delivered this calf live and it plopped on the ground and breathed for a while."

The mother of the calf lay there for a while, looking back at him. The scene became somewhat surreal as the cows expressed their gratitude.

"All these cows were down sniffing the calf and sniffing me and licking my clothes," Al says. "I'm thinking, 'God, this is weirder than hell.' About 30 minutes later, the cow got up and she went over and nuzzled her calf and gave me a big kiss on the shoulder. The calf got up and they both walked away."

The owner of the herd arrived along with his grandfather, a field hand and a vet who worked as a meat inspector. They looked at the new-born calf and said to Al, "Well, gee, thanks. It's all done."

He laughs as he remembers the story.

"That was my one clinical veterinary experience," he said. "You know, it was fun. I actually enjoyed that. You know what? Once a veterinarian, always a veterinarian. Let's face it. Just because you're retired doesn't mean that you forget what you've been trained to do.'"

Anyway, as of January 2007, Amy and I were happily settled in Upstate New York; Ruth and Al Sears were happily retired in Utah. Our dog Dr. Sears had saved had lived for nine years after treatment, having never been bothered by distemper again. Galen rested in peace in the woods along a creek. Dr. Sears had left behind his practice and his canine distemper treatment.

That might have been the end of the story.

Except it wasn't.

A Reluctant Activist

Publishing the distemper story on the Web in May of 2000 set off a chain of events, some good, and some bad. Not everyone who emailed called me a hero. One email came from a gentleman very frustrated with the long-winded tale, which at first didn't offer any concrete advice. He just wanted to save his dog, he snapped, what do I do?

Grudgingly, I made changes. Dr. Sears sent me his protocol for the NDV serum, which I posted. I added the link to a discussion group on canine distemper on AOL, which seemed to be the only active forum out there at the time. But I remained determined to stay out of any active role in promoting the treatment for canine distemper. If this treatment became successful, great, but it was not my job.

My priorities focused on my family, my two jobs and my various writing projects, which included short stories, novel chapters, children's stories and about 10 drafts of the time-travel screenplay. I had a full plate.

With little prodding from me, the distemper story had rippled through the Web and emails, knocking over dominoes on the other side of the world I didn't know existed. The head of an animal blood bank in Korea read my website in 2003, tested out the NDV serum for himself, found it effective and began offering it as a regular product to his clients in 2004. I had no clue this had happened.

On July 4, 2008, I received this email from Dr. Sears:

> "Mr. Bond. After all this time you are still the main conduit of information on the treatment of distemper in the canine. Still cannot get the veterinary literature to publish any information on this procedure. Still many dogs with the acute disease and many more with the neurologic form. Here is a copy of the most recent treatment for the neurologic form, which has been successful in 2 dogs to date. These are the only ones that have been willing to try the procedure. Here is a copy of the protocol for the Neurologic form of distemper. Hope you will be willing to add this to your site. Thanks A. W. Sears DVM (Al)"

This explained a confusing email exchange I'd had with a dog owner in Indonesia at the end of 2007. The owner had contacted Dr. Sears because distemper had killed two of his five dachshunds. The three remaining were sick, two with neurologic problems. NDV might save the one dog without neurologic symptoms, but could the other two be saved?

Dr. Sears dug out his notes on the NDV spinal tap experiment with Dr. Adams at UCLA and sent them to the owner, who found a vet in Thailand to perform the treatment. During the next 9 or 10 months, the dogs recovered.

When the owner emailed me about his case, he assumed I already knew everything about the NDV spinal tap. But I knew nothing. At that point, Dr. Sears had not told me anything about this other treatment. The dog owner threw terms and acronyms at me that made no sense. I knew nothing about the experiment with Dr. Adams at UCLA. I did not trust what this man told me. This contradicted everything that I understood. Dogs who reach the neurologic stage of distemper – such as Tug and Selkie – could not be saved.

He said he wanted to be my friend, to give advice and criticism about my website and complain about the discussion board I had linked my site to. With all due respect, he just rubbed me the wrong way. I had no interest in waging a campaign about canine distemper, didn't appreciate the criticism, and the offer of friendship from a stranger on the Internet set off warning bells in my brain.

My replies were abrupt.

"Good luck with your endeavors, but I've decided not to pursue any further work on this with you."

That's how stubborn I was about not getting involved. However, I did eventually post Dr. Sears' protocol for the NDV spinal tap to the edbond.com website. About a year later, the owner of the dogs treated in Thailand launched his own message board about distemper. It stayed active for a couple of years, but we did not work together.

Starting to believe

In mid-August 2008, canine distemper tracked me down again. I came in for my Saturday shift at the Star-Gazette and found a voicemail waiting for me. A woman named Mada Lixandru had called from Romania. She was desperately trying to save her dog and wanted me to call her back.

No way was I calling back. I had to get to work and didn't want to get sucked into someone's emergency on the other side of the world. She emailed too, and asked if her vet could use the protocol for Dr. Sears' serum off my website. Of course, I said, that was kind of the point. "Most of my information/experience is on my edbond.com Web site. Your best hope is to contact Dr. Sears directly at …"

Then, trying to add a little compassion, I wrote:

"I do know how tough this can be. So, good luck."

"Do you have a cell that I could contact you on, perhaps?" she wrote. "It'd mean the world to me, speaking with someone who went through the experience before…your article meant a lot to me…"

Nope, still not calling her, I thought. I wanted to keep her at arm's length. All the information she needed was on the website. I had nothing more to add. She asked how my dog was, and she wanted to know what Dr. Sears looked like. She couldn't find any pictures of him anywhere. My reply:

> "Galen lived a healthy and happy life for about nine years after he was saved by Dr. Sears in 1997. He had regained his health very quickly after the serum was used, and only needed treatment for a few weeks for his dry pads and dry eyes, which the distemper had affected. He died in Oct. 2006 from liver disease. … Dr. Sears is a personable, compassionate, private man who simply wants to save dogs. He is a big man with white hair. He does not seek the spotlight because he does not wish to be subjected to the public thrashing that someone would face in coming forward with a cure for distemper. Unless vets see his serum in action, they usually don't believe it…. The rest of my experience with distemper is all up my Web site. I do know how painful this can be, and I wish you the best of luck."

That ended the exchange.

By now, we had boosted the dog population at our house back to three. Jack wanted a dog of his own, so we went down to the Horseheads Animal Shelter and he picked out Romeo, a copper-brown and black hound-mix who had been originally rescued from a crowded animal shelter somewhere in Virginia. When we sat at the kitchen table, Romeo would sometimes put his head on my thigh as Galen used to. When I looked down and could only see the front half of his snout, it looked just like Galen's.

Meanwhile, Ithaca College gave me an extra class for the Fall Semester of 2008. I'd be teaching News Writing and News Editing in addition to working nights as a copy editor.

As the 2008 presidential election approached, the economy collapsed. Newspapers have always been fragile creatures in any economic downturn, and this one was devastating. The easiest way for any business to save money is to cut advertising, the life-blood of a newspaper. This time, the loss of revenue struck nearly a death blow to journalism. Newspapers across the country failed or cut back editions. Those trying to survive put more of an emphasis in their online editions but still without knowing how to make money at it. The print newspaper industry dangled off a precipice.

We watched all this from the newsroom in Elmira with growing trepidation. The Star-Gazette's parent company, Gannett, undertook cost-saving measures. The online department in Elmira was closed and merged with our sister paper in Binghamton. This forced Amy out of a job, but they gave her another position in advertising. Not an ideal job for her, but at least something. In the meantime, she started looking for other work.

The company began work furloughs in which we had to take unpaid days off. Layoffs came next. Across the country, we heard distressing news every day of good, experienced journalists losing their jobs. My enthusiasm for journalism – and teaching journalism – took a nosedive. Why teach college students to get ready for jobs that won't be there? I decided Fall 2008 would be my last semester.

The one bright spot amid the gloomy news: Amy landed a job on the website for Cornell University in Ithaca. This gave us much needed security if I got laid off, and very soon I began hoping for that to happen. Better to get it over. I'd grown tired of only seeing Amy at the 5 p.m. switch. But the other shoe took months to drop.

In mid-December, I worked the wire shift, editing national and international news stories for placement throughout the newspaper. As I juggled tasks, I kept a window with Facebook open. Amy had talked me into joining Facebook. I'd find it much more fun than MySpace, she promised. That night, my Facebook tab displayed a group popular with many of my colleagues: "Don't Let Newspapers Die." It had about 50,000 followers.

My chat window popped up.

> **8:05pm Mada**
> hi ed, sorry to bug, you around/
> **8:09pm Ed**
> hi, what's up?
> **8:17pm Mada**
> hi ed, sorry was doing laps around the house trying to put kitten to sleep. =D
> i dunno if you remember me, i'm the girl who kept bugging you about doc
> **8:18pm Ed**
> yes, i remember.
> **8:18pm Mada**
> heh, great...
> well, we did produce the serum after all, and i first wanted to say a big thanks, it wouldn't have been possible without you
> and your article...
> that's one
> and two, i dunno if you remember, but my dog actually died, as she was too far along.... but we did manage to save 5-6 dogs with that serum.

The conversation continued for almost an hour as Mada told me about how her vet made and successfully used the NDV serum. She was trying to get other vets and researchers interested. I kept replying to Mada while switching between wire editing and Facebook. She asked questions about skin rashes on her dogs, and then we chatted about colleges and media.

"So you've really set some potential life-changing things in motion, at least for the pups...;D" Mada wrote towards the end.

"Great, and thanks for letting me know what's been going on. It means a lot to me to know when my posting has helped save dogs."

And what happened, then? Well, in Whoville they say – that the Grinch's small heart grew three sizes that day. By the end of the conversation I'd become a slightly different person.

I knew enough about science to know that results need to be reproduced by other scientists so that they can be confirmed. A vet in Romania had taken Dr. Sears' protocols off of my website, followed them and had the same outcome as Dr. Sears. This saved the lives of at least five dogs. Confirmation?

Except when studies come out, they usually come from one university or institution and then are confirmed by another. Two private practice veterinarians on opposite sides of the world reaching the same result was not as prestigious as two universities. However in a common sense, pragmatic way, the principle was similar. It got my attention.

I suppose, up to this point, I hadn't really believed it. I believed Dr. Sears had saved my dog, but not enough to want to get involved. I had not fully understood what I had been sitting on.

What a stupid asshole I'd been!

Dogs were dying of distemper every day, all over the world. My website described a method that might save their lives. All that was needed was for other vets to do as the vet had in Romania, follow the protocol and make the serum.

And yet, I had done nothing useful about this. I had not made my little website easy to find. I could do so much more to let the world know, and the very tool I needed stared right at me.

My Facebook tab still sat open to the "Don't Let Newspapers Die" group. They had 50,000 members. What if 50,000 people on Facebook knew about Dr. Sears' NDV treatments?

Cold fusion and perpetual motion

The next day, Dec. 15, 2008, I launched the Save Dogs From Canine Distemper page on Facebook. In the first two weeks, it gained 33 followers.[42] I would later try to push the NDV treatments out into the world in every direction I could find – Twitter, Blogger, Wordpress, YouTube, etc.

To me, this was a clear moral imperative.

Doing nothing meant dogs would die when they didn't have to. I could not bear that thought. If I did something, some of these dogs might have a chance to live. Doing something meant possibly sparing other owners the grief Amy and I had gone through with Tug and Selkie. Instead, they might experience the joy we felt when Galen lived. Doing nothing would just be flat out wrong.

This new determination formed with a nugget of guilt in the back of my brain. How many dogs have died of distemper in the past 11 years while I did nothing?

No more. At least not without trying.

The NDV spinal tap treatment had already started to spread without any help from me. A jewelry artist in Georgia named Pippit Carlington contacted me to say her dog Carmella had survived after being treated by her vet there. She had also tracked down Dr. Sears. Hers was the first dog in the U.S. to be treated with the NDV spinal tap since the UCLA experiment. She offered a lot of advice and support throughout those early days.

I sorted through my old emails and reached out to others who had contacted me and I rebuffed. Stories began to pile up. A network emerged, focused on the Facebook page. Via email and other electronic messaging, I would eventually connect with people throughout the world. If this could "go viral," that would be fitting, I thought. Another way to use a virus to fight a virus.

On Jan. 20, 2009, while the newsroom and the rest of the U.S. focused on the inauguration of President Obama, I received emails and Facebook messages from two women with distemper dogs. One lived in Houston, the other in Malibu, California. Over the next few days, the woman in Houston failed to find a vet willing to try the treatment and eventually stopped emailing. The woman in Malibu managed to order the NDV online, but her dog died before it could be treated. She did offer to hold on to the NDV bottles she received in case any other owners needed it.

After these failures, I wondered about the saying attributed to Gandhi that we could "be the change you want to see in the world." It seemed doubtful.

Finding vets willing to try a treatment off the Internet remained the major problem. The principle of injecting a spinal canal with a vaccine for a bird disease just sounded crazy. The idea of injecting a healthy dog with this bird vaccine to make a serum from its blood didn't sound much better. Even those willing to try were shaky about continuing. But at the end of January, I heard a vet in Austin, Texas, used the NDV spinal tap on a dog that survived.

The way I saw it, the best way to treat distemper dogs was to use the NDV serum before they reached the neurologic stage. But so often, the dog owners and vets didn't even realize they had a distemper case until the seizures began. We needed to focus on educating dog owners to recognize the signs of distemper early and act quickly. Since making the serum took time and required finding the right kind of healthy donor dog, some owners were having their vets inject the sick dogs directly with the NDV as an intravenous injection – into the vein.

For that to work, the sick dog would need enough of an immune system left to create the needed reaction on its own. So that was a hit-or-miss, last-ditch effort.

We also had to find a path to acceptance. Having failed to get the story published back in the 90s, I had some idea of the problem. But I needed someone with more experience to put it into perspective. I wrote to a science writer for the New York Times.

"Hi Ed," came the reply. "I wish I could help but this story, as you know, is very difficult to write without more scientific credibility. It's not something I feel comfortable taking on. I'm very sorry."

"I take it then that you would only be interested if it got into a scientific journal first, right?" I asked. "Is there any other criteria short of that that would make it worthwhile?"

"If two or three leading experts in veterinary medicine came out publicly to endorse the treatment, it could make a story," she said. "But they would have to have impeccable credentials. If they spoke out at a national conference in front of their peers, it would be even better."

That's what I had figured. Journalists would stay away from this until publication in a scientific journal happened. Otherwise, they risked their credibility and reputation. This would require scientific studies, carefully documented trials showing repeated successful treatments for a large number of cases. As Dr. Sears knew, that required money and required someone on the research side willing to put the time into an idea, which was "in variance with established knowledge" and not likely to generate a profit. How could we get someone on the research side to listen to a wild claim from a website?

Imagine an amateur astronomer who looks through her backyard telescope, scans the night sky, and spots a comet. So, she calls the observatory for a university and reports its location.

"There's never been a comet there before," comes the answer.

"Well, there's one there now," she says. "Just take a look."

"You're just an amateur," the astronomer says. "That can't be right."

"Just take a look," says the amateur.

"No," says the astronomer. "I won't look because you can't prove it."

"But if you look, that would prove it."

"It's too expensive to look. So, I won't look until you prove it first."

Ridiculous, right? Of course that wouldn't happen in astronomy. But this is essentially the Catch-22 Dr. Sears has faced for much of his life. It would be easy enough for the astronomer to look through the telescope and confirm the comet. What I would learn is that it is not as easy to have a biologist look through the metaphorical microscope and confirm the effectiveness of a treatment.

I put it another way in a message to the Facebook group:

> "Here's the problem: Most vets don't believe this works. That's because their educational system and their professional organizations tell them there is no cure. For some, telling them, 'I know a vet who has found a cure for canine distemper' is equivalent to telling a physicist 'I have discovered cold fusion' or 'I have built a perpetual motion machine.' Those things are impossible."

So, reality check. I am not a vet, a doctor, a scientist or any kind of researcher. No power on earth could compel a veterinarian or a university researcher to listen to me. But the owner of a sick dog could say to a vet, "Please, my dog is going to die anyway, I want to give this treatment a try." In that moment, the vet might shrug and say, "Sure, why not?"

Then what would happen if we mobilized the full power of social media? In Facebook posts and on blogs, I asked those dog owners who persuaded their vets to try the treatment to document their cases. Take photos and video before and after treatment. Then send me the files along with their accounts of what happened. I may not be a scientist, but I knew how to collect stories. Perhaps if we had enough of these stories, someone who could do something would take notice.

The goal was not to bypass the scientific method, but to find a way to participate in it. To get these protocols into the hands of scientists who could evaluate them on their own terms. Hopefully, that would lead to publication in a journal, and then I would walk away.

Granted, that plan relies on a lot of wishful thinking.

In April, the Star-Gazette finally laid me off, and I was thrilled and relieved. I'd enjoyed being in journalism and still had a lot of affection for the Star-Gazette and my former bosses and co-workers. But now, I could focus on other things.

At the end of April, a rescue group in Southern California asked one of its members – an OB/GYN – to save a dog from the South Central Los Angeles animal shelter. Margo, a 1 to 2 year old lab mix, had been about to be euthanized.

After getting the dog home, she worried about the dog's nasal discharge and cough. Could this be distemper? As a precaution, she kept the rescued dog in her garage, away from her two 5-year-old labs. She'd heard about Dr. Sears and his treatment for canine distemper and drove from Orange County to Lancaster only to find out he had retired and the treatment was not available there.

"That was a disappointment," she wrote in a Facebook message. "Any possible vets that you know of out in my neck of the woods that might try?"

I made a mental note to myself to update the website to clarify Dr. Sears had retired. She had already called several vets and could not find one willing to use the protocol. As a medical professional, she was able to discuss specifics with the vets. Also, a friend of hers who researched AIDS had told her the use of NDV to trigger an immune reaction was plausible.

As we tried to figure out options over the next few days, she asked Dr. Sears and me some very useful questions about diagnosing and treating distemper as well as the background on how he made his discovery. These questions later helped me figure out a game plan. She was surprised so few vets knew about the bladder test to confirm distemper.

"Do you happen to have any idea on how many dogs have been treated with the NDV vaccine and the success/failure rate?" she asked.

At that point, I had no idea and no way of knowing. Another mental note.

She followed up with every vet I could suggest and worked several contacts of her own. I contacted the woman from Malibu who had saved the NDV after her dog died. She had given her vials of NDV to a vet so he could give it a try. The OB/GYN contacted that vet and was told, "Since Dr. Sears' treatment did not work on two dogs he tried it on, his opinion is that it is NO BETTER THAN SNAKE OIL." She added, "But at least I learned that it did not seem to cause harm even though it did not help in his case."

For me, "snake oil" stung, but at least it clarified what we were up against.

"Most vets don't understand how it was possible that he just stumbled on to it if he was just a vet in private practice," she said in one of her last messages to me. I did not learn the fate of Margo, and a follow-up email went unanswered.

At about the same time the OB/GYN and I were trying to figure out what to do about Margo, Suzanna Urszuly, an actress who lives in the Los Angeles area, also emailed me about her dog Hunter.

"I have a 5 months old border collie mix puppy who has distemper," she wrote. "She is really sick now, she can't even get up. I don't think we have much time left, and I am very desperate for help."

She emailed me a couple of hours later with "About 10 minutes ago she got up ate and walked around the room. She fell down a couple of times but got up. I am not sure if she has seizures or not but she twitches a little with her head and front legs. Not much just a little bit."

The next morning, I learned my last possible lead for a vet willing to use NDV in California had fallen through. With Suzanna's dog reaching neurologic stage, we were already beyond needing just an injection of NDV. This dog needed the NDV spinal tap, and we had no options in California.

Suzanna wrote back that she'd be willing to drive anywhere in the surrounding states, Nevada, Oregon, Utah or Arizona.

Luckily, Texas came through. The owner of the dog treated in Austin had persuaded that vet to treat two more dogs. Now, that vet – Dr. Liat Zilkha of the White Angel Animal Hospital – was willing to give it a try again. Suzanna got Hunter to Texas within a couple of days.

This email landed in my Inbox on May 19:

> "Thank you so much for checking in. Hunter is doing amazing!!!!! ... She already felt a lot better after her bodily Newcastle shot. Her nose and eyes were clearer and her pneumonia was gone. Now it has been about 9 days since she got her CSF tap. She can walk really well now, she does not fall like she used to. She can see at least 60% now, before she was almost blind. She still has a little bit of the 'head tilting and chewing motion' going on but it is less and less every day. She is such a happy, pretty puppy. I will send you some photos of her soon. She has a lot of energy too. She dug out my flowers and brought them back in the house and then she hid them under her pillow. :-) Thank you again for your help and I'll be sending her pictures soon."

Suzanna sent me before/after photos of Hunter. In the before photo, she looks lethargic, eyes dull and barely open, nose cracked and dry. The after photo shows her carrying the flowers in her mouth, eyes bright and shiny.[43]

After the "snake oil" comment, the photos of Hunter and news that a dog from Florida had also been successfully treated by Pippit's vet cheered me up. Now, if only we could have before/after video as well?

Climbing two mountains at once

In mid-May, my phone rang, and Caller ID displayed the number for Ithaca College. I had not even applied for any positions, so this confused me. When I answered, the head of the journalism department offered me a full-time teaching job on a one-year contract. At the end of the Fall 2008 semester, I felt I was done with teaching. Now, unexpectedly, a full-time professorship at a four-year college had fallen into my lap.

With the drastic changes in the news industry, I had my doubts. Traditional newspaper journalism now stood on a melting sheet of ice, and as it shrunk more reporters and newspapers fell into the surrounding seas. What remained of journalism transformed into new media. If I were to make this work, my classes would have to somehow layer in all the new technology, Web design, video, blogging, etc., on top of the classic skills of journalism. Although I had a taste of these in my professional work, I needed to learn many skills as I went.

Could I do all this and also fight the cause of canine distemper? Could I climb two mountains at the same time?

Had I not taken this chance to teach full-time, I would have always wondered "what if?" So, I accepted the offer from Ithaca College.

At the beginning of the semester, a big boost of confidence about the distemper treatments came from an unexpected place: The Philippines.

On Sept. 18, Clarisse Marcelo-Tanner of Manila wrote me about her dog, Icy:

> "The very day she was diagnosed with distemper, me and my husband kept researching about Canine Distemper. I read many many medical articles about it saying that it has no cure and the prognosis is very poor especially when the Neurological phase sets in. She was tested and diagnosed on August 31 and it progressed really fast. In less than a week, her neuro symptoms first showed on her right front leg, next on her head and then her hind leg muscles started to show subtle spasms. At first it was just bad when she would rest and sleep, then after a day or two, resting or not it was almost non stop. All this happened in a matter of days."

She sent me three video attachments. The first shows Icy, a light yellow Chow mix, sitting up on her dog bed, snuffing and licking the air as if trying to breathe. Icy huffs and gags several times, barely able to keep her eyes open. Their young daughter in the background says, "Icy's sick!"

In the next video, Icy lays flat on some light-colored bedding. Her body rhythmically spasms. Front leg, shoulder and head rise up and down. Her nose twitches. Then the cycle of spasms repeats.

Icy's owners found a vet in the Philippines to perform the NDV spinal tap. The third video shows Clarisse's point of view, which describes: "One morning, a few days after the NDV treatment, I went downstairs and there she was! Greeting me joyfully, jumping, wagging her tail, all excited. She hasn't been this way since she got sick. We can't wait to spread the word and help other dogs."

The video would eventually go up on YouTube and get more than 62,000 views.[44] Icy would live for another six years, passing away in August 2015 from other complications.

Another idea had been forming in my head for a few months. Perhaps, a non-profit group would be the way to go. That way I could avoid seeming less like a snake oil salesman and demonstrate more respectability. Then, fundraising and networking could be taken to a new level.

Looking for advice, I contacted my oldest sister, Jane, in New Jersey. I asked if she had any idea about how to form a non-profit.

That's when she told me she and Karen were already doing that. Karen's habit of rescuing street dogs and finding them homes had grown too much to be just a hobby. So, they were setting up a small non-profit corporation with the goal of helping street dogs. Since canine distemper attacks street dogs and shelters, it made sense for me to join them.

On Sept. 30, the IRS gave its stamp of approval to Karen's application for the new 501(c)3 nonprofit: Kind Hearts In Action. By coincidence, the @distemperdogs Twitter account launched on the same day with: "Dogs with canine distemper can be saved. Ask us how." After creating the Kind Hearts In Action website on WordPress the next month, I switched most distemper pages from edbond.com to the new site – **kindheartsinaction.com** – where I could more easily update information and post stories about cases.

Karen became executive director of KHIA and set up her own project under its umbrella: "Under The Porch," the dog-rescue wing of the group. I took the title of project director for canine distemper and was given free reign to do what I needed to run KHIA's "Save Dogs From Distemper" project. Karen's friends, Casey Hale and Steven Schwartz – who had helped her capture Galen – joined the board of directors. Steven became the business manager.

Mia Shark of Alberta, Canada on October 10 emailed:

"PLEASE HELP!! My puppy was diagnosed (without tests) with distemper. He was a rescue and had kennel cough. He is a husky shepherd bichon mix. He is 3 months old and has phlegm, a slightly runny nose, slightly red eyes. His shakes started in his left back leg then went to the right after the left disappeared. Then the shake came back in both hind legs and is now in the front legs."

Mia would send more than eight minutes of video of her puppies – Kaliber and his sister Lil' Miss – fighting distemper. The video opens with Kaliber lying flat on a carpet, front legs slightly twitching despite phenobarbital. Mia explains on camera he will get the NDV spinal treatment in a few days.[45] She and her boyfriend would be driving from Alberta to New Mexico where they will be able to connect with the vet who treated Pippit's dog. On the video, she narrates: "From today forward, I will be documenting this case to let everyone else know that there is hope for distemper puppies, regardless of what your vet tells you that there is no hope and you should euthanize. There is."

The courage it took for Mia and Clarisse to do this awes me. With a beloved pet dying of a terrible disease, they believed enough in the NDV treatments to take out a camera and record what they saw. Mia described the experience blow for blow: Kaliber's paws twitching, nose dry, eyes red. Lil' Miss had also scratched a raw, bald spot into the top of her head. She often whined and cried in pain from pneumonia.

The video continues on the road to New Mexico, with the two sick puppies lying on dog beds on the floor, doped up on drugs. On the second day of the road trip, the video shows Lil' Miss whining and struggling with pneumonia. She would have to be euthanized before treatment.

The next scene shows Kaliber after the spinal tap operation, with the back of his head and neck shaved, eyes struggling to open from the anesthesia. Mia gives a close-up shot of the small incision from the spinal tap. "He's got a wicked lookin' hair cut right now," she says. "I think it's coming into style, for sure."

In the next segment, as a vet tech carries him out to the lobby at his discharge, Kaliber wags his tail and licks Mia.

The last video, on Oct. 21, 2009, was my favorite.

Kaliber runs in circles, chasing a toy.

"This little monkey is doing sooo good!" Mia says. "You can see his energy has increased like a hundred-fold. He just loves playing and fooling around."

Kaliber latches onto the toy as Mia's boyfriend playfully drags him back and forth on the carpet. Mia laughs. "Look at him go!"

The twitching had stopped. She brings the camera in for a close-up. Kaliber licks the lens. Mia laughs.

"Give me kisses," she says, laughing. "Give everyone kisses and tell them how awesome this was. He got slobber on the lens."[46]

As a journalist, I am skeptical by nature. You can tell me all about something, but I will trust that information only so far. I'd rather see it for myself. In 1997, I saw Galen dying of distemper and then return healthy two days after going to see Dr. Sears. But even so, I only trusted this enough to post the information on my website but not enough to fight for it.

The news from Romania helped me to trust the NDV serum enough to fight for it. Later, the emails and web posts about the NDV spinal tap gave me enough information to at least see what was possible. I remained skeptical. I would give it a chance and treat it fairly in my correspondence. In my heart, I think I relayed the information with an unspoken proviso: "This is what others have told me. I don't know from my own experience." That's why reporters need to attribute sources in news stories. The information doesn't come from the reporter, but who the reporter talked to. That explains the margin for error.

But as with Romania, the videos from Clarisse and Mia changed me again. They helped me believe dogs in the neurologic stage of distemper could also be saved.

Houston

Two days after Kaliber played tug, danced and licked the camera in Alberta, I boarded a commuter plane at the Ithaca airport. I had packed two video cameras, plus a laptop where I stored student projects to be graded over the weekend.

After about a quarter century in journalism, my life now veered into uncharted waters. Had anyone I didn't know called me when I was a reporter to pitch this story, I would have passed on it, very abruptly. Had I pitched a story about an unpublished treatment for canine distemper to a newspaper editor, she'd suggest I find something else.

A task had been placed in the path of my life. I could either walk around it and ignore it or I could pick it up. Because my dog had been saved and I'd received so many corroborating stories in the past year, I picked up the task and tried to do what I could. Dr. Sears never asked me to begin a campaign on his behalf. I chose this challenge on my own.

This entire enterprise went against one of my primary guidelines I followed as a reporter. The lesson came up in countless journalism classes: "Don't get involved in the story."

Too late now. I'm walking a tightrope without a net. And I couldn't see where to step next. As I made my way down the narrow aisle to my seat in the back of the plane, I asked myself why. The answer popped into my head: "I'm just trying to change one small corner of the world."

The Friday afternoon flight would take me to Newark where I'd make a connection to Houston. A rescue group that had battled several distemper cases had invited Dr. Sears to give a lecture and asked me to introduce him. This would be a much-needed education for me because I only knew fragments of information. For months now, dog owners had been writing me with questions I couldn't fully answer. Now I had a chance to get some answers face-to-face.

Dr. Sears and I had not seen each other in 12 years. A twinge of guilt lurked in the back of my brain. It had been there since I'd begun pushing the story through social media at the end of 2008. In a way, I had ruined Dr. Sears' retirement. I'd get hints about this, such as when I invited him to join the Facebook group back in January. His oldest son, Skip, contacted me to let me know Facebook wouldn't work because of the "crazies" who track him down at all hours of the night.

Rather than use Facebook, Skip and Al briefly set up their own website/blog – Treatment4Distemper – but then I got an email from a dog owner that it had gone down. "Two days ago he announced he didn't want to deal with it any longer," Skip wrote to me. For a couple of days, I didn't know if he was done with the website or done with helping dogs with distemper.

"I canceled the Treatment4Distemper because it was inaccurate," Al wrote me a couple of days later. He added later, "You and your Web site are the one true source of information out in cyberspace. Please keep this space active."

Frustration seeped into his messages.

"What always astounds me is that those that have used the technique and know it works will not step forward," he wrote once. "I can now paper walls with rejection letters from the cognoscenti. Go figure."

At noon the next day in Houston, I waited for Dr. Sears at baggage claim with Sherry Parker, a volunteer with the Rescue Ranch Animal Sanctuary. She had arranged for the lecture to happen at a conference room in downtown Houston. He'd have to return to the airport for a 9 p.m. flight to Dallas, where his sister Llona Schaack lived and Ruth would be waiting for him.

Sherry and I chatted about what tech support he might need for his talk. I told her I really didn't know what he would need and didn't know what level of enthusiasm he would bring. I knew he was 73 now and hard-of-hearing and with a memory that occasionally slipped. This would be his first venture into the public about his discovery. Would he be ready for this?

We spotted a tall, white-haired man with a full white beard descending the escalator. He wore a white shirt with an open collar, black pants and had slung his blue jacket over his arm. When he saw me, he gave an understated wave.

I whipped out my Flip video camera.

"My pleasure," he said as he met Sherry. "Let me grab a suitcase. That suitcase is full of information. I brought that along too."

"Ok," I said. "We didn't know if you had a PowerPoint or anything like that. It's all in there?"

"I've had three computer crashes, so this is what's left of what I've been able to resurrect out of my original notes," he said. "I've got boxes of stuff. I went through and filtered out and got what I felt was the most important information. I can go through a whole lot of subjects, distemper, herpes and other diseases as well. If they are interested, I'll cover anything they are interested in."

"The nice thing is we've got cures," he said. "That's what's important."

The baggage claim buzzed and the conveyor brought out the luggage. We shook hands.

"I want to get footage of you coming in the airport," I said as I pointed out the little camera in my hand. He laughed. Any worries about his hesitancy or enthusiasm melted away. Dr. Sears had come loaded with information and energy. He would fill the rest of our day with it.

"It was an interesting airport," he said. "What I'm amazed at is the amount of water that's here. Golly, there were lakes and rivers and it looks like an ocean out on that side. Is that the Gulf you can see from the airplane out there?"

The closest big bodies of water to the airport are Trinity and Galveston bays, with the Gulf of Mexico beyond.

"You're a big fisherman, aren't you?" I said. Until now, the only photo I had of him showed him on a boat holding up a fish. He'd sent it to me a couple of months earlier.

"I am, yes," he said. "But mostly freshwater cause all that have where I am is freshwater."

"Are you feeling good about being here today?"

"I am absolutely thrilled to be here today. I am really looking forward to this lecture. Very definitely."

We headed out the doors.

"And you've come a long way to be at this," he said.

"You know, I gotta tell you, I'm a journalist. I'm not supposed to be an activist," I said. "But I'm an activist for you."

"You know what, I appreciate that," he said.

Out the doors, Sherry introduced Dr. Sears to her son, Bruce, who waited by the car. "Call me Al," he said as he shook hands with Bruce. I shut off my camera as they loaded his bag into the car. Every time I shut off the camera that day, I regretted it because Dr. Sears never stopped talking, and everything was useful and new to me.

Dr. Sears got in the front passenger seat. Sherry and I sat in the back. As Bruce drove us away from the terminal, Sherry bent his ear about a distemper puppy she had recently lost. Bruce, Sherry and Sherry's other son Scott were then also fostering a 2-year-old dog with four newborn puppies, then about two weeks old. They didn't know it, but distemper would later attack that litter. I switched on my camera again as Sherry talked about recognizing the early symptoms of the disease, such as the green discharge out of the nose.

"I've got bad news for you," he said. "There's three other diseases that do that. The most common one is herpes, which I will go over with you. It looks so much like distemper, I got sent herpes cases out of L.A. thinking they were distemper and they were herpes."

"See my puppy that died from distemper this past July never had a discharge from her nose," Sherry said.

"Well, some don't," said Dr. Sears. "Here we are back with medicine again. Nothing in medicine is 100 percent. You can list all of the symptoms of the disease, and not every dog is going to have all of them. Some dogs only have one. Some dogs have none."

He kept talking as Bruce negotiated the traffic into downtown Houston. He touched on the example of dogs like Joe, who had only mild symptoms as a puppy and years later came down with neurologic problems.

"So, there's variations in the virus, and I'll go through the variations that I've seen," he said. "That doesn't mean that's all there is, that's just the ones I've seen. It depends on your area and the breed of dog you have and what they're exposed to as to what you're going to see. So, don't think you have a disease you can tell by looking at it. What drives me crazy is that vets look at it and think they're looking at kennel cough, but they're looking at distemper. Can't tell the difference, treat them for kennel cough and of course the dog's going to die. So, we saw that by the hundreds. We're talking hundreds of dogs. But I'll go over that. I'll go over all of this because it's really fascinating."

One factor that affects the outcome of a distemper case is the genetics of the dog and the strength of its immune system. Sherry and Bruce didn't know it at the time, but about five weeks later, they would lose three of their foster puppies to neurologic distemper. The runt of the litter, Iris, showed no symptoms although a distemper titer test showed she had survived a recent attack. Dr. Sears often talked about how some dogs survive distemper better than others.

"The more you learn about it the more fascinating it becomes," he said as we approached our destination. "Remember everything I say is subject to change. That's the condition of viruses in mammals. As quick as the mammal gets resistant to something, the virus will change and it starts all over again."

Bruce tells him a vet who had been interested in the lecture was not going to make it because of a schedule conflict.

"I would really like to talk to vets because they're the ones who have to carry this forward," Dr. Sears said. "But breeders in my area are the ones who pushed it and kept it going because they were directly involved."

The conference room

We got to the empty conference room, with windows looking out on the nearly empty buildings of Downtown Houston. As it turned out, no other vets did show up. Despite our efforts to spread the word through social media and email, we had only 5 people for the lecture, the four members of the Rescue Ranch and myself.

The head of Rescue Ranch, J.D. Ward, and her husband Mike were bringing Subway sandwiches for lunch and another video camera. While we waited, I showed Dr. Sears the video of Kaliber's treatment and recovery on my laptop.

"That's beautiful," he said.

Since we had no crowd, the plan to have me make an introduction for the lecture switched to recording an intro for a DVD we'd distribute to interested vets. While getting set up, Dr. Sears turned to Bruce and pointed at me. "That man has done more to save dogs from canine distemper than anyone else in the world."

Talk about breaking the rule of not getting involved.

I'd made compilation video of distemper dogs that had been saved. The background music for these videos came from Margaret Owens, the singer who helped us get Selkie to the vet the night we put her down. We played the videos on the conference room's wide-screen TV while I made eight attempts at recording the DVD introduction. Bruce helped me out, suggesting different positions and ways I could keep my notes in view. I'd been a print reporter and not used to working with video. The different takes had various problems with lighting, angles or just me flubbing words.

"Dr. Sears, you were once told to sit down," I said at the end of the last attempt. "Today I am asking you to stand up and tell these people about your discovery."

I stepped behind the camera to switch it off, but then quickly switched it back on because Dr. Sears was already in front of the camera and talking about his time in Lancaster. The video captured a yellowish blurry version of Dr. Sears.

"Our major disease was distemper," he began as I kept adjusting the tripod and the camera angle. "And basically, we were seeing many many many many cases and so it became a major project for me to try to figure out how to get this situation stopped."

My darkened frame slips into the background as I flip on additional lights, and Dr. Sears talks about the boxes of dead dogs, the frustrated owners, the journal article about NDV boosting interferon in cats, the recovery of the dogs from the NDV serum, and the report back from the Cornell lab that his serum did not contain interferon.

"The realization hit us that we had something that was different," he said. The key was his mistake in the timing of withdrawal of blood from the donor dog. "And that particular mistake made all the difference in the world. So from that point forward we had means of treating acute distemper, and I use that term because distemper has many secondary [neurologic] side effects."

But then, he let us know how much more he was ready to talk about.

"We were treating distemper cases and trying this particular material which is a serum on a variety of diseases which we will try to describe today for treatments," he said.

As Dr. Sears told of the rejection from Dr. Ott and got into the story of meeting Dr. Adams, the motorized curtains behind the camera whirr and open. Finally, the light problem resolved and the image improved. I don't think I ever managed to get the camera completely into focus.

"… Those papers never got published, which is a shame," he said about the NDV spinal tap Dr. Adams performed.

"So Dr. Adams believed that this particular form of distemper in the dog was an animal model for MS in humans, which is basically caused by measles virus in the brain of the human doing something very similar to what it does in the dog," he said. "In the human, you also get optic neuritis or blindness, seizing, chorea and I believe you can also see cases of paralysis."

He'd mentioned MS earlier in the car. But I paid attention more intently this time. My sister Jane has multiple sclerosis.

When he got to the point of the story where Dr. Adams died, a sadness fell across his face. "So, let's put a halt there for a minute," he said. I shut off the camera.

Questions and answers

The subject had switched to parvovirus when the camera came back on. Dr. Sears explained how a researcher at the Oklahoma Animal Disease Diagnostic Laboratory – Dr. Sanjay Kapil – could identify particular strains of parvovirus, how they have mutated and spread across the country. This was a problem because the vaccines covered the original strains, not the mutations. But Dr. Sears' NDV serum is not effective against parvovirus.

"Tamiflu absolutely works for parvo," he said. "And we stumbled onto that by accident. The reason is that the serum does not work for parvo. It does not work at all. You can bathe them in it and you get no effect out of it at all. Parvo essentially gets by the serum and gets by the NDV. It doesn't work. But Tamiflu, it turns out, works like a dream."

A few months later, Sherry would get the chance to put Dr. Sears' advice to use when Iris, the puppy who survived distemper attack, fell ill.

"She grew to 40 lbs and was 6 months old when one night she had explosive bloody diarrhea," Sherry wrote to me recently. "I called [J.D.] who told me to put some in a baggie and take to my vet. It was diagnosed as Parvovirus."

With J.D.'s help, Sherry gave Iris amoxicillin and Tamiflu.

"Within an hour of that, Iris tried to raise her head and tried to walk," Sherry said. "After she was given the Tamiflu, within 24 hrs Iris could stand up. Per [J.D.], she was given boiled chicken and potato broth. Within three days, Iris was running and playing again."

Iris' mother would later be used to create a large batch of NDV serum. She is now 12 years old and Iris is 10. "She can no longer jump up on my bed or the sofa but she is very happy and is my best friend," Sherry says about Iris. "I watch for signs of seizures. We have been very lucky so far."

As the afternoon in the conference room progressed, Dr. Sears sometimes would ask us to step closer so he could hear. Or he'd change position to better catch our words. But it never took more than a second try for him to hear or understand us.

Bruce asked: "Can you explain the difference and the meanings of cure, vaccine, booster, and serum."

Dr. Sears nodded at each term.

"A vaccine basically is the virus that you are trying to prevent," he began. "Usually that virus has been changed so that it is not highly contagious and causing disease although in some cases the vaccine can be hot enough to give you marginal effects. But the idea is not to make you sick, but to make your immune system make antibodies against that virus. So the antibodies are flooded into your bloodstream and if later on the virus makes entry to your body those antibodies pick that virus up and destroy it. Or make it available to be destroyed by cells in the body. That's a vaccine."

He paused briefly.

"Now, a booster is usually a second shot," he said. "For some of these diseases a single shot is not sufficient to give you permanent immunity. And where that tends to show up is in puppies. Puppies in most cases will carry maternal antibody against the diseases that you are interested in. So if you vaccinate them too soon, maternal antibodies are able to take that virus and neutralize it so that it can't cause infection. This is what prevents babies from picking up infections."

He explained that the maternal antibodies tend to disappear sometime after 10 weeks of age. Typically, the maternal antibodies disappear completely by 16 weeks of age, but a few rare puppies will still have them after 16 weeks. Maternal antibodies do not help the puppy's immune system learn how to create its own antibodies. That's why repeated vaccinations are needed to make sure a puppy can protect itself from disease.

"So usually, 8 to 10 weeks of age the first vaccine is given," he said. "We feel that you're really immunizing about 65 percent of the dogs at that point. So 35 percent are not being immunized. So, then you wait at least a month, and at 16 weeks when you feel that you've got 99 percent of that maternal antibody gone, you give the second shot and you're picking up 99% of the dogs. You still have 1% that you haven't covered. So those dogs either get sick within that year or they are vaccinated again in a year and at that year you pick up all those puppies again on your booster shots … So that's the reason for the series of shots that are given. That's essentially the timing that we used was, 8 weeks, 16 weeks and a year."

Vets often over-vaccinate dogs, which is an egregious error, he said. Three shots are all that are needed in the first year. No more.

From a review of the academic research:

> "Maternal antibodies are adsorbed in the intestine from colostrum [mother's milk] during the first 2 days of life and are cleared 6 to 12 weeks later. It is recommended that puppies receive a series of 3 vaccinations beginning at 6 to 16 weeks of age to achieve complete immunity to CDV followed by a booster at 1 year of age. Canine distemper virus vaccines impart long-term immunity in dogs. Duration of immunity of 3 years has been reported ... " (Kapil and Yeary 2011)[47]

"Now you talk about serum," Dr. Sears said. "There are two types. There is the serum that has antibodies in it. That is taken from an animal or a person that has already had the disease. Those people that have recovered will have very high levels of antibody in their serum. So for people or dogs that are sick that serum can be injected. And you are basically giving them the antibody to fight the virus. Now, unfortunately it cannot enter a cell. So if you already have the disease that material prevents the spread but it doesn't kill off the disease. Because in virus situations, the virus is inside the cell and the antibody can't get to the virus when it's in there, which is where it does its damage."

Then, Dr. Sears explained his kind of serum "that we really haven't named."

At first he had called it interferon serum because that's what he had been aiming for. But the Cornell test showed it didn't contain interferon. He'd also called it a **cytokine** serum, but other critics had explained that could not be right. He'd also called it **T-cell** serum, thinking these small white blood cells produced by the thymus gland were responsible, but he dropped that name too.

"It's obviously been called voodoo serum, but that's just an appellation which I don't like," he said. He still did not know what material was causing this result, but "This is a viral type material that sets off the immune system to fight the virus. That material can be collected. It can be kept stored in a refrigerator. It can be used and when shot into an animal even in small quantities, it sets off the immune system to go inside the cell and kill the virus in viral diseases where this is possible."

The current in vitro method of making human interferon differed greatly from Sears' in vivo serum, he said. To make human interferon, they would grow human cells in glass tubes – in vitro. An **inducer** – such as a material like NDV – is injected into those cells and at the right time, the interferon is drawn off. Different kinds of interferon are created depending on the type of cell used. This creates a very specific material for a very narrow task, he said.

To explain this, he used barrel size – caliber – of different guns as an analogy.

T-cell – A type of white blood cell produced by the thymus gland. It plays an essential role in immunity by maintaining long term memory to any antigen to which it has been sensitized through vaccination.

Cytokine – A group of proteins that send signals between cells. Interferon is one type of this protein.

Inducer – A microbe such as a virus or bacteria that prompts a cell to create interferon or other desired effect.

"The problem with the in vitro use of this material is it is kind of like using a 22 on a flock of birds as compared to using a 10 gauge shotgun shell," he said, sitting back in his chair with his dark-framed reading glasses folded in his hands. "And so in vitro, you're using a 22. You use it in the living body [in vivo]; you're using the 10 gauge shotgun shell. And that is because there are an infinite amount a number of immune products that are made that to date we haven't elucidated all or understand what they all do in their ability to work in concert. Which is going to knock the most birds down?"

The .22 caliber rifle uses one of the smallest bullets and is not likely to shoot down more than one bird at a time. The shotgun shell fires dozens of pellets.

"As veterinarians, we don't usually pay attention to the little intricacies. What we want to know is 'How do I treat this?' 'What do I do?' And that's what we have come here to try to explain to you."

J.D. and Mike arrive with Subway sandwiches and the extra camera. We take a break to get set up. I use the time to also to fill in some gaps of info. I had a question I could not believe I had not asked him yet.

"How many dogs do you think you have treated for distemper?" I ask.

"For distemper, I think I've treated probably over 600 cases," he replied.

"And all those recovered?"

I knew they didn't, but I wanted the camera to capture how he would put it.

Catarrh – A buildup of mucus in the nose or throat.

Incubation period – The time between exposure to a pathogen and the onset of symptoms.

"No, they don't all recover because some of the dogs are brought to us too late," he said. "Of those dogs we treated that were less than six days of illness, clinical illness, I think our success rate's in the high 90s. ... Those that do survive [without NDV serum] almost 95 percent or more end up with neurologic problems, which now have a secondary treatment. But they also end up with other problems. They end up with hardpad disease. They end up with blindness. They end up with dental problems. They end up with liver problems. They end up with organ failures or a variety of kinds of skin diseases. And some of those things cannot be treated after that period of time."

Nasal planum – The tip of a dog's nose.

"Some diseases have certain stages that they go through," Bruce asked. "What are the stages of distemper?"

Dr. Sears explained:

> "From the time a dog is exposed usually 9 to 14 days of no symptoms and then the dog basically breaks 100 percent, usually with respiratory problems, **catarrh**, which means plugged up nose. Pneumonia accompanies practically 100 percent of dogs that get distemper. Hardpad is one of the problems that you'll see. Vomiting is probably more than half of the dogs. Diarrhea with blood probably in more than half of the dogs. Usually with that particular group death is within the first 10 to 14 days. So you figure from 9 to 14 days from the time of exposure – no symptoms [the **incubation period**]. On about day 14, they begin to show some signs of problems, and the majority of those dogs will die within the next 14 days. Of those dogs that do not die in the first 14 days, some of them will survive out to about a month. And many of those will also

expire. Of those that go on to survive, they will end up with hardpad disease which means they get holes in the pads of their feet from trying to walk with the damage that's done. They end up with pneumonia. They end up with cracking of the nose, the **nasal planum**. They end up with other organ deficiencies internally and of course almost all of them end up with some form of neurologic disease, which we've described already. So, the disease is devastating from A to Z. And if there is a way – which we have discovered – to stop it, we'd recommend using it because the only other option is euthanasia."

"Ok, when you talk about the dogs that have been brought to you that are before the sixth day," Bruce said. "Is that the sixth day showing symptoms?"

"Yes," Dr. Sears said. "What we call clinical symptoms of the first day. The dog has a fever. And usually the fever will run over 102.5, from 102.5 to 105 degrees for dogs with distemper. All of them will get pneumonia. The pneumonia is not viral. It is secondary bacterial, which is interesting. That needs to be treated with antibiotics. Hardpad, dental changes, skin eruptions, diarrhea, vomiting all of these things go with the early stages of this disease."

Humoral – Relating to body fluids.

Mucopurulent – Fluid containing mucus or pus.

Oculonasal – Relating to eyes and nose.

Conjunctivitis – Inflammation of the mucus membranes of the eye and eyelid.

As the disease is described in a journal article:

> "Distemper is a highly contagious disease that poses a threat mainly to concentrated populations of previously unexposed or unvaccinated, susceptible species. In these populations, distemper is almost always fatal ... Robustness of the **humoral** immune response correlates with the disease outcome. Canine distemper virus replicates initially in the lymphoid tissues of the upper respiratory tract followed by immune-mediated progression of the disease over a period of 1 to 2 weeks. A **diphasic** [two-stage] fever is a characteristic feature of the disease, occurring 7 or 8 days after infection that drops rapidly and again climbs by day 11 or 12. Clinical signs of distemper are often unapparent or initially mild during this time, and disease is characterized by **mucopurulent oculonasal** discharges, **conjunctivitis**, respiratory distress, anorexia, vomiting, diarrhea and dehydration, and cutaneous rash ... Weak humoral and cell-mediated responses lead to systemic intracellular spread of virus to the **epithelial** cells of the gastrointestinal and urinary tracts, skin, and the endocrine and central nervous systems causing direct virus-mediated damage. Additional clinical signs that may occur are localized twitching, ascending paresis/paralysis, and/or convulsions. **Hyperkeratosis** [thickening of outermost layer of skin] of the foot pads and nose may be seen. The infection may either prove fatal or persist resulting in subacute or chronic central nervous system (CNS) signs. ... sometimes neurologic impairment does not occur until months later, even without a history of systemic signs." (Kapil and Yeary 2011)[48]

> **Epithelial** – The surface layer of a body
> or of the esophagus, stomach and intestines.
>
> **Hyperkeratosis** – Hardpad and the
> drying/thickening of nasal planum in
> distemper dogs.

As we eat, the topic switches to the difficulties of getting out the word about a cure for canine distemper. J.D. sees an opportunity because she blogs for the Houston Chronicle's website.

"Let's say you have access to the fourth-biggest paper in the country, the Houston Chronicle, that I write for every day," she says. "I have a daily column."

He peers over his reading glasses as he replies.

"Your problem with a medical procedure that doesn't come through the accepted medical literature is it is useless," Dr. Sears said as he gestures with air quotes. "It becomes homeopathic medicine. It becomes Chinese herbal medicine and any qualified veterinarian or physician is not going to listen to that kind of talk. He's not going to listen to it. Why should he? I mean, that's insanity."

"Let's back it up for a second, Dr. Sears," I said. "You've tried to get this published nine times."

"In nine different journals, all at the same time," he said.

"And what happened?"

"One responded," Dr. Sears said. "One responded. And he said 'no.' From the way it was written and the information we had, it was not valid and they could not publish it. So I responded immediately with the information that there was no technique in the literature for the treatment of distemper and we had one that worked, would he please change his mind? And I got back no response."

"What do you think would qualify for veterinary publication?"

"OK," he said. "If you had a lot of money, you could go out and buy a couple of litters of dogs. And you can divide them in half. And you could take half the dogs and not treat them … Well, let's divide them into three parts. You give one set a set of vaccines. You have two others left. One third you didn't do anything to. The third set were inoculated with the virus. So now, you inoculate all three groups with the [hot] virus. So, the group that had the vaccine won't get sick. Historically, won't get sick. The second group gets sick, but you don't treat it. The third group gets sick, and you treat it. Third group survives, the second all die. The first group never got sick."

He looks at me directly over his reading glasses. He's describing experimental controls. Other groups – not treated with the serum – must be documented so that other variables can be ruled out as the cause of the result. This increases the reliability of the experiment by demonstrating the effect had been caused by what the researcher expected and not some other factor.

"It's unethical," he said. "It's unethical. Why would you subject dogs to disease when you know … that's unethical? Think about this for minute. …

He shrugs at us.

"… To make an experiment and use dogs to give them the disease I think you'd be hearing about it for the rest of this century," he said.

Although I did not know about it yet, Laidlaw and Dunkin[49] had identified the cause of distemper and developed the first vaccine by deliberately giving healthy dogs the disease. This was done for the greater good, to save the lives of countless other dogs. I admire Dr. Sears' ethical stance, but it seems others in the scientific world see the ethics differently.

"What about as dogs come in, confirming they have the disease, treating them for the disease, documenting that they've been cured? And get a big enough track record?" I ask.

"You have done that," he said. "I have done that. And the answer to that question is our controls are all the other dogs treated with the standard procedures in the literature, which are antibiotics and fluids and supportive therapy. OK? How many of those dogs are dead? How many of them went on to die? How many went on to have neurologic problems? But that is our control. So you and I don't have to set up a control. Every veterinarian in the United States has set up your control for you. To be honest with you. Ask them what they did. Ask them what happened. ... So there's your controls. Will you accept that? The guy I wrote to didn't accept that."

The view of academia

This is the crux of the problem. In discussions of canine distemper at the time, there seemed to be two camps in the resistance to searching for an effective treatment. On the one hand, distemper is often portrayed as a death sentence from which there is no escape. Euthanasia gets proposed as the most humane way to deal with it. On the other hand, it is also described as being survivable. How survivable appeared to be in dispute.

In the first camp are vets who did not spend much time trying to save dogs with distemper. Very often, I heard from owners who say their vets don't know if they have a distemper case on their hands until the neurologic stage begins. For them, nothing could be done except to wait for that stage and then euthanize.

In the other camp, I read comments and reactions online to the stories of dogs surviving after being treated with NDV serum as "no big deal." Dogs can survive distemper. So what if dogs treated your way survived? When I was in the midst of this fight, I felt as if the critics wanted to have it both ways. But since then, I have had a few years to do some more research.

What I found was that the view of distemper in academia is very different from what Dr. Sears describes of his 40 years of clinical experience, and very different from the descriptions I received through my social media, websites and email.

A study at Cornell University in 1984 – which used three groups of puppies in a similar way to what Dr. Sears just described – sheds some light on the disagreement. (Summers et al. 1984)[50] In the study, 3- to 4-month old Beagle puppies, bred to be pathogen free, were infected with one of three strains of canine distemper.

- 6 were given Snyder Hill strain
- 11 were given Cornell A75-17 strain
- 12 were given Ohio strain R252

About half of these pups developed neurologic problems and died, but all were eventually euthanized for the study after two months. The Snyder Hill strain, which struck faster, caused a "moribund state" within 14 days and half died from the virus. But some of the Snyder Hill dogs that survived beyond the third week recovered. In the A75-17 group, some dogs reached the moribund stage between the 29th and 38th days. "In both A75-17 and R252 infections, neurologic defects were detectable in about one-half of the dogs."

The study included clinical observations, antibody tests of blood serum, cerebrospinal fluid, loss of myelin, central nervous system lesions and brain damage. In the discussion:

> "Characteristic of CDV-SH infection is that dogs follow 1 or 2 courses. Approximately one-half succumb to their grey matter disease whereas the remainder recover. … The Cornell A75- 17 and Ohio R252 strains behaved quite similarly and clearly differed from CDV-SH in the disease pattern they produced. Dogs followed 1 of 3 clinical courses: terminal sub acute disease after 28 days (cf., earliest with CDV- SH was 14 days), chronic persistent CNS infection, or total recovery."

The paper goes on to report: "From further studies with larger numbers of dogs infected with A75-17 [one of the viral strains] we have found that approximately one-third succumb, another third develop persistent infection, while the remaining third recover. In any litter of dogs, however, the outcome is quite variable and depends upon animal age, stress (for example, repeated bleeding for immune function studies) and possibly even upon genetic factors."

In a later collection of papers on paramyxoviruses which cited the Cornell study, "It is claimed that chronic **encephalomyelitis** with inflammatory demyelinative changes develops in about one-third of dogs experimentally infected with CD virus." (Randall and Russell 1991)[51]

That surprised me when I read that. In my very small sample of three distemper dogs, the result had been the exact opposite of what the researchers describe. Amy and I lost two-thirds of our dogs to neurologic distemper. Dr. Sears' experience with his "many, many, many boxes of dead dogs," where he estimated he lost 90 percent or more of his patients to distemper before he found his serum also paints a very different picture from what those researchers discovered.

One point I'd make is that conditions in a laboratory do not reflect what happens out in the street. As quoted earlier, when distemper hits a concentrated, unvaccinated, vulnerable population – perhaps a shelter full of puppies – "distemper is almost always fatal."

Encephalomyelitis – Inflammation of brain and spinal cord.

An outbreak at a shelter differs quite a bit from a controlled study at a university. The puppies at an infected shelter are being attacked from many directions as their fellow shelter residents shed the virus in multiple ways. In a study, the infection can be given in a controlled way, such as via a single nasal injection and the researchers can take steps to avoid cross-infection from other dogs in the study. Shelter puppies are also likely being attacked by opportunistic infections, such as pneumonia.

Of the three strains of distemper studied at Cornell, the impact on the dogs' health and survivability varied from group to group. And the strains of distemper still evolve and change. From the veterinary literature:

> "The major vaccine strains were isolated in the 1930s and it is not known if they continue to circulate in nature as they have not been detected for many years. Although CDV vaccine strains have not changed in the past 60 years, there is potential for newer antigenic variants of CDV to emerge around the world. However, the current vaccines have largely provided adequate protection against clinical disease when properly administered to healthy domesticated dogs in this country." (Kapil and Yeary 2011)[52]

Genotype – The genetic makeup.

Studies have identified "12 distinct geographically separated clusters of CDV **genotypes**: American-1 (including most vaccine strains), American-2 (North America), Arctic (Arctic region and Europe), Asia-1, Asia-2, Asia-3, Europe, European wildlife, South Africa, Argentina, Rockborn-like, and a new **genotype** of primarily Mexican strains. Serengeti isolates are distinctive from CDV isolates from other parts of the world. In the United States, genotypes that have been identified in dogs and wildlife in addition to the American-1 and America-2 strains are the European wildlife, EdoMex, and Arctic strains in domestic dogs." (Kapil and Yeary 2011)[53]

While some critics have shrugged at a treatment for canine distemper, there are two kinds of shrugs. In the first kind, the vet does not know whether they have a distemper case until the neurologic stage begins. That vet can simply shrug at the NDV-serum treatment in a pre-neurologic dog and say, "Well, that wasn't distemper."

The second kind may come from a vet who is aware of the studies like the one at Cornell and shrug at the NDV-serum treatment in a pre-neurologic dog and say, "Well, not all distemper dogs go into neurologic stage. Some dogs will recover on their own."

I get it.

But when Galen came home after treatment, he was strong, hale and hearty. As Dr. Sears would say, the virus had been shut off. The damage by the virus remained, as evidenced by the dry eyes and nose. But this was not a dog who would struggle with a virus over a matter of weeks. Not only had he survived, but also the course of the disease had been cut short. He had beaten distemper on that two-day trip.

However, I'm not a scientist or a vet. That's just my opinion as a dog owner. And saving one dog does not prove a treatment.

But now that I have read the Cornell study and other literature, and this is years after the Houston trip, I can see that any proof that a treatment works would have to account for the variations in the viral strains, age of dog and other conditions. Any study would have to show the treatment dramatically outperforms the known survival rates on distemper from university studies.

As of 2020, Cornell's Wildlife Health Lab website reported that canine distemper "is often fatal with a mortality rate of 50% in adult dogs and 80% in puppies." [54]

So, the main question of a NDV serum study should be whether this material can prevent distemper dogs from reaching the neurologic stage of the disease, shorten the course of the disease and ultimately save more lives than the traditional supportive methods. In other words, more happy endings as we had with Galen.

Pictures worth a thousand words

Getting back to the conference room in Houston, the conversation about Dr. Adams and his search to help humans with MS lead to a question of how people would be treated for measles.

"Now, we've been treating dogs with this problem," he said, leaning back in his chair. "The question is: Can you treat people? Well, maybe, maybe not. All species don't respond the same way. Could you use the serum? Make serum in humans and use it? Because these things are very species specific. You can't use human stuff in the dog; you can't use the dog stuff in the humans. But you could certainly make the stuff in humans."

"Do you think you could make the serum in humans the same way?" J.D. asked.

He leans forward.

"Exactly the same way," he said. "The timing is identical because you're talking about a system in the mammalian system. And in the mammalian system, it doesn't matter whether you're a monkey or a dog or a rat or a mouse or a human."

He leans on his armrest. His fingers grip the tips of the temples of his glasses so the lenses suspend in mid-air.

"My contention is with measles with this stuff, you should be able to wipe it out like you can [distemper] in dogs," he said. "You should be able to cure it in 12 hours. Who's going to try it? Do you have any physician who has the guts in the United States to look a lawyer in the eye and say I'm going to give this to somebody and I'm going to take the serum and I'm going to shoot it into the next kid who walks in with measles? Give me a break! It isn't going to happen. Any more than I'd take my sister with her walker and put her out on the freeway and tell her to go to the movies. It isn't going to happen."

So, the subject of human treatment dropped. J.D. switched the talk back to dogs.

"What would make a vet go from a non-believer to a believer?" she asked.

He raised his arm, pointed at me.

"This man's e-mails or his blog out there, showing cases – which he has one here he'll show you – showing cases recovering," he said. "A picture's worth a thousand words, and when you see these animals recovered you say 'God I don't have any of those.' "

"And a video is worth a thousand pictures," I said with a laugh.

He turns to his laptop, which he had set up on a chair, and sorts through his files to get set up for the presentation on making NDV serum. Mike and I get our cameras into position. The sun has changed and cast a glare on the TV screen. It takes several minutes to figure out the balance between enough natural light while limiting the glare. As the room buzzes, Dr. Sears has his first slide up and I can see he is ready to start. The title of the card reads: "Procedures for making Anti-Viral Serum."

> **Procedures for making**
> Anti-Viral Serum
>
> - The following protocol
>   is for the production of
>   anti-Viral serum.
> - This serum is used
>   S.Q. for the control of
>   distemper virus in
>   dogs.

"What are we looking at here, Dr. Sears?" I ask.

He stands in front of the camera, hand on his hip with the screen behind him. He talks with his hands and poses questions to us throughout that he immediately answers.

"Basically, what we doing here is we are giving you a picture postcard, comic book if you will on how to make canine NDV-induced serum. It's relatively simple to do. The reason we set it up this way is we have a word system on how to do it. But that gets confusing. So this is it in pictures, and it really is pretty simple."

He taps his laptop to change the slide.[55]

> Anti-Viral Serum
>
> - Dog- use an 8-12
>   month old mixed
>   breed dog 60-100 lbs,
>   young and healthy.
> - Do full lab work up to
>   eliminate all possible
>   health problems.
>
> - Vaccinate against all
>   local diseases.
> - Do not use breeds or
>   individuals known to
>   have immune
>   deficiency problems.

"So using an 8 to 12 month old mixed breed dog 60 to 100 pounds," he said. "Why that age? For us it just seemed that at that age their immune systems were intact, they were functional. We made sure these were not spayed or neutered animals because spaying and neutering, which we will get into later, interferes with their immune systems.

"We like the dog to be between 60 and 100 pounds because there's no sense doing this in a 10-pound dog, you can't get enough blood. You need to get as much blood out as you can. So, you get 8 percent. A 100 pound dog 8 percent will give you about 80 CCs. Well, it gives you more than that, about 250 CCs. You spin it down and you get 110 CCs of serum. So you can only do this once, you can't do this more than once in any dog."[56]

"Why is that?" asked Bruce.

Dr. Sears leans in.

"Because [after that] you get antibodies to the Newcastle Disease Virus. You have vaccinated the dog to a chicken virus, OK? At this particular period of time – 8 to 12 hours – this is not [antibodies]. This is an immune storm that you have created inside that dog. That dog has been shocked with a virus, and the immune system if it's intact is responding. And the response is incredible."

Demodex – Mange. A mite that infects the skin of animals, especially dogs. It impairs the immune system.

Diluent – A fluid used as a medium to inject or apply the vaccine particles. Newcastle's Disease Vaccine often comes with a bottle of blue diluent.

However, the term "immune storm" would later create a lot of problems for vets who saw the video. To them, it sounded as if he was describing a cytokine storm, which is a potentially fatal immune reaction. (Tisoncik et al. 2012)[57] A cytokine storm can cause a host of symptoms such as redness, swelling and pain as well as organ damage. But that is not what the NDV reaction causes or what Dr. Sears was attempting to describe. He continued.

"So, do full lab work to eliminate all possible health problems. You don't want a dog with heartworms. You don't want a dog with Babesia gibsoni [a blood parasite]. You don't want a dog that is carrying any kind of immune problem. Vaccinate against all diseases. So you don't have them carrying something cause you're going to give this to a dozen dogs. You don't want to be spreading disease out there. OK? Do not use breeds or individuals known to have immune deficiency problems. Any dog that's got **demodex** you don't want to use. By definition that dog has an immune problem. Why use it? You don't want a dog that has ascarids [roundworms] because they shut down the immune system also. OK?"

"Why not heartworm?" J.D. asks.

"Because it's floating around in the serum. It's not in the red cells. You're pulling the red cells out."

"You don't want to transfer heartworm to the dog?"

"Sure! Of course."

He taps the laptop and brings up a slide showing a bottle of Newcastle Disease Vaccine.

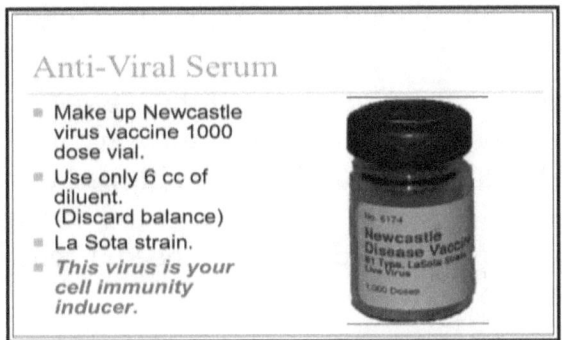

"So, this is your inducer. This is the one that we had. There are several I have in my files now that you can have. But this is Newcastle Disease Virus. This happens to be the LaSota strain. Why that one? Because that's what the chicken place we bought the vaccine from had. It seems to work very well. OK? What was the cost? A box of six cost us about 10 bucks, so you're talking about 2 dollars a bottle. Comes with 20 CCs of **diluent**, usually 1000 virus particles in these things. We usually made it up with 6 CCs of diluent and threw the rest of the diluent away. Why? Because that was how much the bottle held. The bottle holds about 6 CCs."

So, the NDV vaccine arrives in a small bottle as a dry powder, but it must be reconstituted with a liquid so it can be applied in an injection. Very often, the virus bottle would come with a blue liquid – the diluent – which is combined with the virus powder to make the mixture. Sometimes the vets would use saline or sterile water instead of the blue diluent.

"So, please understand this was back in the early days. We didn't even understand what the hell we were doing."

He raises both of his hands over his head.

"We didn't understand the immune system. It was totally out of our understanding. Certainly, nobody else knew anything about it. Okay?

"OK, so that's basically what you use, and there are several sources which we have in the files now. And you can buy this overnight in the United States and have it shipped to you."

He taps the laptop again. The slide shows a needle being inserted into a dog's front leg.

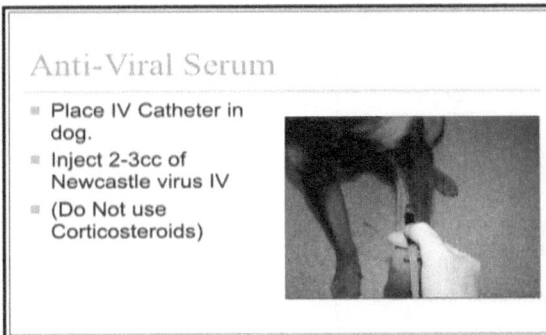

Anti-Viral Serum
- Place IV Catheter in dog.
- Inject 2-3cc of Newcastle virus IV
- (Do Not use Corticosteroids)

"OK, so we place an IV catheter in the dog. We inject 2 to 3 CCs in about 100 pound dog. Why that much? Because that worked pretty well for us. It's all a priori, just what we've developed.

"Do not use any cortical steroids. Why? Because that interferes with your immune system."

Another tap.

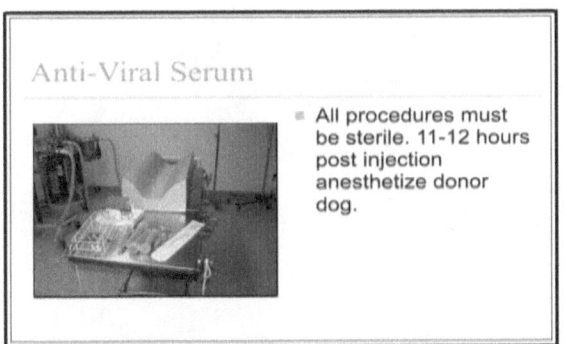

Anti-Viral Serum
- All procedures must be sterile. 11-12 hours post injection anesthetize donor dog.

"OK, there's our surgery. We recommend you do it as sterilely as possible. The bottles were given to us by the local lab. Those are 20 CC syringes sitting on the table with 18-gauge needles. They have what looks like a splint lying out there. That's a table we put them on their backs to stabilize them. And the dog is of course anesthetized."

ED BOND

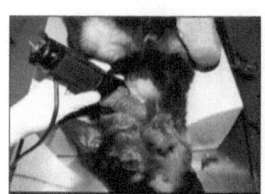

Anti-Viral Serum

- Timing is essential. Take blood 11-12 hours post injection
- (11-12 hrs post injection= Anti-viral factors=Very effective against distemper Virus in VIVO.)

"And timing is essential. Timing is everything when you're dealing with immune materials in the body. In you stimulate it with a virus and you pull it off at 6 to 8 hours, you are pulling off interferon. Interferon does not cure distemper. OK? Does not cure distemper ..."

"Eleven to 12 hours post injection put the dog to sleep get an IV running on them, shave their necks, and what we did was ..."

Tap.

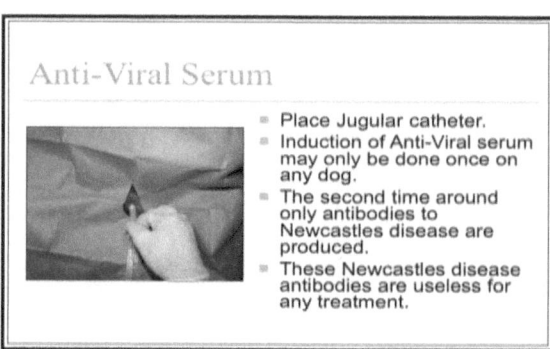

Anti-Viral Serum

- Place Jugular catheter.
- Induction of Anti-Viral serum may only be done once on any dog.
- The second time around only antibodies to Newcastles disease are produced.
- These Newcastles disease antibodies are useless for any treatment.

"Put an IV catheter. This is a jugular catheter. Why did we use that? Because you can pull a lot of blood quickly out this dog. If you tried to do this out of the cephalic vein [in the limb] you'd get really slow as you tried to get the blood out, takes you almost 45 minutes to do that. You can do this in 15 minutes.

"And so on the one line, you're giving fluids. On the other, you're pulling blood. You pull blood until the dog looks like it's going to go into shock. You get as much out of the dog as you can because you only get one shot at this."

For example, the gums blanching – turning white from a lack of blood – is a sign of the onset of shock, when not enough blood is flowing through the tissues. Shock is a dangerous medical condition, so the procedure has to end before shock takes hold.

"So place the jugular catheter 11 to 12 hours after you have given the vaccine. The second time around, you can't use it because you have antibodies then. Antibodies block what you are trying to do. These Newcastle Disease antibodies are useless for any treatment. They don't do anything. OK? And then you take blood. 20 CC syringes."

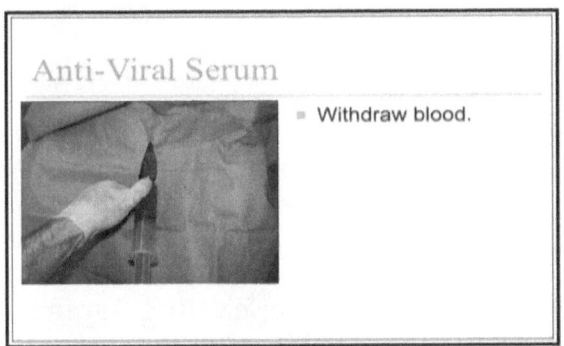

Anti-Viral Serum

■ Withdraw blood.

Tap.

"It's immediately put into bottles. OK? 10 cc vials, sterile. No additive. Nothing. Just spin down bottles. The lab usually will give them to you. Allow the blood to clot. In the dog it takes about 30 minutes. In the cat, it takes about 10 minutes. If you don't take the blood off immediately, what happens is the red cells begin to lyse [break down]. Then you have hemoglobin in there, which you really don't want. You want it clear, so…"

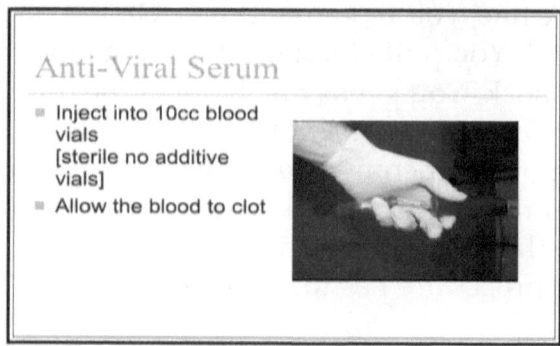

Tap. Brings up a photo of the centrifuge, the mini-carnival ride that separates serum from red blood cells.

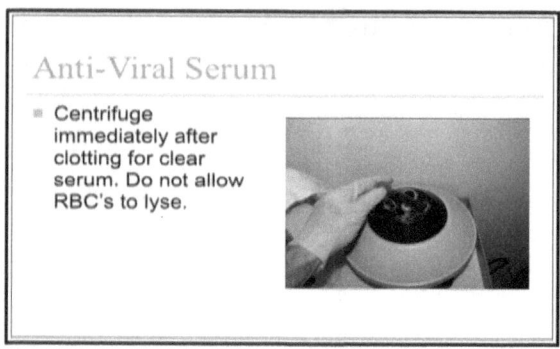

"As soon as it clots – immediately after clotting – spin it down. You want to get the red cells out of there. Why do you want to get the red cells out? Because if you give red cells to a dog that doesn't have the same blood type you're going to get a reaction. If you use serum, there's no reaction."

He holds up a finger.

"Species to species. Species to same species is critical. OK?"

Tap.

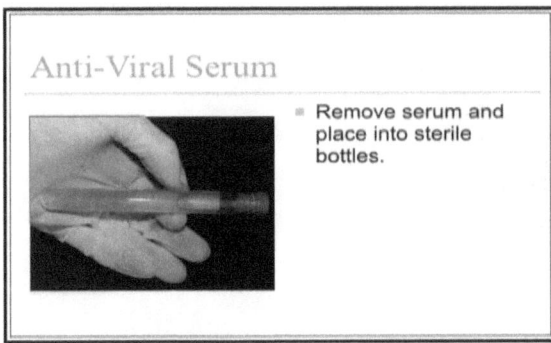

Anti-Viral Serum

- Remove serum and place into sterile bottles.

"That's what it looks like when you take it out. Pull the serum off. Red cells are left behind. It's put into bottles like that, which are sterile. 10cc bottles, OK?"

Tap.

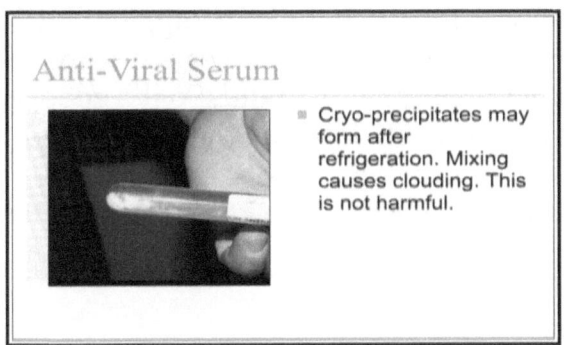

Anti-Viral Serum

- Cryo-precipitates may form after refrigeration. Mixing causes clouding. This is not harmful.

"When you refrigerate this, there are very large proteins in that serum. They are called cryo-precipitates. They make absolutely no difference. You can leave them in there or you can filter them out. We found over time that they made no difference. They were white precipitates at the bottom, which you can see. And if you shake the bottle basically what will happen is it will sort of make the serum cloudy. So, you can clear it."

Tap.

Anti-Viral Serum

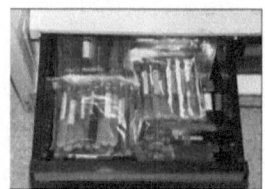

- Place serum bottles in baggies and store in refrigerator.
- Bottles of serum can be stored for up to five years in a refrigerator.

"This is how we stored this stuff. This is the crisper in the refrigerator. These are the bottles in Baggies. Make sure the tops got alcoholed off, so that they are clean, you don't have any blood left or you're going to get secondary mold. You've got to be careful of that. But then you just stick them in Baggies and put them in the refrigerator. We used stuff five years old and it had every bit of the control the original stuff did. So it's good for, we feel, up to five years, probably longer. Somewhere along the way, I read you could freeze this stuff and it's good for 30 years. Go figure. I never froze any of this. We kept it this way in the crisper, in the refrigerator."

Tap.

Rx of Individual Sick Pups.

- Weigh pup 1 to 10 lbs
- Give 1 cc of ANTIVIRAL SERUM per 10lbs + 1cc per dog to dogs very 12 hrs for 3 treatments

---

"OK, how do you treat them? Sick dog. You want to get them before the sixth day if possible. If you get them before the sixth day, they're easy to treat. Here's the treatment. Weigh the dog. One to 10 pounds. You give 1cc of the material [per 10 pounds] plus 1cc for the dog, three times. Give it 12 hours apart, three treatments. By the time you give the third treatment, they're already well. You could probably get away with one treatment. But we used three.

"Don't ask me why we used three. That's just what we set up. That was the way it was. You could probably do it with one.

"What is amazing is – look at the amount of material you're talking about. You've got a 10-pound dog. You're giving it a CC of this material, which is nothing."

He points to a can of Coca-Cola on the table from lunch.

"A CC of Coca-Cola wouldn't even wet your whistle. And that is enough to set off whatever the immune stuff that's in this stuff to get into the dog and trigger all the cells that are necessary to kill the virus intracellularly."

He leans in for emphasis, pausing dramatically.

"Now, I say that to people that have medical training and they say 'Oh come on. That's not possible.' There it is."

He swings his head back at the slide.

"You're looking at it. It does. It works. And this is what we did for the first [few] years. Until people would write to us and say, 'How do you get we serum?'

"Well in the meantime, we had a problem. The FDA came along, and it said, 'Hmmmm. We're not going to allow veterinarians to ship serum for anything except blood expansion. Any serum that is shipped to treat a disease in the United States is illegal and it is to be subject to a fine and jail time. Period. So we stopped shipping serum to anybody. You could come to the clinic and we could treat you, but we could not ship serum. I didn't want to spend time in jail. It didn't make any sense to me, but that was the ruling. So we stopped shipping serum, period.

"So about that time we realized that we've got a problem. What do you do with somebody, say, in France. You can't ship serum. Or somebody in Texas, you can't ship serum. 'Why don't we try just shooting the dog with the NDV straight?' Well, all right, well here's the problem."

He fingers his pinky, as if counting.

"Distemper can cause immune failure. It's why you have the disease in the first place. It got in around the [immune system]. So you have a dog with immune failure, you hit it with NDV; it doesn't make the materials that are necessary. It doesn't clear the disease."

He holds his hands open.

"Conversely, you get a dog with demodex..."

He raises his right hand.

"...we know that dog is immune deficient. You hit it with NDV, and nothing happens. It dies of distemper. It didn't work."

He keeps moving and talking with his hands.

"You get other dogs that have genetic problems, combined immunodeficiency problems, you can't treat those dogs.

"You also really can't treat a dog that's less than puberty. Because they haven't gotten to the point where their full T-cell system has developed until they go through puberty. Why is that?"

He raises his hands above head, opens his fingers broadly.

"I didn't do it. God did it."

"But when you get your sex hormones developing that's when your immune system comes to full fruition."

He drives both index fingers down for emphasis, and then they spin back up in a circle.

"So you spay a dog at four months, you're leaving 'em susceptible to all kinds of problems.

"But the pounds all spay dogs at four months. Down in California they spay them at 12 weeks. All right. They can't get pregnant, so they don't have more puppies for the pounds. But now, they've got the biggest damn problem in the world with distemper.

In his practice, Dr. Sears says be came across many dogs adopted out of the pounds that had some kind of disease or respiratory problem. He counts on his fingers, starting with the thumb.

"They've got distemper. They've got herpes. They've got parainfluenza. They've got influenza, now, you have flu. And you've got parvo. They've got five diseases walking out the door."

All five fingers have gone up.

"When do they show up? Five to six days after they walk out."

"Why?"

He points around the room at us.

"Why? … Because they hold them five days. What's the incubation period for a virus? 14 days."

His hands spread wide.

"So five days. They're fine. They're spayed. They're shot."

He goes pfft, mimics an injection with a syringe.

"Spaying gives them a hell of a kick in the head as far as their immune system is concerned. They're also puppies. They don't have one to begin with. Now, you hit them with the vaccine and spay them and you run them out the door."

His arm swings as if shooing out a dog.

"And a week later, here they come."

His arms go wide open.

"Full-blown disease. Which one do they have?"

He raises a single finger.

"Ah, that's the key!"

Tap.

Anti-Viral Serum

- Serum does not stop Parvo
- Serum does treat interstitial cystitis (call or write AWS)
- Serum does treat acute distemper.(call or write AWS)

"Okay so here we are. It doesn't treat parvo. We bathed dogs in with the stuff. I mean we gave hundreds of CCs and it had no effect. But … years later along came Tamiflu, and it clears parvo. So, there's no problem there."[58]

He went back to his laptop, searched through his files and pulled up another group of slides. The first one shows a yellowish cocker spaniel, looking haggard and uncomfortable. The fur has lost its luster.

"Here's a dog. That's day one, hour one, distemper case?"

"How do we identify this? What is this? How do we know this is distemper and not herpes? OK, that became the major test."

From this, he described the Brush Bladder Smear to find signs of the distemper virus in the bladder cells. He also named fever as a key signpost in a distemper diagnosis.

"If he's got a fever, it isn't kennel cough," he said. "Kennel cough does not give you a fever. Three diseases give you a fever. Distemper, herpes, flu … Dog flu. Starting to show everywhere. Looks like distemper, got a fever, runny nose, cough."

He makes a cough.

"Is it distemper or is it flu? How do you tell? Well, you can't tell herpes or flu, but you can tell distemper. So, what you do is you do the bladder test, and if they're not there, it's either herpes or flu."

Too often vets draw the wrong conclusion and say, "You've got kennel cough," said Dr. Sears. "He gives you an antibiotic and sends you home. Two weeks later, you're back and your dog is still vomiting and his nose is worse. Now, he's got pneumonia. 'Oh,' he says, 'Maybe it wasn't kennel cough. It must have been distemper.'

"Too late," Dr. Sears said, leaning in dramatically. "Too late. … Now, what are you going to do? If you treat, you may get rid of it. You may not. The dog is probably going to get neurologic problems, and he's going to say to euthanize it. By that time, you've spent $700. OK? Maybe more."

He points back at the screen with the sick cocker spaniel. He taps through a series of photos, and in each one the dog's condition worsens. On the last photo, the dog has receded into a ball into the corner of its cage looking sad and hopeless.

"So you asked me, 'Where are our clinical proofs?' " he said, pointing at the screen. "Don't treat that dog. That's a clinical proof. That's legal."

He makes air quotes with one hand at the word, "legal."

By doing nothing beyond the typical supportive care, he would be safe from legal action. But what about the dog? Treating the dog opens him up for repercussions.

"If I did this, and the owner got mad at me and called in a lawyer could I protect myself against that?" he said. "You think so? You know how much it's going to protect myself even if I'm right?"

He turns back to the sick cocker spaniel.

"Antibiotics and fluids going to help that? You going to wipe its nose with Kleenex? You going to give it a kiss on the head?"

He makes little kissing noises in the air.

"You going to feed it special food? You going to give it a big IV? You going to give it vitamin B12?"

He mimics an injection into his arm.

"Vitamin C?" he said. "That dog's going to die. Alright, here we are. Now what?"

"Call Dr. Sears," J.D. says under her breath.

"OK, so, you want to know where the controls are?" He waves his arms out in a broad circle. "All those other cases, treated by all those veterinarians, across the world are your controls."

He turns back and taps on the laptop, brings up another picture of the yellow cocker spaniel.

"I sent that dog home within 24 hours," he said. "And then they take this dog to another vet and they're going to say they treated him for distemper, and they're going to say, 'Oh, come on!' He didn't have distemper. That's what they're going to tell them. The doctor used voodoo medicine. OK? If voodoo medicine works, why not?"

Throughout the afternoon and into the early evening, Dr. Sears jumped from topic to topic as he answered our questions and tapped through the files and photos on his laptop. Sometimes we needed to have him go over material he'd already covered, to make sure we understood. He answered our questions patiently and repeatedly. And when he didn't know the answer, he let us know. Some of the topics he covered:

Using straight NDV

J.D. asked whether the straight NDV vaccine should be given sub-Q when NDV serum cannot be made or acquired in time.

"It has to be IV," Dr. Sears said. The intravenous injection of NDV vaccine is a shot directly into the vein. "Why the difference? I don't know. But sub-Q doesn't seem to work as well."

He leans back, raises both index fingers.

"And if you're going to use the NDV virus straight, the dog must not be immunocompromised," he said. "It must be old enough that it can respond properly, preferably unspayed up until it had a heat cycle so that you have an intact immune system … any dog under the age of 16 weeks it probably won't work, although it does work in some. But not all because those dogs just can't respond properly. And so if you don't have access to serum, that's the next best thing to do.

"Now, if you're talking about [straight] NDV, it doesn't work all the time," he said. "[Straight NDV] is not as good as using the serum, and you can only do it once. So if the dog develops a problem later on, you can't use NDV again. You have to use something else. But you can use the serum multiple times."

NDV serum vs. the distemper vaccine

"But right now at 8 weeks, we give them the distemper vaccine," Bruce said. "Would you rather us use serum instead of vaccination?"

"No!" Dr. Sears said, alarmed. "Serum is only used to treat infected dogs showing symptoms. All the serum does is kill the virus. Gives you a chance to recover. "[The distemper] vaccine is supposed to prevent it.

"So in between prevention and treatment, you've got that space of time," he said, with his hands opposite each other twisting back and forth. "When the dog is infected maybe and no symptoms. Now if you know that it's been exposed, and you know it's going to break next week. That would make you prescient. And I've got news for you. I don't have that kind of ability."

He rests a hand on the side of his head.

"I have to see a symptom. Runny nose, pneumonia, fever. That's the first one to show up. Crappy eyes and crappy nose, that's the two that show up immediately. When you see a dog with its nose all gummed up, the chances are he's got distemper. But, could have parvo. Could have herpes. Could have flu. Could have parainfluenza. Do you know which one it is?"

He shakes his head.

The importance of diagnosis

At one point, he repeated something he often wrote in emails to me.

"But you haven't solved your original problem," he said, waving a finger dramatically. "Unless you identify your original problem – diagnosis – if you don't have diagnosis you haven't got anything."

Other causes of neurologic problems in dogs

He puts a list of diseases and conditions on the screen.

"Now, here are causes of seizures in dogs that are not distemper. So, everybody that seizes isn't distemper. These are causes of seizures in dogs. Do you see that? How many cases do you have on there? 40? At least.... "

Some of the conditions on the list include meningitis, necrotizing encephalitis, spongiform encephalopathy, toxoplasmosis, hepatitis and tick-borne encephalitis.

"... So when you say, 'Ah the dog is seizing, it must have distemper.' Pfft! Not a chance. Now, if it's four months old and it hasn't been vaccinated and it came out of the pound, I'll give you odds. OK, but if you get a 5 or 6 year old dog, that was in a kennel for three days and it comes out one of those? How about walking through any of the mountain areas in California or Colorado for four days?"

From the veterinary literature:

"Canine distemper infection can be challenging to diagnose because many diseases can cause symptoms resembling canine distemper. The respiratory symptoms of canine distemper may be mistaken as canine respiratory disease complex. Canine parvovirus, coronavirus, bacterial, and internal parasite infections should be ruled out as causes of vomiting and diarrhea. Often, CDV-infected animals that exhibit neurologic signs are mistaken as having rabies. Neurologic symptoms must be differentiated from other infections, trauma, and ingestion of toxins. Vaccination history of the affected animal, clinical symptoms, and laboratory testing support a probable diagnosis of CDV infection. State and commercial veterinary diagnostic laboratories offer testing for canine distemper and advice practitioners on appropriate specimens to submit, tests to order and the limitations of test results given the circumstances of each individual case submitted." (Kapil and Yeary 2011)[59]

Best practices for a rescue or shelter to keep disease from spreading

"In other words, how do you keep a population clean?" he said. "You vaccinate it. That's the key, that's the gold standard. Vaccinate it on time."

His index fingers and thumbs form circles as if conducting an orchestra.

"Before exposure. How long before exposure? At least two weeks."

He holds up two fingers.

"Two weeks, but only dogs that are immune competent. You do it to a puppy or a dog with ascarids or a dog with demodex, you haven't covered them."

He points to imaginary dogs.

"It's not covered. Ok, so you give them the shot. You think hey, I had my shot. And they get sick and you say 'what happened?' They had demodex. Or he was loaded with ascarids. Ascarids block distemper antibodies."

He waves his hands flat in a blocking motion.

"Block them."

Further info, from the veterinary literature:

> "Reasons that a vaccine may fail, in addition to the presence of maternal antibodies in puppies, are incomplete immunity due to failure to complete the puppy booster vaccination series, stressors in the physical environment, the animal's immune competence and specific responsiveness to CDV **antigen** or intercurrent exposure to other virulent viruses such as canine parvovirus or coronavirus or even parasites, and improper storage and handling of vaccine." (Kapil and Yeary 2011)[60]

Antigen – A substance that prompts an immune response within a body.

"We do rescue," J.D. said. "We have a huge rescue. We get them from the shelter."

"The first thing you do is isolate the dog," he said.

"I isolate for two weeks."

"Yup. Ten days is enough."

From the literature:

> "In addition to immunization of domestic dog populations, hygienic measures are necessary. Unvaccinated puppies should be isolated from

dogs other than their bitches. Strict isolation of dogs infected with CDV is the most important step in controlling the disease. Virus is shed in all body secretions and excretions during the acute systemic disease. Direct dog-to-dog contact and indirect aerosol transmission are the main routes of viral spread, but CDV can be transmitted from **fomites** at room temperature or lower for several hours. Disinfection of CDV in the environment, particularly in shelters and kennels, is important. Inactivation of canine distemper virus with benzalkonium chloride (0.05%), a quaternary ammonium compound, occurs in 10 minutes at room temperature. Similarly, 70% ethanol is effective against CDV." (Kapil and Yeary 2011)[61]

Timing of vaccinations

He advised that no vaccine should be used within four months of a dog about to be bred. The vaccine could kill the entire litter, he said.

Titers, IgG and IgM

"We're talking about antibodies. Remember when you get sick, you got macrophages [white blood cells] that break it up ..."

He mimes with hands going from step to step.

"... give it to a T-cell. The T-cell then makes a cytokine tells the **B cell** to make an antibody. The antibody then goes to a **plasma cell**. The plasma cell explodes ..."

He mimes with hands waving broadly as if an explosion.

"... antibodies into the body, makes tons of antibody, and that's what you're looking for. So in an active infection, you've got very high titers of antibody."

Titer – The amount of antibody in the blood.

Fomites – Objects or materials that are
likely to carry infection, such as clothes,
utensils, and furniture. Dust and fine
particles in the air can also
transmit pathogens.

B cell – A type of white blood cell
not made by the thymus.

Plasma cell – A kind of B cell that
produces a specific antibody.

His hands go up as high as possible.

"But the disease will usually drive it higher, so you're talking 1 to 10 IgM which is the first five or six days of antibodies. That's the first one. Then IgG comes in and it will climb higher than 1 to 40. And I've seen 1 to 16,000."

"What's IgG and IgM?" I ask.

"IgM is a circular form of antibody," he says, forming his hands together to make a circle. "That shows up first in the body to try to isolate the virus. Remember, it cannot get into the cell where the virus is. It simply keeps virus from floating around in the body. That's all it does. It's the first one to show up.

"The second one to show up is IgG."

Fingers make a tent on the table as he demonstrates.

"And there are multiple IgGs. But IgG, basically the measure is just that. It shows up and it will go very high in a street infection. "

But veterinarians seemed to be struggling with telling the difference between antibodies from a "street" infection vs. vaccination. So, a test within 3 to 4 weeks of vaccination would result in a false-positive. As the experts say:

> "Diagnostic testing for CDV and anti-CDV antibodies presents a special challenge because results do not distinguish between naturally acquired CDV disease (wild-type strains), infection with attenuated virus vaccine strains used in modified-live (MLV) vaccines, or immune response due to the **recombinant**, virus-vectored vaccine. Canine distemper viruses are of a single serotype (monotypic), thus the various genotypes cannot be distinguished using classic serologic techniques … A negative result does not rule out distemper. Immunization for CDV with modified live virus (MLV) vaccine interferes with **PCR** testing for approximately 3 to 4 weeks, creating a false-positive result." (Kapil and Yeary 2011)[62]

PCR or polymerase chain reaction – Another method of detecting viruses by making a copy of a piece of genetic information from the virus and then making thousands to millions of copies.

Recombinant – Created by combining other genetic material.

Variations in distemper virus he encountered

1)   "OK, let me read this to you," he said. "The most common type of distemper that we saw routinely – young unvaccinated dogs or dogs recently vaccinated from pounds. Pound dogs will show up seven days after release dogs with all recognizable symptoms of pneumonia, catarrh, KS – which is the dry eye – fever. Diarrhea, collapse, inclusions in the bladder, elevated anti-distemper serum IgG IgM and in some cases from pound dogs there may be no titers. In other words, less than one to five IgG and IgM usually these dogs have very high titers when checked two weeks later. They are distemper cases and should be treated even though previously vaccinated."

He spins away from his notes on the screen to talk to us directly.

"So, dogs who got out of the pound came with full-blown symptoms. I mean what's distemper? That's a distemper case. You look at it and say, 'A-hah. That's a distemper case.' But they had dogs that came out of there that didn't have titers. In the early days we did titers on everybody. So anybody with more than 1 to 10 IgM and 1 to 40 IgG was considered a distemper case."

These numbers, though, rely on the results of a laboratory, and sometimes the lab can be wrong, he said. He knew one lab just always reported the same levels on its reports. "So, I put in here," he said, turning back to his laptop. "Let's see here. Some labs will return an IgG of 1 to 350 whether vaccinated or not, sick or not, young or old so if this data comes back from the lab, ignore it. It's not valid. Do a bladder cell study instead. I had to put that in there. Cause, God, that means everybody is sick," he shrugs. "That's not possible."

2) "OK, the next one down is a mild, nondescript disease, shows transient signs often not regulated or recognized in early stages. Quick recovery. Can be confused with kennel cough. The secondary symptoms appear later, up to eight years later. And you can even see chorea, demylenation, hardpad, nasal symptoms, pneumonia, ocular dental symptoms, KS, Old dog encephalitis, see neurology below."

He turns back to us to explain

"So that's the disease we were talking about from the other part of the desert where they got sick for two days. He didn't know it was distemper. Then it got better. Then 6 to 8 years later, bang, here comes the neurologic form of it. OK, we saw lots of those cases because they all came out of one triangle out there in the desert."

He draws a triangle in the air. Lancaster to Mojave to Boron.

"So, those dogs whether vaccinated or not broke with this little mild symptom, which their owners didn't even bring them into the hospital and later on they got neurologic problems and we saw a lot of those."

"That's the 7-year-old dog I took down to Dr. Adams."

He turns back to the laptop.

3)   "A new form of distemper relatively rare, older adult dog, fully vaccinated multiple times ..." he raises finger to punctuate "...breaks with some symptoms of distemper. The exposure factor is unknown, possibly wild species exposure, may be a new strain of distemper, see distemper in lions and felines."

Turns back to explain

"We feel that might have gotten into the coyotes. This came up with some of my breeders that had multiple dogs up against the National Forest and being enclosed. And they would all be thoroughly vaccinated and one or two dogs would break with symptoms of distemper."

He holds up one, then two fingers.

"Now you walk into a vet and say I've got an 8-year-old dog that's been vaccinated every year for distemper. What's the matter with it? You look at it and say. Oh my God ..."

He looks at the palm of his hand as if it is a case file.

"... It's been vaccinated. It can't be distemper. Scratch"

He makes a scratching with an imaginary pencil.

"Distemper. No. ... But yes it is.

"How do you know? The bladder won't be positive. [laughs] It's an older dog. It's vaccinated. No bladder signs. It's going to have pneumonia. It's going to have a fever. Looks like distemper. Treat it like distemper and it'll get better instantly. Don't treat it and it'll probably die of encyphilitic lesions within a couple weeks. OK? I saw probably eight of these cases. Only eight in 40 years, but they made us wake up and pay attention because they were unusual.

"Is that a new virus?" he asked, pointing to the laptop.

"Why not call it a new virus? Coming of the wild animals in that area, maybe the forest of California? I don't know. Can't answer the question. We never had it typed because in those days we didn't have the ability to do the genomes. We didn't know."

4) "Vaccine type. No pneumonia. No inclusions in body or bladder. Seizures. Inclusions in brain. No other pathology found upon autopsy. ELISA test for distemper antibody and the CSF are positive."

He turns to us, holds out hand to demonstrate snap test

"In the early days, we had a snap test for distemper antibodies. It came out. So you take a dog and you could take it's blood and put it in and snap it, and if it came up positive it had distemper antibodies. That was a great test. We figured we could do it with the CSF. So, we drew CSF, put it in the test snap it. When they had ODE, it went positive. And when they didn't have it, it went negative.

"The problem is they pulled it off the market. Then we didn't have it anymore."

Back to reading.

"OK, so distemper types, vaccine induced. You have no inclusions anywhere in the body. Not in the bladder. Not in the lungs. Not in the kidneys. Not anywhere. The brain, yes. Usually showed up two to three weeks after a shot. It still happens in my opinion; it's a genetic screw up in the dog some way. They can't handle the vaccine. It gets through the blood-brain barrier. I don't know how it does it. It's rare. I personally have seen a bunch of cases. ...

"I've heard of from one from Ireland. I heard of one from France and I think I got one from Korea and that's what I heard.

"A lot of those, I'm sure are either misdiagnosed or they are put down as being street virus, but it's the vaccine that does it. And there's no way to know who this is going to happen to. But it does happen. It's probably only about one in 3,000 or 4,000 dogs. It's not common. But it happens."

The blood-brain barrier

Al leaned forward and moved his hands parallel to each other as he made this point. "The body is made of two compartments as far as the immunology is concerned," he said. "You have the systemic body."

The two hands form the walls of a container. Then they move to the side to indicate a different container.

"And you have the neural compartment. They are not connected when it comes to treatment of the viruses. You cannot take antibody from the body and put it into the brain."

One hand travels from to the other, mimics putting it into a container.

"Doesn't work. It doesn't go there.

"So you have roaring distemper and you have an antibody count of 1 to 16,000. If you check the brain before the virus gets there, it's negative."

"You can have no antibody in the body, and have seizures with distemper, check the brain and there you have antibodies. Okay? So the two are not connected because of the blood brain barrier, unless that's disrupted."

Years earlier, he believed combinations of vaccines for parvovirus and distemper had resulted in dogs getting immediate neurologic distemper without showing the respiratory symptoms. He concluded the combination somehow allowed the distemper virus to be carried straight into the nervous system. So, he began separating the vaccinations for parvovirus and distemper and the problem went away. After he retired, he went back to visit his former clinic and learned that the vaccine combination had improved and did not cause these problems.

Dr. Adams published papers on MS and distemper

"Old dog encephalitis. This is Dr. Adams published information," (Adams et al. 1975)[63] he reads from the screen, which includes photos published with Dr. Adams' article. Then he reads: "Number one. **Intranuclear** inclusion body in the brain of a dog with old dog encephalitis. That's a virus inside the cell there. OK?

"OK, B. This one here," continuing to read. "Intranuclear inclusion body in to the brain of a person with subacute **sclerosing** panencephalitis."

He turns to look at us with each picture.

"See the virus, right in the middle? Can't miss it. This is Dr. Adams, OK?"

Intranuclear – Within the cell nucleus.

Sclerosing – Causing the overgrowth and/or hardening of tissues.

Necrosis – Cell death

Atrophic – Wasting away tissues.

"C. Internuclear inclusion in a person with multiple sclerosis. Imagine that. Is that distemper? No, that's measles."

"Guess what guys?" he says, with a gleam in his eye. He points at the laptop screen. "There it is, right there. OK?"

A tap brings up another image from Adams' paper, displaying damage to brain cells. The damage includes demylenation, damage and changes to the cells. The images compare the brains of a dog with distemper and a person with MS. "Looks damn similar, doesn't it?" he said.

"Number 4. Cavity formation and severe **necrosis** in an **atrophic** brain from a person with neuromylitis optica," he draws out the term so we can understand it better. Damage to the myelin of the optic nerve, which connects the eye to the brain. "Neuormyelitis optica. ... N.O. ... O.N. ... optical neuritis. You get two species that do that.

"The dog with distemper," he said, counting on his index finger. Dogs in neuro stage distemper often lose their sight because of the damage to the optic nerve. Then he counts on his thumb.

"People with measles. How about that? In the dog, I wonder how many cases we have now that have been treated. But the case that we treated [at UCLA] was blind and got its sight back. The case that we had there [in Indonesia] got its sight back. And I'm sure most of the ones that are blind, within four or five days get their sight back. Nobody's treated on the human side."

As an aside, I'd realized at this moment a very good 7th-grade teacher helped me sort through all these medical terms. He spent a semester teaching us how to break down and understand the language of science through visualization. Often, these terms are based on Latin. For example, "cerebra" means brain. To remember that, he would say, "Imagine a zebra. But instead of a head, it just has a big brain. Cerebra ... zebra ... brain."

Most medical terms can be understood better like this. For example, "neuromylitis optica." Break it down.

Neuro – nerve or nervous system.

Myl – itis – damage or infection to the myelin.

Optica – related to the eye.

Many medical terms just explain the condition in Latin.

How viruses damage the brain and nervous system

Dr. Sears turns back to laptop.

"OK, let's go down from there." He taps again.

"So here's a brain. That's what we're talking about. That's a brain."

A journal illustration pops up on the screen.

"OK? Here's a neuron. The white stuff you see around the edges is the myelin insulation, fatty material. What it does is insulates the electrical currents going down neurons, so they can go very fast from the tip of your toe to your brain takes less than a microsecond."

He points, looks directly at me.

"You pinch your toe. Oh! It hurts. Why does it go that fast? It's traveling all the way up and all the way back."

He shows the path by pointing with finger up and down his body.

"Makes you jerk your foot back. That's a protected neuron. It's got insulation."

Holds up hands to indicate covering on a nerve.

"Take the insulation off, and you can't do that," he said. Just like stripping the rubber or plastic off a copper wire, making it susceptible to shorting out.

He pulls up an illustration from Scientific American, which demonstrates damage to a neuron.

Oligodentrocyte – The cell that produces myelin in the central nervous system.

Lymphocytes – A type of white blood cell in the lymphatic system.

Plasmids – Small strands of DNA that float and replicate in the cytoplasm of the cell.

"This is MS," he said. "All right, what's missing in this picture? This is **oligodentrocyte** or a cell Schwan. It makes the myelin. This is myelin that's being destroyed. These are T cells or macrophages that are activating **lymphocytes**, which are making **plasmids**, making antibodies and destroying the myelin. Bang! It's just a big mishmash of horrible inflammation."

He waves his hands in the air dramatically.

"What's missing in that picture? C'mon guys. I just showed you. C'mon. Do you see a virus in there?"

He pauses to let his point settle in.

"No virus! Where's the virus?"

He leans into us.

"This is human. Where's the virus?" he said. "This didn't start because you walked into a hotel the wrong way."

He repeatedly points to his laptop as he talks.

"This was started by a virus. This is a response to a virus. This is an inflammatory cell that killed that cell, which is the oligodendrocyte, know as the Schwan cell that makes the myelin..."

He brings his hands up, fingers interlocked, and then spreads them away from each other to mimic things coming apart.

"So the myelin is starting to disintegrate, the cell is disintegrating. ... The only thing you see in this picture, though, is only the myelin is being destroyed. That cell dies. [the oligodendrocyte] Why did that cell die? It had a virus in it. It had a measles or a distemper virus in it."

"Is there anything to reverse the demyelization?" J.D. asked.

"Yeah, there are a variety of materials that are being done at this point in time that replace myelin. There are about five materials, which I was going to read you off that last sheet. That are on the human side, and what they are trying to do is put the myelin back. But they are looking at that picture."

Points to the journal illustration.

"They're going to put that myelin back. Well if you can't put that cell back, you're not growing any new myelin. That cell is the one that does it. Now, when you put NDV into the brain, you kill the virus. In the ventricles, there are stem cells for the brain.

"Really?" he poses the question for himself. "Yeah, really! What do they do? They replace cells that die. So stem cells in the absence of the virus can make that cell back again, which then makes myelin because that's what it does."

His hands stretch out along an imaginary nerve.

"How interesting can that get? Isn't that fascinating? That's the human view of MS, right there. ... All the research that I've read so far, and there's five medications that have come out recently try to replace the myelin. None of them address the virus. None of them." However, others will have a different interpretation of the effects of the NDV spinal tap.

How to use the NDV spinal tap

"Ok, you've got a dog, comes to you," I said. "Diagnosed with distemper. Having seizures. What do you do?"

He nods.

"Take us through it, step by step."

He leans back.

"The sooner you treat it, the better chance you have of control," he said. "Wait till later and there's enough damage, the dog's going to die regardless. You've got four kinds."

He holds up four fingers with the back of hand facing out.

> **Thoracic** – Relating to chest cavity
> between neck and abdomen.

"The one coming up the backbone, you've got to do pretty quick because once it reaches up into the **thoracic** area it'll turn off the ability to breathe."

He points his glasses at his chest, moving back and forth.

"And you're not going to be able to do anything to save that dog. The optic neuritis [blindness] it turns out it treats it really quickly. We're talking sometimes less than a week. These dogs go back to being sighted. And I find it extraordinary. OK?"

He's holding up two fingers now.

"The seizing dogs, I think it would take a little bit longer."

Down to one finger.

"The ones that we treated in Indonesia, the seizing dog was also blind. It regained its eyesight within about a week or so. The seizing took about 4 to 6 weeks to come under control. The dog with chorea..."

He shakes his hands in a spasm.

"I'm trying to think about the time. I think it was four to six weeks also, and the chorea stopped on that dog. That dog was paralyzed in its hind legs when we treated it. It could not walk. And it did walk. The dog we treated there..."

Points to his files from UCLA across the room.

"Could not walk, could not see," he said. "Was sighted and walking within a matter of weeks, the one we treated in UCLA. So that's been documented, but never printed, never published."

Later, he popped onto the screen the lab reports on the dogs from Indonesia, which confirmed they had distemper in their cerebrospinal fluid.

"But what are the steps for treatment?" I ask.

"You want to tap the brain, you want to give it an anesthetic, prep it for surgery. Tap the brain."

He reaches behind his head and touches the top of neck/base of skull.

"You do that by doing it through the foramen magnum," he said. "You want to pull some of that [CSF – cerebrospinal fluid] material off. You want to get some."

He mimes the needle draw with his fingers.

"Then you take the same needle, leave it where it is and you put in about half a CC, depending on the size of the dog, of active NDV the virus into the brain. Then you follow it with a flush of saline. Why that? So that essentially you flush the needle and you get it all in there because otherwise the needle's going to have probably two tenths of a CC stuck in it, and you don't want it left in the needle."

He holds up fingers to indicate how much in the needle.

"Now, I had somebody write me and say they made the NDV up with saline rather than distilled water and they didn't get any seizures. My experience is that every time you put NDV into a dog, you're going to get seizures."

These are not seizures from distemper damage, but instead from the shock to the system as with Joe at UCLA.

"So, you need to have a catheter into him for fluids," he said, miming a catheter line going into his arm. "And you need to have them anesthetized when you do it. But this individual wrote to me and said we gave it with saline mixed with the NDV. It worked just as well and we didn't have any secondary effects from it. So, yeah, I would do it that way."

I'd been getting many questions about this on the Internet. Often, I'd been told a vet with ultrasound equipment needed to do the spinal tap.

"Now, you're talking about putting a needle into the spinal canal?" I said.

"Spinal canal. Yes," he said, nodding. "Not the spinal cord, but the canal."

"Now, a big concern is whether you might nick the spinal cord," I said.

He laughs. "Yeah, that's called pithing."

He leans back, smiles.

"Somebody who knows how to do that needs to do it," he said.

"Do you need ultrasound to guide the needle?" I ask.

"I did it without an ultrasound for years without a problem because I also did spinal surgery. We dropped needles in, and you can close your eyes ..."

He closes his eyes, demonstrating on imaginary dog's head in front of him. One hand holds the dog's head and one finger on other hand pushes in and out gently at an imaginary needle.

"And you've got the dog in position and you've got your fingers on it and you've got the needle right where you want it and you can feel your way down the bone and ..."

He makes a pfft sound.

"... pop right through. There's a thick membrane there. You can feel it pop right through that and you don't have to go any further. You're there. And what happens is the fluid comes up through the needle."

His finger shows the path of the fluid up the imaginary needle.

"So we would put a catheter on the needle and pull the fluid off because that way you didn't bother the needle. Then we would pull the catheter out and inject the NDV into the needle.

"Now two-tenths of it is stuck in the needle, probably one tenth because you are using a very tiny needle. And then flush it with a little saline and just pull the needle out.

"The whole thing takes five minutes, two minutes."

He mimics moving the needle in and out gently.

"The trick is to walk it down, walk it down until you feel it pop."

"... Now, I've had people who weren't quite as adept injure the neural cord. Some guy in the Philippines, apparently pithed a dog. And the dog had trouble walking. It just cut its legs off literally.

"And then I had another case where the dog had been in a field with cows and so had cow shit all over it. And apparently the guy didn't clip it and prep it for surgery and the dog got tetanus when he put the needle in.

"So, the dog had tetanus. Does NDV cause tetanus? No it doesn't, but that doesn't mean you can't get tetanus if you don't do it cleanly. It requires that you do this in a surgical manner."

Using NDV serum in the spinal tap?

"Now, the question is, would the serum work?" he asked. "I never had a chance to try it. I don't know. Probably. What I would do in that case, I would put a catheter in, run it up into the brain and shoot it with serum two or three times a day for a week. You don't need much, just a CC a day. Should work, but I don't know because I never had a chance to try it. Most of the cases I treated for ODE were done long distance, with other vets doing the work."

"If you had a chance to try it, would you?" J.D. asks.

"Sure, certainly, damn right." He picks up his glasses from table. "In an instant."

What this could lead to

It had dawned on me these protocols could help someone in my family. "I just want to make sure I've heard you right," I said. "Because I've had a dog with distemper and a sister with MS."

There was no connection between those distemper and MS cases, he said. But the connection between measles and MS had my attention. "There's a possibility that this treatment you've come up with might address MS," I said.

"Yes," he said, raising a finger. "You find a physician that will take your sister and give her a shot of NDV into the brain and I will buy you dinner for a year."

He leans in and smiles. I've been made a believer in the NDV serum. I've slowly become a supporter of the NDV spinal tap for dogs. But I did not know whether I am ready to make the leap into using NDV to treat multiple sclerosis. We'd be a long way from proving that, and we still need to prove NDV can save dogs from distemper. One battle at a time.

Other research into measles and MS

I later learned that Dr. John Adams was not the only researcher who believed measles could be the cause of MS, as "an autoimmune disease possibly induced by a virus infection." (Randall and Russell 1991)

Studies about measles and other viruses causing MS have been conducted for decades. Some experiments demonstrated how viruses could induce neurologic problems in hamsters and rats. However, despite evidence of measles infections in the brains of MS patients, some researchers eventually began to doubt the connection. They debated and contradicted each other in their conclusions. "For example, it has been suggested that silent invasion of the brain is a fairly common event in uncomplicated measles infection. … However, in this respect it is of interest to note that measles virus-specific sequences have been detected in brain autopsies from MS patients." (Randall and Russell 1991)[64]

A review of the research posted online in May 2017 summed up the findings at that time:

> "Whether viruses in MS are principally causal or simply contributory remains to be proven, but many viruses or viral elements-predominantly Epstein-Barr virus, human endogenous retroviruses (HERVs) and human herpesvirus 6 (HHV-6) but also less common viruses such as Saffold and measles viruses-are associated with MS. … We argue that it is crucially important not to interpret 'absence of evidence' as 'evidence of absence' and that future studies need to focus on distinguishing correlative from causative associations. Progress in the MS-virus field is expected to arise from an increasing body of knowledge on the interplay between viruses and HERVs in MS." (Mentis et al. 2017)[65]

Treating cancers with NDV

Dr. Sears leans back in his chair, holds up one hand.

"Let's go back a minute...," he said. "A young physician in Hungary who is an intern gets a chicken farmer in who has stomach cancer."

Dr. Sears slaps his stomach.

"...He says to the guy you need surgery now if we're going to save your life. The guy says, 'I have 10,000 chickens that need to be processed and sent to market. I'm not about to be taken into surgery.' He says, 'You're really ill and you're going to die.' The guy says, 'Can't do it.' So he goes out to his chickens, and low and behold the chickens get Newcastle's Disease Virus and he loses half his flock. And he's in there working with the birds and they're blowing stuff, sneezing and he's sucking it up."

He makes a fake sneeze, sucks it back up, gestures with hands.

"He gets a little bit of conjunctivitis. Gets his chickens to market. He empties his place out and goes back to the doctor says, 'OK, I'm ready for surgery. The doctor examines him. The cancer's gone." (Csatary 1971)[66]

Dr. Sears leans his head back. His eyes go wide with wonder.

"It's gone," he said. "The doctor says 'not possible.' Can't happen.

The doctor, Laszlo Csatary, develops a variation on the Newcastle Disease Virus – MTH-68. This variation went on to be used in research to treat other disease and cancers, such as in brain and breast cancer.

"It's being done in Europe. It's being done in Israel. I don't know of any cases being treated in the United States.

"The corollary to this is I treated one case," he said. "Stomach cancer, successfully. The dog died last year, nine years after we diagnosed it. We diagnosed it with an ultrasound and a biopsy. So, we knew what we were dealing with."

The dog had thickened stomach lining and was vomiting blood.

"So I said to the guy, look I just read this article. Are you willing to try? One of my breeders. He said, 'if you think it will work. Let's do it.' So, the trick was to give a shot of the NDV virus vaccine every day for seven days. The dog stopped vomiting. We did an ultrasound; the stomach went back to normal. The dog lived nine more years."

"One case," he said, holding up a finger. "Does that make a reason to start the world afire? … No…. But if I had stomach cancer, I would sure as hell pull my NDV virus vaccine bottle out, and I would give myself a shot tomorrow."

He went on to discuss other cases he'd read papers on.

"A child with brain cancer," he said. "And I can't remember which one he had. Had half his brain removed, and it had spread into the other half. The kid was still functional. They said he's going to die, let's give it a try. They injected him with NDV. Stopped it and the kid lived." (Csatary 1999)[67]

"… And so when [Ted] Kennedy got sick, I thought, you know he needs a shot of NDV," he said, shaking a finger. "It would probably save his life. But are they going to listen to a vet from Lancaster, who's retired, who has these crazy ideas about using a chicken virus to do what?" (U.S. Sen. Edward Kennedy D-MA had died a couple months earlier of a malignant glioma brain tumor.)

He makes air quotes at "crazy idea" and forms a puzzled look on his face.

The possibilities of NDV as a cancer fighter have also been reported in several papers for decades. According to the National Cancer Institute, NDV may be more likely to attack and destroy tumor cells rather than healthy cells. "NDV-based anticancer therapy has been reported to be of benefit in more than a dozen clinical studies, but the results of these studies must be considered inconclusive because the study designs were weak and the study reports were generally incomplete."[68]

In Israel, researchers still see the potential in using NDV against cancer after some issues can be resolved. (Tayeb et al 2015)[69] A study in Mexico tested NDV against human and canine lymphoma cells and found it may be a promising treatment. (Sánchez et al. 2016)[70] Other researchers have had success reprogramming viruses such as the common cold to attack cancers. (Alonso et al. 2012)[71] This appears to be a possible method of fighting cancer that could be more thoroughly explored.

Diagnosing and treating respiratory herpes

I have to admit, this topic had confused me. I was aware of herpes. I knew a version of it was what gave me a cold sore on my lip now and then. I knew it could hit the genitals, of course. But I didn't understand how this disease could mimic distemper in the dog.

Necropsy – An autopsy on an animal.

"Herpes! Here we come," Dr. Sears said after popping up the first slide on the topic. "Okay so I'm going to run down this and you guys, I'm telling you, are going to see a lot of **[necropsies]**."

I brace myself. I'd visited human anatomy labs, so I understood the frame of mind I needed. "Bring a wall" was the advice I once learned. Separate what you see from your emotions. Still, I had never seen so many dead puppies split open. [72]

He hovers over the laptop as he taps through slides that appear behind his head.

"Let me stand over here where I can see what we're doing," he said. "I can see it here and talk to you as we go. OK, diagnostic procedures. Herpes, a viral disease of the dog. Respiratory reproductive, but we only know the one virus. It is not known whether there is more than one. Almost every species has more than one."

He ran into respiratory herpes in dogs frequently during his work with the dog breeders of the Antelope Valley.

"Now, I was lucky enough to have breeders that cooperated with me," he said. "Marvelous people, knew their breeds. God, I loved them to death, cooperated with me in every way that they could. There are certain breeds that just went crazy with this disease."

A respiratory disease had been killing new-born puppies. When he performed necropsies on them, he would find the lungs completely consolidated, filled with fluid. When he sent samples off to the lab, the results came back as "pneumonitis," a broad term that simply means an inflammation of the lungs, usually caused by a virus.

"Diagnosis, pneumonitis," he said. "What the hell does that mean? You're a veterinarian. You've got dead puppies, and you're going to send off a box that costs you 100 bucks. It comes back, pneumanitis. What killed my puppies? Pneumanitis? What the hell is that? What is that? I don't know. You don't know. The lab doesn't know."

After digging through the veterinary literature, he found the answer he needed from a 1965 article by L.E. Carmichael of the Baker Institute at Cornell University, where the first definition of respiratory herpes had been published. Some of the information he read to us:

- Fatal illness occurs in pups less than one month old; some as old as four months.
- Sudden death of apparently healthy puppies occurs after an illness of no more than 24 hours.
- Viremia [virus in the blood] is associated with the period during which the puppy's temperature is optimal for Herpes virus replication.

Because the disease could not be diagnosed until after death, Dr. Sears would have to wait until a litter of newborn puppies died. He'd perform necropsies on them to determine what killed them. He showed us how he did that. With slide after slide, Dr. Sears taught us the difference between respiratory herpes and other conditions.

"Look at the lungs, they look like liver tissue. See them? OK?... Intestines look beautiful, they're fine. Just the lungs are consolidated on this guy. ... Now here's one where you have splotchy lungs, died before he had a chance to get consolidated, but look at the spots on those lungs. This is not postmortem death this is antimortem damage to these tissues okay? Now, the stomach is here somewhere ... Here's the stomach right here. See it, all bloated up?"

These pups endured terrible pain in their very short lives.

"These guys, people always say they roll up on their backs and they cry," he said. "Well hell yes, if your stomach got that big and round and your lungs were not working properly, and you're trying to get catch their breath in lungs that aren't working, and the stomach is pushing up into the diaphragm, shit that's a crappy way to die, guys. That is not comfortable. And they cry until they die. OK?"

He taps through more photos.

"...Look at the consolidation on these lungs. Now that's a dead piece of intestine, but that's inconsequential that happened secondary. ...Okay here we go again. These intestines begin to look a little nasty, but look at that lung. That lung is fully consolidated. OK?... Okay now there's a kidney with lesions.... See all those spots on those kidneys? There is virus in those kidneys, OK? ... Okay here's one, and again, you're looking at lungs on this puppy. Look at the stomach all bloated out. Remember, the vessels to this the intestines coming out of the stomach are damaged. So that part of the intestine has no peristalsis [the movement of muscles that move food along] so the stomach just fills up and especially if they are trying to force milk in the puppy because it's crying. They're just blowing that stomach up. It's not going anywhere. OK?"

If the **necropsy** showed the pups had died from respiratory herpes, he'd then know what to do to save the rest of the kennel. His NDV serum worked against this disease too.

"By the time we identified a kennel with herpes, we didn't give them a chance to die after that point," he said. "We hit them with serum at the day of birth. And we stopped deaths, 95 percent, if it was herpes. Herpes. Now, you've got to identify herpes. You've got to autopsy the puppies. That tells you the mother's infected. If the mother's infected, the kennel's infected."

"How far out?" J.D. asked.

"Within twenty-four hours of birth," he said. "For every litter that's born. Forever."

"Adults too?"

"No, you're not going to treat the adults. They show no lesions. None, zip, nada. Nothing. Once they've had a heat cycle – except for Mastiff breed – no lesions show up."

All that was needed was 1 CC of the serum, usually.

"These are little tiny guys," he said. "These are four ounces. Little teeny, teeny ones, I give a half a CC sometimes. It stops the virus!"

He drives his hand down like a knife.

"Bang! And they live. Now, there's never always. Every once in a while, you lose a puppy. But the great majority makes it. You're not losing whole litters at a time, and we had kennels that couldn't save dogs. Let me tell you."

I ask whether the serum he used is made the same was as for distemper.

"Yes, same stuff," he said. "We just had it in the refrigerator and said, 'OK, it treats that virus, let's try it on other viruses.' "

He keeps going through the slides, and by now we could all recognize the bloated stomachs, the consolidated lungs, and the non-functional intestines.

Then, he finally reached a photo of six healthy golden retriever puppies.

"Now, golden retrievers die by the numbers," he said. "My breeders either came in and got shots or they brought me dogs to make serum. We gave them half. We kept half. They gave their own dogs shots. Most of them came in to have me give them shots. If they did that, they brought their own serum, we gave the shots. We shared the serum with them because they brought us the donor dogs."

Then he put up on screen another treatment for respiratory herpes using Acyclovir and an incubator to raise their temperatures. The treatment had not been published in a veterinary journal. A breeder had found it in the International Labrador Digest and brought it to him.

"Everyone believed that if you heated them to a temperature of 110 degrees they would survive," he said. "Uh-huh. Didn't work. OK? Give fluids orally. .... Having saved the pups from certain death does not guarantee that you will not see reproductive lesions in dogs before puberty. Good old puberty again. Why puberty? It's when the immune system goes solid."[73]

He puts up a photo of a puppy (below).

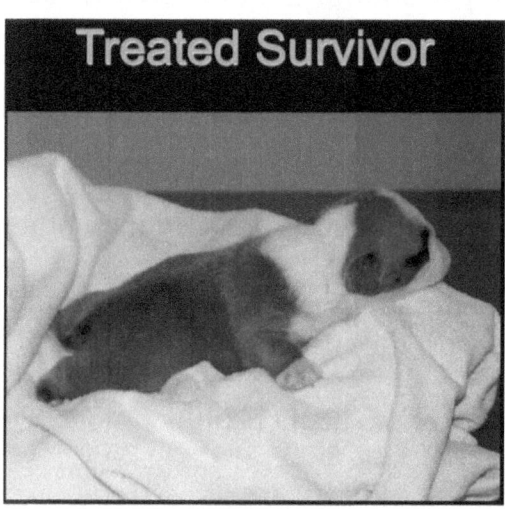

Treated Survivor

"So, here's a treated survivor," he said. "One of the first that we had. The dog was sick when he came in, crying. Obviously it was herpes. Other puppies probably already died. So, we tried to treat him, and we actually had some survivors. I figure you're going to save about half. The reason for that is you don't know what stage those puppies are in. If you catch them early, you're going to save them. If you catch them later, you're not going to because they die quickly. If you can get those lungs clear, you've got a chance to save them. If you can't get their lungs clear, you're toast. You're done. OK?"

He then launched into slides and a discussion about how to avoid genital lesions in dogs with herpes. His answer: Don't spay the female dogs until after their first heat cycle and do not neuter male dogs until after the equivalent time.

"Never?" asks J.D.

"No, after you have a heat cycle, the virus goes into remission and you never find it. Where is it? In humans, it's supposed to be in the dorsal nerve root **ganglia**."

He points to the back of his neck.

Ganglia – A structure of nerve cells.

"In animals we have no clue where it is. They don't get the secondary diseases like you do in humans. We have no clue where it goes. Do not spay, not till they've had a heat cycle. When we told that to the pound, they said, 'We'll have a lawyer on your doorstep tomorrow morning.' You can't tell people that."

He reads from his notes:

"Always allow at least one heat cycle before spaying. No effective treatment for herpes after spaying. Cannot tell if they are infected if no lesions appear. Many veterinarians will not agree.

"Oh boy, you'll find all kinds of attitudes out there."

He continues to tap through his notes.

"Could the lesions be anything else besides herpes?" J.D. asked.

"That would cause a vaginal lesion like that?" he said. "We hadn't found anything. Yes, it could be, but we hadn't found it. If you've got hundreds of cases that turn out to be herpes, you have to believe what you see.

"One of my old guys used to say if it walks like a duck, sounds like a duck, it's gotta be a duck. So, don't be calling it a giraffe if it looks like a duck. I'm sure there are giraffes out there that walk like a duck and sound like a duck, but that's going to be the exception to the rule.

"And when you have this many cases, trust your instincts. Because you are not going to be able to identify it in normal ways that you would identify other diseases. It can't be done. I call this the hidden disease. It really is a monster."

Another tap. "This is ..."

"Sir," Bruce interrupts. "It's 8 o'clock."

"This is my rejection, by the way from the literature."

The screen displays the 2002 letter from the editor at JAAHA.

"But you have to leave, though," J.D. said.

"I know, but I still want to show this to you."

He taps again, and keeps going, pouring as much of his experience as he could into our ears and the cameras. But all the while, our time with him was running out.

The message to the vets

"Can I ask you to say one very important thing?" J.D. asked. "If you were speaking to the vets that we're going to distribute this DVD to, could you tell them why it's important?"

"You could try."

"No," I said. "How would YOU tell them?"

"What would I say to the vets?" he said, turning to look directly into my camera. "Give it a try because you don't have any other choices to treat some of these diseases and these things work. So, the best thing you can do is follow the advice that you're getting from your breeders and your protectors of dogs. Let them take the serum and try it. Then I want you to go back and see the cases they treat and see how they handle this. If you don't, you know what the consequences to the dogs are because in distemper cases, you're probably losing 80 percent of your cases. In herpes cases, you're probably missing all of the diagnosis and certainly all of your puppies are dying. So, have some serum made. Give it a try. Don't be afraid. It won't hurt you. It doesn't affect any of your staff if you use it properly. And it does some marvelous things. Make some serum. Give it to your breeders. Give it a try. How's that?"

"Excellent," J.D. said.

"Thank you," I said.

He kept going until he finally stopped about eight minutes after 8 p.m.

Saying goodbye

We drove him back to the airport and got him to the check-in counter before his flight took off. But the airline would not let him go through to his gate. He missed his flight. Instead, I offered to let him share my hotel room for the night. Then, we'd take the hotel shuttle back to airport so he could catch the earliest flight in the morning.

We had dinner at the hotel. He talked about his role in the world of medicine.

"I'm a veterinarian, OK?" he said. "I'm a clinical veterinarian. And clinical veterinarians are looked down on like privates in the Army. We're the field people. You've got generals and captains and colonels and all that, all the way down from universities and people that work in the states that control the licensing. You get all the way down to a clinical veterinarian. We're the lowest people on the totem poll, so to speak. Physicians look at all veterinarians the same way. You're the tail of medicine, and the dog doesn't wag its tail all the time."

We rose early and got ready for the airport shuttle in a rush. We arrived unshowered at the curb in front of the hotel in the early morning darkness. Dr. Sears had barely had time to brush his hair. His voice, coated with morning phlegm, sounded an octave deeper.

As we chatted while waiting for the shuttle, I switched on my Flip video camera.

"What basically I'm saying is, I'm grateful for what you've done because you've kept the system alive," he said. "Basically, eventually somebody is going to pick this up and run with it. And we know we control it in animals and so we have an animal model for this."

"What we're talking about is measles and MS, and we need somebody on the human side to pick up on this, get excited about it and run with it. The problem is it is going to take a couple more years, maybe decades before that happens. The reason for that is there is reluctance to practice anything like this on humans. But we have an animal model. We've proven that you can treat and cure these diseases in the animal model. If we can do that in the animal model, there's very small reason why it shouldn't work in the human. So, we need to get this material out, not only to treat animals, but hopefully at some point in the future to treat humans with the same condition."

I asked what was by now an obvious question, but I wanted to make sure I had it clearly explained on video.

Neonate – Newborn.

"And this would be treating humans with what disease?"

"We'd be treating humans for measles and for MS and for herpes, that's in **neonates**, which apparently is a bigger problem than I even knew. But an article showed up last week in the New England Journal of Medicine about herpes in women, and it turns out that we are losing probably 2 or 3 children per hundred to this disease and in an animal model we can control this very nicely. So, this information needs to be transferred across the species line, so to speak. So, that's what we're interested in. And again, I thank you for keeping this alive because this all developed back in the early 70s, and here we are in 2009 and it hasn't progressed hardly at all in that period of time."

"What can people do to thank you?" I said.

"To thank me?" He shook his head. "Make it available to everybody. Make sure that people know about it. Make sure people are using it. Make sure they stop this disease. That's how they can thank me. I'm only giving back what was given to me over the last couple of decades. One, it gave me an education from the state of California, which I have always appreciated, and two, all the breeders have worked with me over the last 40 years with this because this didn't happen instantaneously. Breeders helped dramatically with this. Thank God for breeders."

We boarded the shuttle to the airport and I walked him to his ticket counter. I was flying out of a different terminal to catch a connection to Detroit, and then home. Something still bothered me though, and on the train that took me from his terminal to mine, I pulled out my Flip camera and pointed it at myself.

"Well, here I am on the train, the inter-terminal train going from B to A," I said. "I just dropped off Dr. Sears at the ticket counter at Continental Airlines. I shook his hand and he had a tear in his eye as he thanked me again for what I had done for him. And I told him I finally figured out why I am doing all this. I tell my students, 'Never get involved in a story. Don't join the cause.' What I realized was that in my 25 years of journalism, that story I wrote back in 1997 and put on the web in 2000. That was a story that became a cause. And I realized that unless I did something about it that entire treatment would disappear. So, I became an activist for a cause."

On my way home, I spent most of my time grading student work on my laptop, either in terminals or in an airplane seat. In the back of my mind, I tested out ideas for the DVD I would be editing. I kept thinking about one thing Dr. Sears had said: "Eventually somebody is going to pick this up and run with it."

That's what we needed to get credibility and acceptance for these treatments. One person. The right person who could see the potential in this and who either had the means to make it happen or could give the guidance we needed to do it ourselves.

That became my new goal.

Open and Closed Doors

      The Park School of Communications sits among the buildings of Ithaca College on South Hill. From my office window on the second floor, I could look out on Cayuga Lake, the city of Ithaca, and the esteemed buildings of Cornell University jutting up from the slopes of East Hill.

      Somewhere out there in the Collegetown neighborhood adjacent to campus, Amy worked on the Cornell University website. Somewhere out beyond that – and a separate world from hers or mine and beyond my line of sight – lay the College of Veterinary Medicine at Cornell. The proximity of this school had not been lost on me.

Early on, I had decided not to ask Amy to push the cause of canine distemper at Cornell. Her job on the website had enough challenges, and she was a new employee. I'd also learned how much a cause drained you emotionally. To some, my websites may have been a godsend, but to others, I was a snake oil salesman. The only way I could maintain my sanity was to ignore both the praise and criticism because either could tear you apart. I tried to buffer Amy from the roller coaster craziness of my canine distemper activism. Occasionally, I'd tell her about the highs and lows of the cause, the successes and failures, but most of the time I didn't bring home my work.

In December 2009, Amy pointed out to me a link on the College of Veterinary Medicine website at Cornell where vets could submit possible treatments for clinical trials. As far as Dr. Sears was concerned, he had made his attempt to get Cornell's attention years ago and he was not interested in trying them again.

However, I felt it might be worth it for me to give it a try. Perhaps things had changed. I composed an email to the address Amy had pointed me to, fully aware I had no standing as a veterinarian, scientist, researcher or expert.

My email, from my official Ithaca College account, began with a few points I hoped would reassure the recipient I was at least no madman. Not only was I a college professor right here in Ithaca, but I also represented a small but accredited 501(c)3 nonprofit. Kind Hearts In Action now had a website where we posted information on the NDV treatments as well as stories, photos and videos from dog owners and vets. I wrote:

> "Canine distemper is becoming more common in the U.S. and Asia. From the e-mails I have received, it is clear that despite the success of the canine distemper vaccine, this disease is still common in shelters, strays and young puppies.

There has been a spike in activity in Texas, Florida and California in the U.S., and it is also more active in Asian countries such as The Philippines, Indonesia and India. However, our group believes there is a solution. Veterinary science can save dogs with canine distemper."

To be honest, I have to say I was overselling my case by declaring a "spike" in activity. I had only been doing this long enough to know there were cases in these regions. I did not know if what I was seeing at the time was any worse than any earlier period. Then again, neither did anyone else because no one was keeping records. I then explained the background of Dr. Sears' discovery and the rejections he encountered, including how he could not pay for a study back in the 1980s. I continued with:

"Thanks to the technology of Facebook, Twitter, Blogger and Wordpress, many more dog owners have found out about Dr. Sears and his discovery, and we have established an informal track record, which includes testimonials from dog owners, photos and videos. Our group has saved dogs in Florida, Georgia, Texas, California, Canada and the Philippines using the protocols developed by Dr. Sears. But of course, that's not enough to prove Dr. Sears' case. His ideas need to be proven through scientific trials. Kind Hearts in Action is committed to finding a way to make these trials happen, either through the acquisition of grants, fundraising or other methods. We are hopeful that after seeing our Web site, Cornell may now be interested in conducting clinical trials. We are confident that when such trials are conducted, they will validate Dr. Sears' work and other vets across the world will be able to use this life saving treatment.

"Please contact me as soon as possible with the information on the current requirements for pursuing this research."

The email received no reply. Can't say I was really surprised. But I had to try. Two possible conclusions:

- The content of the message did not compel a response.
- The credibility of the messenger fell short.

Of course, it's always possible my email got caught in a spam filter or was accidentally deleted somehow, but by now I'd become gun shy about rejection. I decided not to try Cornell again until the credibility of either the message or the messenger could be improved. I did not blame them for my failings in measuring up to their standards.

Since I began the canine distemper crusade, I'd run into more closed doors than open ones. Repeated attempts to connect with the vet in Georgia who had treated Pippit's dog had been rebuffed, even though he had also treated Mia's dog in New Mexico. My phone calls and emails to him went unanswered. But I knew he was talking with other vets who were curious about the treatment. In October, I had written him an old-fashioned letter and received no reply.

I'd also dropped off a copy of the protocols to my vet clinic in Horseheads to see whether the owner had any interest. What I heard back from the staff was that he worried about endangering his clinic. Again, malpractice insurance does not cover cases when vets try experimental procedures.

Fair enough. I didn't press the issue with him any further. I also didn't expect to find many allies here in Horseheads because canine distemper is controlled so well in Upstate New York that few vets even encounter a case. Very few people I knew in the Northeast had lost a dog to canine distemper. The need for a treatment did not seem so critical as it was in California, Texas and Florida.

The "snake oil" term used by the vet in California back in May still weighed heavily on my mind. This had happened after many failed attempts to find a vet willing to treat Margo, the lab mix rescued from the South Central shelter. In the midst of this, I had tried calling possible leads around the San Fernando Valley and ran into an unexpected problem. Panic seized me every time I dialed.

As a reporter, making phone calls had been a piece of cake. If I needed info, I called the person with the info, I then asked questions, and then I may or may not get answers. If I didn't get the answers to my questions in one call, I'd just keep making calls until I got the information I needed. In a way, it was like being an actor in a well-rehearsed role. A comfort zone. I knew what I needed to do and had few surprises.

Now, my role had changed. I would not be calling to get information, but to pitch an unpublished treatment. As I'd told the Facebook group, the veterinary community as a whole considered a cure for distemper to be as impossible as a perpetual motion machine or cold fusion. Also, professionals generally don't like non-professionals telling them how to do their job. I needed to offer the information tactfully. In my gut, I knew I did not belong in the world of veterinary medicine. But I still felt ethically compelled to try.

When I called the first vet's office, the woman who answered the phone was receptive at first, but later the clinic would back off. When all these leads fell through and the only response I got from the most promising lead had been "snake oil," I lost interest in any further phone calls. This later developed into an aversion to using the telephone.

Rejecting a treatment for canine distemper made sense for many reasons. You'd want your vet to use the best information, right? You'd want your vet to rely on the latest, published techniques. You'd be wary if your vet was willing to use some unproven, unpublished treatment off the Internet. You'd understand if your vet didn't want to use a technique that would not be covered by malpractice insurance and could put them out of business. All those calculations make sense.

So, I respected vets and dog owners who didn't want to try the protocols. There are also rules against veterinarians having an "unprofessional alliance" with a non-veterinarian. Courts have ruled against vets using an "agent" to treat an animal remotely and then split the fees. Perhaps some of these vets feared I aimed to set up such a scheme, which would cause them to lose their license. I never had any intention to make money at this, and I never treated a dog myself. The 501(c)3 status might have helped answer one question about my motives, but I still ran into many who were cautious. "What's the catch?" they'd wonder.

"Thanks for your help," wrote a dog owner from Texas. "I am curious...what do you do? Let me ask a better question. How are you connected with distemper in dogs?"

Yeah, why is a journalism professor involved in canine distemper anyway?

Cold calls didn't work. People who owned dogs dying of distemper opened more doors than I ever did.

The view from a vet's office

"The first time we learned about Dr. Sears work, was when [the dog owner] came to us and asked if we will be willing to do the treatment for her dog," Tal Shohamy wrote to me in September 2009. Tal is the manager for his wife, Dr. Liat E. Zilkha, who owns White Angel Animal Hospital in Austin, Texas. They had treated and saved their first dog at the end of January, and in May successfully treated Hunter from Southern California.

"The first question that my wife had was why do other doctors refuse to do it," Tal wrote. "I read everything that was on the net on it – only your site and [the message board by the owner of the dachshunds in Indonesia.] … I got to tell you that only by ignoring the message board were we able to even go forward. This protocol was presented as a CURE for everything and that guy … was giving instructions regarding medication online. The biggest two red flags a vet can have were right there on page one."

What Tal explained, and I would read more about later on, is that using the term "cure," implying a guarantee of success could get a vet into a lot of trouble. "A careful veterinarian never guarantees to cure an animal." [74] Veterinarians have lost lawsuits when an animal dies after a recovery has been promised. And malpractice insurance may not cover them if the vet had made a promise of a cure.

"The only thing that kept us reading was the idea that if we don't try – the dog is dead..." Tal wrote. "When we looked at the Veterinary Information Network (VIN) which is where vets go to exchange information and ask each other for their opinions, we only saw ridicule for this."

That explained a key problem.

"I've been dealing with a pattern where vets would show interest in the treatment, and then later completely back off from it," I wrote to Tal. "Now, it becomes clearer."

Obviously, "snake oil" had only been the tip of the iceberg. The information about Dr. Sears' NDV treatments had already been circulated on the Veterinary Information Network and dismissed out of hand. My social media campaign had been negated by a competing campaign.

The remedy to the skepticism came down to having three things reach the right vet: 1) A dying dog. 2) A willing owner. 3) A bottle of NDV. Confronted with a dog that would probably die, some vets became open to giving the protocol a try. Getting those same three things to a veterinary college was probably the only way to open the door to a study of the NDV protocols. But I did not have the means to make that happen.

White Angel only went ahead with the treatment after protecting themselves legally. They performed the treatment after establishing a veterinarian-client-patient in which the client grants "informed consent," saying that they understand the risks and dangers of the procedure.

As Tal wrote, "We talk to each client before Dr. Z agrees to take their case, and we inform them about the science behind it and the history of Dr. Sears' protocol. We then inform them about the risk that may be associated with CSF taps & with an experimental procedure. We have them sign a page-long legal waiver. If they still want to go ahead and they understand that this is not a guaranteed cure, then we can perform the protocol."

Because of Tal, I replaced most references on my websites to "cure" with the word "treatment." Through my emails, I began to emphasize that we offered hope, not a guarantee. "There is hope" became the slogan for the Save Dogs From Distemper project.

Tal told me that even when the dog died after the procedure, the owners will often say, "It's not about the money. You know what, I'm glad we tried to do everything that we could."

"Every family that got their pet back is a success," Tal said.

Messages and media

Sharing information became my best way to be useful. Often my role became more like a librarian than journalist or activist: answering questions from emails, digging out info, networking and finding contact information. Often when multiple people from the same part of the world asked for help, I'd encourage them to connect and work together to find solutions. When I could, I'd encourage them to have their vets call other vets who had successfully used the treatments.

Whether the dog could be saved or not, many of these dog owners just appreciated having their questions answered by someone who had been through the same traumatic experience. Still, most of the heavy work happened out there in the real world while I mostly sat at my computer in Horseheads or Ithaca answering email. In various parts of the U.S. and the world, volunteer dog owners stepped forward and knocked on doors or shared information with others near them.

In a way, I also saw my job as an enhancement of vet-to-vet communication. The whole point was to transfer Dr. Sears' knowledge and experience into the hands of other vets so they could decide how to use it. The emails, websites, blogs and videos simply put a megaphone on the message. The protocols and experience of Dr. Sears went in one end of the megaphone. Vets willing to listen received the information on the other side, with the help of their clients who found the websites. If I could keep myself out of the message, all the better. But that became impossible.

As someone who had studied and taught mass media, I knew the old adage from the communications theorist and philosopher Marshall McLuhan: "The media is the message." By this he meant that HOW you received the message was as important as WHAT the message was. So, a message of "treatment for distemper" loses much of its impact if the source of the message is "guy on Internet." Another reason our task had been an uphill battle.

And even as just a messenger, terrible mistakes can be made.

At the end of September 2009, I had enthusiastically sent out an email to my contacts in Southern California. A vet had been found to join the "Coalition of the Willing," as I called it. In August, this vet in a practice south of Los Angeles had performed three NDV spinal taps at the urging of his clients. While all three dogs eventually died, he noted the distemper symptoms had begun to reverse. Pneumonia had killed them, not distemper. He was willing to try again.

"I wanted to let you know about this so that you can spread the word through your groups there that there is a California vet that distemper dogs can go to," I wrote in my email, which included his name and contact information. It would not be for a few months before I realized what a mistake this was.

The cause appeared to be on an upswing. Three vets in the U.S. were willing to treat dogs, and I had a connection with two of them. The vet in Georgia would not respond to me, but for now was still accepting patients sent his way. At least in some parts of the country, the desperate scramble to find a willing vet in the midst of crisis got easier.

In mid-November, Jeff Wells of Houston sent me a dramatic set of videos of his 4-month old boxer mix, Max.[75] The first shot zooms in on Max's profile, as he lays on a blue blanket, nearly unconscious. His black jaw and snout twitch. The next shot shows his full, light brown body as all four legs slowly spasm and move involuntarily. His back paw rhythmically taps.

The light dims for the next part of the video, showing Max asleep on his side and wheezing with every breath from pneumonia. The lungs rise and fall like bellows as the air fights to enter and leave his snout. Another shot shows him sleeping with his head on his paws in the same condition. With each video, his mass shrinks slightly. He's wasting away.

In the next videos, Max has curled into a ball of skin and bones on a bed. His eyelids flutter. "Max ..." Jeff says gently. The eyelids struggle to spread open, then close. "Max ... Max ... Max..." The third time, a little louder, the eyes open again. Then close. "Max!" Open, close.

Jeff strokes his back as Max opens his eyes fully, then lets them close. Then open again, letting the light reflect off the eyes. Then closed again. As Jeff takes his hand away, Max opens his eyes one more time, then lets them shut heavily.

That image brought back memories. When Amy and I fought to save Tug with 24-hour nursing care, sometimes she'd just stop breathing. Then we'd call out her name, and she'd breathe again, as if she needed to be reminded how. She only survived a couple of days after that.

Jeff's next video happened after Max's treatment at Dr. Zilkha's clinic in Austin. He hardly looked like the same dog. Max sat up on the living-room floor, his eyes locked on a pink dog toy. Excitement builds in his throat and snout.

"Yap!" Max said, the back of his head shaved from the NDV spinal tap. "Yap!"

"Get it, Max!" said Jeff. "Get it! Get 'em!"

Max looks at the camera, then back at the toy.

"Yap! Yap!" said Max.

Max lays flat with paws forward, challenging the toy to play. His yaps jump up and down in pitch, trying to find which sound will bring the toy to life.

In the next video, the camera hovers over Max as he bounces playfully, tail wagging.

"Who wants to play, Max? Who wants to play?" Jeff said. "What do ya got?"

Max lays flat on the floor, wagging his tail. Then he leaps up and charges forward, rubbing against Jeff's leg as he receives pets on his side.

"Oh, what a good boy, good boy," Jeff said. He scratches his rib cage. "Tail wagging. Jumping up and down. I've never seen him jumping up and down like that before."

In his email with the videos, Jeff wrote on Nov. 14:

Re: Max

Hi Ed,
he certainly seems to be doing a lot better. I took him yesterday for his second 'nebulization' treatment (enclosed humid kennel with gaseous antibiotics) to help his pneumonia.

I think his breathing has improved after these. Dr. Zilkha said the pneumonia is probably his biggest risk now.

He is like a different dog now that he actually has energy to get up during the days …

Thank you, again, for your help, and for having created the cause and websites. I'm looking forward to being an active member, and to Max being a poster-puppy for it :)

Jeff

Twitter posts:

"Now trying to help a 3-month-old puppy in India."
Nov. 23

"We just received word that the puppy in India died before the owner could do anything about it."
Nov. 25

Emails came in from all over the world: India, Argentina, China, Florida, Texas, Colorado, Arizona, California, South Africa, and especially from the Philippines, just to name a few. Although we had a better chance of helping a dog in Texas or California, in other places the dog owners struggled to find a willing vet. Treatment in Florida became hit or miss. A vet might be persuaded to use the NDV shot in one case, but not in another. Vets worried about bringing distemper dogs into the clinics, and I would hear stories about owners in South Florida paying a vet $50 to give the NDV injections in the parking lot.

Often the owners would email back to say their dog didn't have distemper after all. Other times, the vets would just shrug and say they would not know for sure until the neurologic stage began. Very often, the dog owners had found the websites too late.

With the mix of outcomes, I couldn't be sure whether successes were ahead or behind the failures. I'd answer these emails and then clear my head and get back to my job as a journalism professor as quickly as possible. I had no time to stop and count outcomes.

Answering distemper emails became what I did when someone else might be checking sports scores or watching cat videos. Only highlights stood out in my mind.

Meanwhile, J.D. Ward launched her own effort to promote the NDV treatments among vets in Texas she called Project Hope. Her story could probably make a book on its own, but I don't think I could do that properly.

However, she recently sent me a snippet of what she had gone through in 2009:

> "Little black Great Dane puppy, Emmy, was first. Her mama and two litter mates survived with no symptoms despite complete exposure. She came with a cut under her eye from the shelter. The virus snuck in then... Baby Hope's litter was ten puppies big and mama, Cherry. Cherry was eventually treated with serum with Hope but was never symptomatic. I struggled for months with the litter, doing everything for kennel cough and the upper respiratory infections, vet after vet kept diagnosing...until they ALL, except for Hope, went into neuro distemper. Thanksgiving, 2009. It was the closest thing to a disease-caused holocaust I've experienced and I was left, after three days in complete isolation caring for them, completely broken after the ninth pup in a row died in my arms. I had only Tramadol to ease their symptoms.
> My friend, Sherry, lost three of four rescue puppies, too, that weekend, after her Coco died months prior. The fourth was a natural survivor with no symptoms still seven years out and her mother was an unspayed donor dog.

Cherry and Hope lived together in isolation until I heard the familiar beeping bleat hiccup noise that only people who had tiny puppies with neuro distemper starting recognize. I thought they had beat it. It took a split second after I heard that to act. That was it! I packed up, left 20-30 dogs and headed to Austin to make the first batch of Project Hope serum ... I have four survivors here now, seven years out."

Amy, the boys and I drove down to my sister Jane's house to spend Thanksgiving weekend with her and her boyfriend Alan in New Jersey. I told her about Dr. Sears' lecture and the possibility of using NDV against MS. Her response: "I don't want to be the first one."

Fair enough.

As we settled into the guest room that Friday night, a woman named Agneza in Croatia emailed me about seven cases of distemper she had on her hands: five puppies from one litter, one puppy from another and an adult dog. Ultimately, all of the puppies died, but the adult dog survived after she found a vet willing to use the NDV spinal tap. She would later help other owners in that region of the world get their dogs treated.

In December, a vet in Alberta treated a 4-year-old German shepherd who survived, and White Angel treated Tigger, a 12-week-old puppy from El Paso, Texas, in neurologic distemper. The owners sent photos and video for the website.

At the end of December, a Los Angeles area woman named Bronwyne Mirkovich contacted me about a dog named Dante, who had been found in Hancock Park three weeks earlier and adopted out of a shelter. Dante had been diagnosed with kennel cough, but as his head began to tilt from neurologic trouble, the diagnosis switched to distemper.

Neither Dante's new family nor Bronwyne could risk keeping him, for fear of their other dogs getting distemper. This time, my sister Karen swung into action in her role as director of "Under The Porch," the dog-rescue arm of Kind Hearts In Action and got him into her vet's clinic.

A few days later, the story of Dante ended.

From Karen:

> "Dante didn't make it – he passed away in the night after the last bed check at midnight and before the 6 am rounds. He appeared to have gone in his sleep not all twisted from a seizure. The vet techs had all spend time with him petting and talking to him and trying to make him comfortable. It was just too late for him ... Sorry guys, we tried ... We will save the next one is what we have to hope."

At the L.A. Times, I'd written a column about a fire chief celebrating 50 years in firefighting. He told me too many stories to fit in the space I had. In one story that stuck in my head, they responded to a child who died in a hanging. Sadness loomed over the station after they came back from the run. The chief told his crew to let go of the sadness. They wouldn't be ready for the next call if they didn't. The other firefighters took the advice, and on the next call, they saved a life.

The point: You can't succeed if you dwell on the failures.

Obstacles and challenges

In early January, a vet with a blog called Skeptivet took notice of the treatments because a client had asked about them. I was described as "someone named Ed Bond, who apparently has no medical or veterinary background, but who thinks his dog was cured by Dr. Sears' treatment." The blog went on to say that Dr. Sears and I appeared to be honest and not making much money on this. Then continued with:

"While this idea is not impossible, there are several things about the claims on the various websites that raise red flags for me. These include; 1: claims for effectiveness with absolutely no data presented to back up those claims, 2: hints that most dogs still experience the usual complications and sequelae of the disease, 3: a lack of information about side effects or mortality from the treatment or in the dogs used as serum donors, 4: the claim on the page about Dr. Sears that he has developed treatments for a wide variety of diseases but has never published anything about these treatments, 5: finally there are several reasons to be concerned about potential problems with this treatment that are not related to it's effectiveness or lack thereof... **Anytime someone makes claims such as the claims that are being made for this treatment, they have an obligation to keep good records of both the positive and negative outcomes.** At this point there are hints that the treatment may not be as effective as it's supporters would like, but by focusing on the positive outcomes, and minimizing the negative, there is no way to tell if the treatment is effective, ineffective or just downright dangerous. ... When some patients get better, it is easy to attribute their improvement to whatever you did, but some dogs have always survived distemper."[76]

All valid objections. But we had little means of responding since Dr. Sears had retired and was no longer treating dogs, and I was just a guy on a computer in Horseheads who would not and could not treat distemper dogs. I barely had time to answer the emails coming in.

As to keeping records of positive and negative outcomes, I had to mostly rely on what owners told me and also the intermittent reports from vets willing to reply. I filed the criticism from Skeptivet away in the back of my head. Somehow, I would have to find a way to respond.

At about the same time Dante died, I received this email from the vet south of Los Angeles:

> "I am very sorry I could not respond to your previous mail, as I was in and out of the office most of the time due to the holidays. I have used the serum in 14 puppies for a rescue group. These puppies were diagnosed with canine distemper at another hospital and were showing all the symptoms of distemper but not the neurological signs. The last I heard was four of the puppies were euthanized, rest of them were doing ok for now ... I have been receiving lot of calls for the information and possible treatment for canine distemper, it seems like you are working overtime. I will keep in touch and if you need any more information please let me know."

So, for those of you keeping score, that's a 70 percent survival rate in that group. Also in January, a vet in India made the NDV serum and used it to save a dog named Muttu owned by Kaveri Uthaiah in Bangalore.[77] The same day Muttu's story went up on the Kind Hearts In Action website, a TV station in Austin filmed a report on an NDV spinal tap performed at White Angel on a dog named Cahokia, owned by Donna Lochmann of St. Louis.

From the story by Ashley Porter of News 8:

"There are no proven cures for the virus, but veterinarian Dr. Al Sears has developed an experimental treatment that a few clinics across the country are testing ... It took several attempts for the injection to work successfully. The next day, Lochmann was excited to see Cahokia lift her head, devour food eagerly and even walk. ... 'She was hungry, she was alert, trying to walk, as wobbly as she was, looking like she had a few too many margaritas,' Lochmann said."

Three days later came an email from Karen Hall, a math teacher in Broomfield, Colorado, who was trying to save her shepherd-mix puppy in neurologic distemper named Selena. She would persuade her vet to perform the NDV spinal tap, but the dog ultimately died four months later, after a difficult struggle. Not every dog was being saved. Some died.

"Is anyone keeping a spreadsheet of the stats from the procedures?" she wrote me during one exchange, raising an issue that the OB/GYN had raised a year earlier.

"You know, the full stats are probably stored right here in all my e-mails," I replied. "I just have never had time to tally everything up. But I do post the highlights on either Twitter or the kindhearts Web page when we have news."

In early February, some confusion about my email address caused a minor crisis. I'd created multiple Yahoo! accounts but then closed a couple to streamline things. Dr. Sears got a bounce back on an email, saying my account had closed. "Has this become too much for you and are you closing down?" he wrote to my other account. "I sure hope not. Doc"

I wrote back, "I am with you until you and your treatments get the recognition that is deserved."

"Good," he replied. "I was worried that this was becoming a drag on your time and efforts. Thanks for hanging in there. Doc"

We had made clear our commitment to the cause and each other. He had not asked me to do any of this, but he was glad of it.

About this time, a vet in Mexico near the border with Brownsville, Texas, contacted us to say he was willing to use NDV. Then, Vickie Novak, a nurse from Central Florida, wrote me about her dog with head spasms and chewing gum seizures. After taking her dog Sookie up to the vet in Georgia for the NDV spinal tap, she became another invaluable ally. She wrote me afterwards:

"Well Sookie is doing well, today she actually did a little gallop — now this is a dog that was severely weak … The head spasm and jaw tremor are about the same but the arm tremor is just off and on now and Sookie is only 48 hours post spinal — so it is pretty remarkable! … I saw the pic of your Selkie and when I send pics of Sookie you will see how very much Sookie and Selkie look alike – Sookie a labby mix too! I am so sorry for yours and your families loss of your precious furbabies."

"It always hits home when I see a pup that was saved that reminds me of one I lost," I wrote back. "I don't mourn the ones I lost so much now. But they are the ones who inspired me to do this."

Vickie's local vet continued treating Sookie for pneumonia after the spinal tap treatment, and he took an interest in using the NDV treatments. Sookie would live for another four years.

Twitter:
"I'm using a free online translation program to try to help someone in Uruguay."
March 5, 2010

"Sadly, the puppy in North Carolina did not make it. We couldn't get him to treatment fast enough."
March 11, 2010

The momentum in California fell apart on the Ides of March. A dog owner who I'd been trying to help emailed with: "When is the last time you were in communication with Dr. [from south of Los Angeles]? One receptionist is telling me I have to talk to him first which I can not get a call back. Another receptionist who just answered is telling me he does not do this treatment anymore."

"Sadly, I just got off the phone with his office and Dr. [name omitted] has discontinued the treatment for lack of good results," she wrote a few minutes later. "The air just went out of my tires."

Stunned, I sent an email to the vet:

"I've received word that you've lost interest in Dr. Sears' NDV treatments. I was confused by this because I thought that you'd had good results from this. Also, this comes at a time when more vets from around the country and the world are starting to pick this up…. In any event, what you decide to do is up to you. You have to do what you feel is best for your practice and the animals that you treat. But I hope you could reconsider."

The next day, while waiting for the reply from California, I received an email from Vickie's vet in Florida: "I am excited to try the treatment. It's giving hope to these poor dogs." That cheered me up, until the vet in California wrote to explain why he stopped using NDV:

> "Main reason for this is, one of the clients with a puppy showing neurological signs was very unhappy with the treatment. I have explained to this gentleman at length the procedure and he was also told that there is no guarantee that his puppy was going to be fine, and he was also told that he need to give a few months for the twitching to get better.

"He was agreeable to all this. The puppy was in our care for one week. Even though the puppy was twitching, he was still eating well. When the owner picked up the puppy he was very unhappy that the puppy was still twitching. When I told him he was explained about the same thing, and he need to give a few months to see improvement in the twitching, he picked up the puppy but he still did not look happy.

"When my receptionist called him a few weeks later to see how the puppy was doing, he said the puppy was euthanized the very next day, and he was accusing us of running a scam and was going to take legal action against us. My receptionist did send him the copy of the release form he signed. With the way the things are, I don't need any headaches of this kind. Even though we use totally different anesthetic tubing and baralyme (CO_2 absorber) for these patients during the procedure, and they are kept in isolation room, still I am concerned about the transmission of the disease to our other hospitalized animals. Once I get these things straightened out I will be more than happy to pursue this treatment ...."

This left me feeling sick. A costly lesson, which more than dampened the good news of a new vet in Florida. I relayed the message to Dr. Sears.

"Ed, just as I thought, California and the law," he replied. "Vets are always looking over their shoulders and still get sued. I do not blame Dr. ... for stopping."

We had not only lost a dog, but also the only vet using the protocols in California. I blamed myself. The mistake was in pushing the vet's information out into the world too aggressively. My thinking had been that so many dogs were being lost because they weren't getting the treatment early enough, within the six-day window. The owner of a dog needed to know right after a distemper diagnosis what to do and where to go. I'd figured that sending that information out to every contact I had in California, we'd improve our chances of success.

This plan fell victim to a version of the old game, telephone. The email information got passed along, copy/pasted, transcribed and scribbled down until someone, somewhere handed the contact information for this vet to this dog owner and said, "Here, this vet will cure your dog."

So, even with all the warnings and explanations from the vet and his clinic staff, the dog owner still held a promise of complete recovery in his head. Then he felt betrayed when the reality did not meet expectation. To be perfectly honest, it's likely this is why the vet in Georgia kept me at arms length. Often vets don't want to draw a lot of attention to themselves if they are using an unpublished treatment. This is also why I am not publishing the names of some of the vets who have used the treatments.

Picking up the pieces

Fortunately, a new tool to recruit other vets became ready. I finished editing the video of Dr. Sears's lecture in Houston. Learning to splice footage between the multiple cameras, plus adding graphics and captions had been a challenge. J.D. Ward found a supporter who burned dozens of copies to disc. Her husband Mike did much of the work sending out DVDs beginning in early March. [78] "He's an unsung hero," J.D. says about Mike. "He took a good four months or more to get this out to everyone."

Boxes of DVDs went to contacts in California, who hand delivered them to vets. "The names of the vet or vets that we work with need to be kept confidential," I wrote in an email to my California contacts. "The people who need the help need to find us and be referred to the vet through us, and as we make the referral, we need to educate them about the realities of the treatment. But we can also share with them our stories, photos and videos so that they know this is not a scam, only an effort to save their dogs. However, we should remember that in medical science there is never a 100 percent guarantee of success. However, we can say that there is an excellent chance of recovery."

By the end of March, a new California vet – in Westlake Village, Ventura County – had started treating dogs with NDV.

Back in Florida, a couple of notable cases included Romeo and Basher. A volunteer with Dachshund Rescue South Florida wrote me about Romeo, one of their dogs with neurologic distemper. The new vet in Central Florida treated him. His recovery was difficult, but he finally turned the corner in April.

The Central Florida vet also treated Basher, a lab-Dachshund mix, with NDV serum before the onset of the neurologic stage. The owners gratefully sent me video of Basher playing in a park after recovery.

Twitter

Please say a prayer for Nanook, a California dog with neuro symptoms. Vet gave him the spinal treatment on his day off. What a vet!
9:06 AM - 3 Apr 2010

19 of 20 distemper dogs treated with NDV in Tennessee are recovering. The last one is struggling, but there is always hope.
12:37 PM - 3 Apr 2010

Cookie, the momma dog from Northern Virginia, was in too much pain and had to be euthanized.
9:18 PM - 18 Apr 2010

Nanook was put to sleep after a long battle.
http://kindheartsinaction.com/2010/04/19/nanook-treated-with-ndv/
1:01 PM - 11 May 2010

Just heard of case of neuro distemper from Upstate New York (near Vermont). This is a first for us.
4:44 PM - 15 May 2010

Pup in upstate New York died. Owner could find no one in New York or Boston who was willing to try NDV treatment.
6:15 PM - 18 May 2010

The email:

> "It is with great sadness that I inform you that our puppy Samba had to be put down yesterday. Her seizures were relentless, she was seizuring even under phenobarbital and Valium combined and every vet said that they could only maintain her but not do anything to cure her. We were not able to get anyone, and I really mean no one in the state of NY or in Boston to administer the NDV vaccine on her. They all told us that this is a procedure with no scientific basis and that actually the documentation on it through the orthodox medical publications says the results were not good at all. So I am just trying to understand all this because I can very well understand that most people are not willing be pioneers, after all it takes balls and commitment to reasons larger than a pay check and a comfortable

lifestyle for a vet to want to take the risk and stick
their neck out there, but what I can't understand is
the disparity of information in between what we
saw on your web site and the medical literature on
the same subject. They told us there were no
successful cases with this treatment, and you guys
have in your web site what seemed to us
documented cases of many success cases.
So what is it with this matter?
If you can explain it I would greatly appreciate!
Best regards and thanks for your support!"
Filipe Pinheiro
Greenwich, NY

In a way, the point of this entire book is an answer to this
email, explaining why things are the way they are. But the main
disparity between the success stories on the website and what
may be found in a scientific journal is that our website stories
are only considered "anecdotal evidence." Results needed to be
documented professionally by a researcher and reviewed by
peers in the scientific community to be considered credible.

During my year as both a full-time college professor and
volunteer advocate for the NDV treatments, I received or wrote
thousands of emails about canine distemper. Too much to
include them all here. The chain of events and connections
made by all the other people trying to help spread the word
about how to treat dogs with canine distemper would probably
make a fascinating book on its own. But I can only focus on my
experience, and what I knew through the window on the world
I had: my computer screen.

By the end of the academic year, my overall strategy had evolved. Rather than push the treatment out into the world, I'd set a system up so the interested and willing could find their way to my websites, blogs and ultimately my email address. The approach became passive, not aggressive. This made acceptance a little easier. If someone approaches you offering something too good to be true, you'd be smart to doubt it. But if you come across useful information in your own research and choose to follow the information to the source, you might be more open to what you found.

In mid-May, Tal and I checked in with each other. Despite the progress, my outlook seemed grimmer. Too many dogs were dying after the NDV spinal tap.

I wrote:

> "Overall, worldwide there had been bad news. Vet in Romania who had a lot of success with serum, says that most dogs who he tries the spinal tap die. He just had a case die, and I believe he had tried this a couple of dozen times. One treated by [vet in Georgia] recently was having a very bad time and is hanging on. One in California had to be put to sleep after a long struggle, but there have been some successful cases in California. And a vet in Hong Kong tried this, and the dog was fine for a while, but then after going to sleep it would not wake up. That owner has not updated me recently, but I fear the worse. Oh, and there was a dog with a spinal treatment in Virginia that also had to be put to sleep.

Stepping back and looking at the big picture, I'm wondering what's going on. Actually, Dr. Sears and I were asking each other about this last week. It could be just a learning curve for some of these vets. ... The thought occurred to me recently that perhaps the virus itself could change – in which case we're screwed – or perhaps something has changed with the NDV, how it's made or where it is coming from. Or it's just a bad string of bad luck. What do you think?"

Tal's reply:

"We had a few that had to be put to sleep too after a CSF Tap. However we did have great results with stopping the outbreak in the shelter and we saved about 60 some dogs. My wife thinks that it is possible that the Virus changes... I don't think that this is the end of the game. We gathered enough evidence to show that there is something to it. Once my wife publishes her paper, the next step is to get this thing to the next level. It's time for the treatment to move on from the domain of the rescue people to the Universities and the big Pharma. I know that there is an interest in Texas A&M – once of the leading vet schools in the country – in what we are doing in WAAH: We just did a CSF tap and we are fighting on the life of a small Corgi, that had been seen by the Neurologist from Texas A&M. That specialist had given the owner a no chance of survival when he diagnosed it with distemper. The dog was tested positive with the test we send out to A&M.

"However it is a week after the CSF tap and the dog is doing better!!! ... I really hope that this dog will survive, because that will convince some people. You see – once they hear about it from another doctor and not from rescue people, some of the other doctors are showing open minds. So, keep positive, we are making progress and I am very hopeful for publishing this year!!!"

As we wrote this exchange, my year at Ithaca College came to a close. I had not made a successful transition from part-time adjunct to full-time professor. My attempts to layer the new technologies into my old-fashioned courses had failed. In the 1990s in California, I did better as a teacher because I had recently been an L.A. Times reporter, so my lessons carried a relevance. As a part-time news editing teacher in the mid-2000s, my lessons came straight out of my job on the news desk, often from the night before. The class worked. The students appreciated learning a useful skill.

By 2009-10, the value of print newspaper skills had tanked and so had my enthusiasm. My knowledge of the latest digital technology was shaky. My plans to bring in the new technology had been too ambitious, with not enough time in the semester to really cover what the students needed. My anecdotes about my professional career lost relevance. In the evaluations, the students described me as unhelpful and difficult. Perhaps I might have been able to pull back and plan it all out better for the next year, but I didn't get the chance. I didn't apply for a long-term full-time position that had become available. Instead, I offered to teach as a part-timer again. Teaching the one class would have been a better fit for me. However, the department did not ask me back.

One cannot climb two mountains at once.

While it is true I might have been more successful as a professor had I not had to answer five emails about canine distemper from the Philippines or India or California every time I stepped out of the classroom, that would still be a cop out. I also realized I had been on the wrong path in my life. Perhaps I was not meant to be a professor, or even a journalist, or even an advocate for dogs with canine distemper.

My brain took the death of my teaching career with a shrug. "I'll find something else." But later on I would realize emotions have their own response, no matter what your rational mind wants you to do. The full impact of my educational and journalism careers ending so abruptly would hit years later.

Something better awaited me, but I would not find it for a couple more years. It would be revealed in a dream.

Taking Stock

"…Also, I know she is being treated with Sears' Serum, here in Korea…" – Sarah W., July 20, 2010

[record scratch] Huh, what?

Korea?

"I had not been aware that Dr. Sears' serum was in Korea. Could you get me the info on where it is available there?"

Sarah wrote me about a dog she had rescued from a shelter in Korea with a head tilt and diagnosed with distemper. In the following exchange of emails, she wrote:

"The Sears serum, as far as I know, has RECENTLY been introduced into the Korean market. I have actually not heard about this type of treatment until a couple of months ago when a dog with pneumonia was being treated with it… The Sears serum seems to be only in use at big vets which cost around 50,000 won (about 48.00$) per treatment!"

I relayed this to Dr. Sears and received the reply: "Ed, years ago I had contact with a Vet Professor at the University there. They did make some up and use it and found it adequate. Never did hear anything more."

By now, I'd bought a ledger from Staples and begun sorting through all the distemper messages on my Yahoo! email account. I'd gone all the way back to the first email on January 20, 2009, noting name of dog, owner contact info, when the first email was received, whether the case was pre-seizures, seizure, used serum, NDV as IV or spinal tap, whether it was later determined to be another disease and outcome. The criticism from Skeptivet still lurked in the back of my mind, and the ledger began my first attempt to build a response. At the very least, I might have a better idea of whether I'd been wasting my time. On the entry for this day, I wrote in all caps: "KOREA IS USING SEARS SERUM!!"

I wrote back to Sarah:

"I would really, really like to get in touch with someone who speaks English and who can tell me particulars about how recently the serum started being used, how it is made there, how many cases have been treated in Korea and what outcomes they have had. I am the canine distemper project director for a U.S. charity called Kind Hearts In Action."

It would take several months to track down this mystery. Meanwhile, just compiling the ledger took weeks. At the time, Yahoo! emails remained stubbornly disorganized. Each message came in separately, and a separate search of a correspondent's address was needed to find out the outcome of each case.

In September, my frustration from the distemper and personal emails all coming to the same account and the disorganization of Yahoo! at that time, led me to create a new Gmail account dedicated only to distemper cases. I found Gmail much better organized for keeping track of the outcome of cases because emails could be organized into conversations, something Yahoo! would do later on.

Finally, I got through all the Yahoo! emails, 30 double-truck pages of notes on more than 400 cases. Ten percent came from the Philippines. But way, way too often, the column under "Outcome" remained blank or marked "unknown." Often, dog owners never responded after getting the info.

At the kitchen table, I jotted down the totals on a scrap of paper as Amy sat nearby:

> Yahoo email
> Serum/NDV
> Survived = 23
> Died = 20
>
> Spinal tap
> Survived = 26
> Died = 32
>
> Died before treatment
> 29
>
> Total survived: 49
> Total died: 52

"Forty-nine survived, 52 died," I said, disappointed.

"Well, that's 49 dogs still alive," Amy said.

Not a very convincing number. Not enough to tell whether NDV had really made a difference. On the other hand, so many dogs were being treated late or inconsistently; it was too soon to know NDV was useless either. In the back of the ledger, I wrote: "8757 emails in Yahoo!; 6005 with distemper." Then I jotted down a list of when emails first came from a state or a country. These included:

> Virginia: 3/31/10
> Tennessee: 4/3/10
> South Africa: 4/13
> Serbia: 6/9/10

Puerto Rico: 5/25
Mexico: 4/11
Dominican Republic: 5/19
Brazil: 4/10

On the side of this list, I wrote: "Must contact school in Korea about their use of the Sears serum." However, all the information about the Sears serum in Korea was written in Korean on Korean websites. This would take time.

For the next few months, the priority became compiling numbers. Follow-up emails went out to every case where the outcome was not known. I drew up an address list of every vet around the world rumored to have used NDV for distemper.

The Coalition of the Willing kept changing. The Humane Society of Puerto Rico helped vets there to use NDV in May, and in June a vet in Mexico successfully used the NDV serum on a dog named "Hope." Vets were also using NDV in the Dominican Republic. Agneza in Croatia helped someone in Serbia get their dog treated with the NDV spinal tap in June. However, the vet in Georgia completely dropped the treatments. I learned this from a dog owner through a Facebook message in mid-June.

Then in July, a dog owner in Istanbul persuaded her vet there to perform the NDV spinal tap. Vickie Novak gave a lot of help and advice through this and many other cases of neurologic distemper. Since I had not personally experienced having a neurologic distemper dog survive, I usually went to someone like Vickie or J.D. Ward to give advice to other dog owners in that situation. With her background in medicine, Vickie's advice was especially useful. J.D. Ward often had a lot of practical, hands on advice for dog owners. One of the most useful tips was that a tablespoon of corn syrup in 8-ounces of drinking water could help a distemper dog regain enough appetite to eat. Survival often turned on whether these dogs ate. J.D., Vickie and I copied each other on countless messages.

Twitter

News from Gallup, NM: "Amazingly the pup has
rebounded and is eating well. Her fever is down and she
looks like a different dog."
11:27 AM - 15 Jul 2010

The question of money

In August came word that a rescue group had persuaded
a vet on the west coast of Southern Florida to make the NDV
serum and treat dogs there.

Vets in different cities and different parts of the country –
and world – charged differently for their services. When I could,
I would let dog owners have a general idea of what to expect
the procedures to cost. For example, in the U.S., an NDV spinal
tap could cost anywhere from $500 to $1500, but those numbers
could go up depending on the demands of a particular case. Vet
clinics calculated their costs for making the NDV serum
differently, but from what I heard the vet bill for an NDV serum
or NDV as IV treatment could run $100 to $300, depending on
the weight of the dog. "Nobody makes money from this," said
Tal Shohamy at White Angel.

The vets using the treatments also took on a risk to their
practices. Those who did use it told me they did so just because
they wanted to try to save these dogs. I have to admire that
courage.

When a question about patenting the treatment came up,
Dr. Sears had no interest. The treatment was meant to be his
"gift to the world." He did not plan on making money on his
discovery. Neither did I. Neither did J.D. Ward, who continued
her campaign to promote the treatment among vets in Texas
through Project Hope. Our common goal had been to see the
treatments accepted by the veterinary community and at the
very least for Dr. Sears to get credit for what he had found.

My wish in particular would be to see the acceptance of NDV serum being used before the onset of the neurologic stage. That seemed to be the easiest and most reliable way to save the most dogs. Once they reached the neurologic stage, survival became more difficult.

From Texas, California, and elsewhere around the world, I continued to receive a mix of reports on dogs in the neurologic stage of distemper getting the NDV spinal tap. Some would live. Some died.

In October, an email came in from a transport driver for an animal hospital in Korea, who had copied my inquiry to a vet in Seoul. The vet replied to my email on Nov. 5 with "So what can I do for you?"

"We are trying to document the effectiveness of Dr. Sears' serum around the world. I'm trying to find any studies, surveys on how it is used in Korea and what record of success/failure it has shown. Can you help me track down that information?"

Then, no reply.

Encouraging news

In mid-December, Dr. Sears copied me on an email from the Shelter of Szekszárd in Hungary. Szilvia Fiáth wrote to tell him their vet had made the NDV serum and used it to save 5 dogs.

"I am very happy your vet had the temerity to try the procedure," Dr. Sears wrote back. "Congratulations on your success. Sounds like you have followed the protocol to the very best of ability."

Ten minutes after his email, I replied very excitedly.

"I would like to use the pictures and your story to put together a page on our website – kindheartsinaction.com – to demonstrate the effectiveness of the serum. Would you be willing to work with me on that?"

She would send me several before/after photos and videos and case reports for the website on these and on their later use of the NDV spinal tap. [79] The other shelter dogs barked constantly in the background of these videos, a joyful sound. The barking of dogs at a Hungarian shelter sounds identical to an American or Indian or Filipino kennel. Dogs possess a universal language, and people who love dogs can be found in every country of the world.

Two days after the Hungary email, I tried again with Korea, and got no immediate reply. Meanwhile, I sent out surveys to vets using NDV and more follow-up emails to dog owners.

Very often, even vets who were willing to use NDV could only give intermittent replies and minimal info on cases. I'd sometimes suggest elaborate plans where the NDV vets could combine their efforts, share information or build a central file on the treatment of cases to make an argument for the effectiveness of NDV. These plans never went very far.

Why?

Because vets are busy! Not only are they dealing with a constant flow of cases with a wide range of illness, injury and species, they usually have to run a business, plus handle emergency calls on top of all of that. This had been one of the main obstacles Dr. Sears had faced when he first discovered the NDV serum in the 1970s, while working 12 hour days, six days a week with Chuck Whitt. Time remains a luxury clinical vets do not have.

"Sorry I didn't get back to you sooner, I have been quite busy," wrote the new vet using NDV in California. "But anything you need me to do to help the cause just let me know. I don't have a lot of free time but I'll help in whatever way I can."

But I usually did not get any kind of response. Since I have no standing within the veterinary community, they have no reason to work with me.

When I sent out a survey to 37 vets who may have been using NDV, I tried to keep the impact on time to a minimum. Each letter included a card with YES/NO or simple questions:

> Do you use NDV to treat canine distemper? Do you use NDV-induced serum?
> How many dogs have you treated with NDV serum?
> How many of those dogs survived?
> Do you use NDV as an IV injection?
> How many dogs have you treated with NDV as an IV injection?
> How many of those dogs survived?
> Do you use the NDV spinal tap treatment?
> How many dogs have you treated with NDV spinal tap?
> How many of those dogs survived?

The vet in Korea made contact again at the end of December and promised to help track down information about any studies leading to the use of Dr. Sears' serum in Korea. But then I heard nothing for another month.

In mid-January, the office manager to a Houston-area vet who had worked with J.D. Ward's Project Hope emailed a reply to my survey. She reported in a brief message that the NDV serum had been used on 150 distemper dogs with a 90 percent survival rate. They also tried the NDV spinal tap on 23 dogs, but only two of those dogs survived. When J.D. began the project, she said her understanding had been it would conclude with a detailed report on the cases treated, but the clinic did not come forward with any further information. Later, I would learn for myself all the challenges a working vet clinic must overcome to document a treatment's effectiveness.

This veterinarian had kept me at arms length but also never turned away a client with a distemper dog. I always heard good comments from dog owners after their visits. So, I was grateful they stayed with the treatments even when they did not respond to calls or messages from me. As long as they kept accepting dogs, I kept them on my list of willing vets. This list was not posted publicly, only given out privately as a reply to emails from owners of distemper dogs.

To get on the list, I would ask the owner of a dog who lived following an NDV treatment to ask the vet whether they would be willing to have other referrals and what contact information they would want to be sent via private emails. When a dog owner told me a particular clinic had said they were no longer using NDV, I took them off the list.

After getting the email about the 150 dogs treated in Houston, I took Romeo for a walk in the woods. The path we took came within a few yards of where Galen had been buried and ran parallel to the little creek where we had scattered Wanda and Shadow's ashes. Wanda had died in August 2010, Shadow on March 26, 2009, exactly 13 years after Tug died. All the pets we had brought back from California had now died. Our family had reached our second generation of pets, Romeo and two cats.

On the walk, I took stock of where we were. Responses from vets using NDV were still coming in, and so were the replies to the follow-up emails from dog owners. All this information remained sketchy. What we had fell short of "good records of both the positive and negative outcomes." We had survival rates but we had to rely on each vet's say-so that these were distemper cases. The methods of diagnosis varied. Sometimes they came from lab reports, but sometimes distemper was assumed because the clinic was in the middle of handling an outbreak. We had raw numbers, not details.

In a note from Dr. Sears, he reminded me, "Diagnosis critical. Cannot prescribe for what you don't know. Guessing usually fails."

Compiling the numbers and stories from vets and dog owners simply created a mound of anecdotal evidence, not hard science, and I knew that. But a goal at this point was to at least give other dog owners enough hope and courage to ask their vets to give it a try. Then hope the light bulb would go off in the head of some researcher who could take a closer look. However, getting the numbers from Houston had been a huge relief for me. Had I never gotten an answer or been told most of the dogs died, everything might have ground to a halt. Just like the news from Romania and the videos from the Philippines and Alberta, this became a checkpoint. Another vet had followed Dr. Sears' discovery and had similar results with a substantial number of dogs. I had enough to still believe. As I trudged through the snow with Romeo, my muscles let go of a tension that had been building for months.

I wrote an email to J.D. and Dr. Sears on Jan. 14, 2011:

"There are at least 135 dogs who are alive today because of all the work you did. The work of Project Hope and all the others out there who found vets and persuaded them to try this has laid the groundwork for the full scientific trials that are to come. Today, I feel more confident than ever that they will become a reality."

Later, J.D. would report that by working with the vet in Houston and others, Project Hope had saved more than 200 dogs. After I received more responses to my survey, I wrote up a summary for Dr. Sears at the end of January:

> "So far, vets responding to the survey reported treating 221 distemper dogs with Newcastle Disease Vaccine. Of those, 169 lived, a survival rate of 76 percent. The survivors include 160 treated with NDV serum, seven treated with NDV spinal taps and two with NDV as an injection to the body ...

"We've also surveyed dog owners and have received the outcomes of 219 distemper dogs treated with NDV since December 2008. Of those, 131 lived, for a survival rate of 59.8 percent. The survivors include 35 treated with NDV serum, 44 with NDV as an injection to the body and 52 treated with the NDV spinal tap. We also received reports on 115 other distemper cases not treated with NDV in which 17 percent of the dogs survived."

I made a few points to Dr. Sears:

"1) These numbers are not performing as well as we know they can. Obviously this is a result of the delays that often happen. Owners and vets often do not recognize they have a distemper case until it is late in the game, then the vet recommends euthanasia, but then some owners will get on the Web looking for alternatives, but by the time they find us, it is nearly too late to help them. 2) Even so, when compared against the group that did not get any NDV treatments, the NDV performs dramatically better. Without NDV the survival rate is only 17 percent. With an NDV treatment, the rate is either 60 percent or 76 percent, depending on the group. I was surprised that so many dogs survived without NDV. 17 percent seemed high to me, but one thing to bear in mind is that the group of people in this survey are more likely to go to great lengths to keep their dogs alive. They are the ones who chose not to trust their vets and to find alternatives on the Web.

3) It looks like the NDV injection is out-performing the serum, but I would attribute that to the fact that by the time people find this information it is almost nearly too late. There is not enough time to get the serum made and so they opt for the NDV as IV. There has been a lot of luck with it.

4) These numbers are not scientific, but they do put a foot in the door for us. This can make it possible for media and potential donors to get behind these treatments and push for scientific trials."

Ok, I wanted to talk about the book, too. But this e-mail is already too long. I will put it in the next e-mail."

Dr. Sears had been working on a book about his treatments and earlier that month sent me what he had. He'd asked me to help edit his book, but I realized he needed more help than just an edit.   So, I suggested he tell his story to me through a series of phone interviews.

"I'm going to let you do it because obviously you're someone who works with words," he said during that first phone call. "I'm not. I don't consider myself a writer at all. That's another reason why it probably didn't get out there. I tried to give it to the world, and they didn't like the way I wrote it."

My original plan had been to help him create a book of only his words and only his story. But by now, our lives and our goals had become intertwined. I'd find it difficult to separate my story from his. We began working as co-authors.

Meanwhile, I'd sent the preliminary information about the reported cases to some of the vets who had responded. I received this reply from Istanbul:

"Hi Ed this is Dr. Sinem Karsli Parmaksizoglu from Turkey,

I've got your e-mail about the preliminary number, and am still in shock about the fact that the numbers are so few. We have too many stray dogs in Istanbul and that's why we have thousands of distemper dogs. I have seen many of them die and some of them survive till today. The NDV treatment is a big hope for dogs in my country. I hope the numbers would increase soon so that you can push for scientific trials as much as you can. Today I will welcome one more distemper doggie to my clinic, and tomorrow another one is coming. The word goes around really quick. So please tell me how I can help about the survey? best wishes"

I replied to thank her for her help and to just keep updating me on the outcome of cases. At the end of January, I tried again with the vet in Korea. This time, he had found for me the website and email for the Korean Animal Blood Bank. On a page of mostly Korean characters, I found the words in English "anti-distemper serum." Scrolling further down the page, I found a collection of the success stories from my original website, posted in 2000 and 2001, including the email from Dawn H. to me about Cookie.

On Super Bowl Sunday 2011, I checked my email before we headed over to my brother-in-law's house to watch the game. This message from Dr. Kim Hee Young, senior researcher of the Korean Animal Blood Bank, waited for me:

"Dear Ed Bond

I am sorry to be late for response.

We have used Sears plasma (serum) in Distemper cases and found it works wonderful.

Actually, some of vets had already used Sears plasma and they recommended to produce this drug. At the first time, we did not believe that Sears would treat infected or moderately affected dogs with distemper.

On our first trial (2003), Sears plasma was sent vets to test in Distemper cases. After sending, we contacted the vets again.

They were good responses about Sears and are still ordering it.

In moderately affected case, we have recommended to use anti-serum with enough Distemper-antibody together.

Their successful rate were more than 60 % (until 2004.... after then, we did not collect data).

We can make good things to save animals.

Please let me know if I have something to help you."

Even though the Steelers lost to the Packers in the Super Bowl that day, this email lifted my spirits. With the news from Houston, Hungary, Turkey and now Korea – plus the other stories and numbers coming in from around the world – success seemed to be only a matter of time.

Dr. Kim Hee-Young had found out about Dr. Sears through my website in 2003 and "felt like that I found a golden drug." He had left Korea in 2006 and become a professor at the University of Texas at Galveston. However, he still maintained his position at the blood bank and asked his staff to look up the records. A few days later, he emailed:

"In 2003, 102 dogs (from 12 vets) were diagnosed by ELISA[80] as Distemper infection. Of them, the 54 dogs (52 %) were recovered completely on the check-up 6 weeks after Sears treatment. In Korea, the success rate of conventional treatment in case confirmed as Distemper (ELISA) was usually lower than 8 %."

I told him about the numbers, stories, photos and videos I'd been collecting on distemper cases. He said those might lead to publication in a veterinary journal, but of course "it would be best if you have details."

As of Feb. 14, 2011, 10 veterinarians from Florida, Texas, California, Puerto Rico, Canada, and Romania had answered my survey and the outcomes of nearly 300 distemper dogs cared for by owners, rescuers, fosters and shelters around the world had been received. A chart from those numbers along with reports from dog owners is on the next page.

In these numbers, the survival rate for dogs in neurologic distemper getting the NDV spinal tap never got better than the upper 40s, but Tal Shohamy still puts the chances of survival at 50-50. White Angel saved about every other dog who received the spinal tap, he said, but the numbers from vets trying the treatment for the first time could throw off the average. Many clinics trying the NDV spinal tap would have a learning curve at first, so they may have been losing more of their earlier cases. "I don't even know if they injected it in the right way," he said.

REPORTS FROM VETS

10 veterinarians treat
234 dogs with NDV

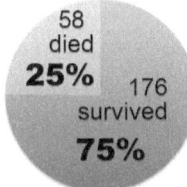

58
died
25%   176
survived
75%

191 dogs treated
with NDV serum

7 dogs treated
with NDV as IV

36 treated with
NDV spinal taps

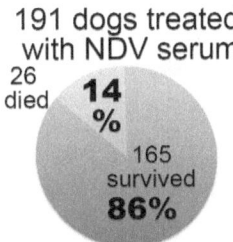

26
died   **14
%**
165
survived
86%

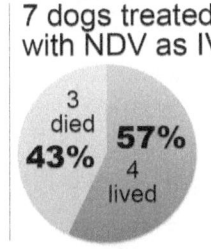

3
died   **57%**
43%   4
lived

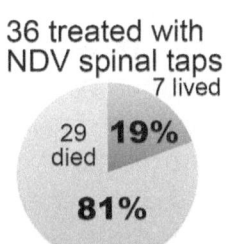

7 lived
29   **19%**
died
81%

Kind Hearts In Action website
Feb. 14, 2011

REPORTS FROM
DOG OWNERS/CAREGIVERS

288 dogs
with distemper

166 treated with NDV

122 not treated
with NDV

33
died   **20%**
80%
133
survived

100
died
82%   **18%**
22
survived

57 dogs treated
with NDV serum

57 dogs treated
with NDV as IV

109 treated with
NDV spinal taps

37%
21 died   36
survived
63%

21%
12   45
died   survived
79%

52
57   lived
died   **47.7%**
52.3%

Kind Hearts In Action website
February 14, 2011

The more info collected, the better the numbers. But we needed details. Even though he had been keeping me at arm's length, I tried again with the vet in Houston, explaining that a professor at the University of Texas could be interested in compiling data on cases into an academic paper.

I received no reply.

Days later, Dr. Sinem Karsli Parmaksizoglu in Istanbul sent me before/after video of a beagle named Hector treated with the NDV spinal tap.[81] She wrote:

> "Hector was having a happy life, until one day he started crying with pain. He wasn't able to go to sleep or stand still because of the nervous symptoms. At nights he was screaming in pain, and the owner was in shock because he had two distemper shots before.
> He was treated with NDV spinal tap on Feb. 10. Eighteen hours after the spinal tap, he was depressed but you can see that he is looking hopeful, still shaking the legs but much better. On Feb. 16, he was much happier, alert and started putting the front legs on bed. he is again sleeping with his owner in bed. ☺
> With all my best wishes"
> Vet Sinem Karsli Parmaksizoglu
> Istanbul, Turkey
> Feb. 17, 2011

During the next couple of months, more emails went out to the vets who had replied to the survey, asking for specifics on cases this time: "We need details such as dates, with breed of dog, ages, initial symptoms, how diagnosed and treated and what outcomes you found."

In March 2011, Joyce Burton-Titular posted the story of her dog Bailey, who survived after being treated with NDV serum and the NDV spinal tap. Joyce had been crowned Ms. Philippines Universe in 1985, and has been an actress, news presenter and celebrity in the Philippines. Her blog, "Adventures of a Beauty Queen," had more than 3.5 million hits, and the story about Bailey filled up my Inbox with hundreds of comments. To be quite honest, I believe Joyce is a big reason why so many people have written me from the Philippines. Since since began talking about Bailey's story, I've had more than 1,300 people write to me from that country.

The vet in Southern Florida sent me copies of two cases and wrote:

> "I was only able to remember 2 of the dogs. The serum wasn't in our computer as an invoice item initially so there is no other way to search for it. But I can give you the details on the 2 dogs I found.
>
> 1.   Rey from a Rescue- 10 year old miniature poodle. Rescue from Miami, FL shelter- came in with symptoms of URTI (lethargic, not eating, not active, congestion, and sneezing)- treated with serum 4/24/2010 and antibiotics- no diagnostics were done on this patient. Rescue has other confirmed cases of distemper from this shelter around this time. Patient recovered- no other symptoms developed. Patient was unfortunately later euthanized due to aggression.
>
> 2.   Astro from the same rescue- 4 ½ year old miniature poodle- also rescued from Miami- shelter. Came in 5/12 with mucopurulent nasal discharge and respiratory symptoms. Treated with antibiotics and serum. Patient developed GI symptoms lateral 5/19 treated supportively - patient recovered."

Maritza Rodriguez of the Humane Society of Puerto Rico wrote:

"With the serum we treated three pups. On March 2010 we treated: Pi, female, Miniature Pincher Mix, 10-12 weeks, she had fever, nose and eyes secretion, cough. Brownie, litter of 5 when we found they had distemper, 4 of them died before I found Dr. Sears method and try to save Brownie (the fifth). Brownie is a corgi-shar-pei mix, also 10-12 weeks, he had high fever, also nose and eyes secretion, hard pads, he started neurological like chewing gum, but after the serum it stopped. Pi and Brownie were treated NDV (IV) and Serum both recovered.

"January 2011 - Lolita - mix dog, 12 - 14 weeks old when diagnosed. We also proceeded with direct NDV and only a small dose of serum (we only had available 1.5cc). She got neurological in her back legs, she bounces. She had high fever, anorexia, nose/eyes secretion, cough, hard pads and chorea. She also lost most of her teeth and the one left are brownish. We treated her with direct NDV also and serum. She is alive and kicking, fully vaccinated. Just hope she can be adopted!"

As much as I appreciated the additional details, these were but a handful of the potential number of cases. This fell far short of what would qualify for a journal. Obviously, trying to capture information after dogs had been treated would not work. By the time we requested the information, the vets had already moved on to a hundred other cases. These busy vets did not have the time or ability to maintain their records on NDV serum separately. Somehow, we'd have to get ahead of the curve.

Seeing a finish line

Geography remained a problem for me. On one hand, I was lucky to live in a region that did not have a lot of distemper. But I knew I could make progress if there were a lot of cases and a willing vet near Upstate New York. Trying to compile this information remotely and through the efforts of others – as grateful as I was for their help – added to the challenge.

By May 2011, I'd transcribed 35,000 words from phone interviews with Dr. Sears plus another 40,000 words from his Houston lecture. I'd also plunged deep into my research on the history of the disease. I sent him the transcriptions for his review, but I knew this story missed something essential.

When I had been a newspaper reporter, about 80 percent of my day focused on gathering info. Only about 20 percent went to writing. The writing came easily if I had all my facts by the time I sat down at the computer. It worked best if I knew where the story would end. Right now, the story of Dr. Sears ended with a treatment that had not been accepted or proven. I didn't like the ending.

Inspiration on how I might change that came from an unexpected direction.

At a family picnic the previous summer, my niece, Sarah Wigsten, took a photo of a group of us, which caught me from the side. When it was posted on Facebook, I didn't like what I saw. The bathroom scale had been telling me for years how much weight I had gained. I had stopped running after my injury in the L.A. marathon. Mathematically, I knew I'd slowly become obese. But numbers are one thing. Seeing myself how others did was another. The photo showed the weight had all gone straight to my belly. I looked like a tugboat.

"If I'm not giving up on distemper dogs, I'm not going to give up on myself either," I said to myself. My feet and my knees yelled when I resumed jogging that summer. I overcame this pain by wearing drug store joint braces. By the spring, I deemed myself fit enough to run my first 5K in eight years and entered in the Twin Tiers Race for the Cure in Elmira. On a cool, drizzly Sunday morning in May 2011, I joined a sea of pink and white at a starting line a half-block from the Star-Gazette building to support Susan G. Komen for the Cure and their efforts to defeat breast cancer.

The runners were encouraged to wear signs to honor the memory of friends or family who had died from breast cancer. I didn't have anyone who had lost that particular battle, so on my sign I wrote the names: "Ingrid Bergman, Bette Davis, Rosalind Russell, Molly Ivins." My drug-store braces and I survived the 3.1 mile route through Elmira without stopping. But as I approached the finish line and the banner emblazoned with the words "Race for the Cure," an idea hit me.

"All these people," I thought as I crossed the finish line, panting hard. "All this effort for a cause just trying to FIND a cure for a disease. Kind Hearts In Action already HAD a cure [OK, treatment] for its disease. All we had to do was prove it."

Simple, right?

Not so simple, but this clarified everything. If time and data were major obstacles to the goal of "good records of both the positive and negative outcomes," what could be done?

As a writer, this led me to ask a dangerous question:

What would it take to change the ending of this book?

Over the next few days, I mulled this over. On my jogs through my neighborhood, the situation, the interviews, the research I'd been doing on the history of distemper and Newcastle Disease rolled over in my mind. When I ran track in high school, I never learned to run hurdles. Now, many hurdles lay between us and the goal of getting Dr. Sears published. Maybe I could clear some of them. More likely, I'd trip and stumble. I could wipe out and get hurt. Most likely, there'd be hurdles I did not even know about.

And yet, crossing the finish line was all that was needed.

This new project forming in my head needed a focus, a name that summed up the struggle. Finally, as I made the last turn onto my road on the way home, I remembered the Frenchman who identified the cause of distemper even though most of the scientific community did not believe him for years. The words popped into my head:

Project Carré.

Project Carré

About the time Project Carré was forming, I asked Dr. Sears, "What is it like to have distemper?" His answer:

> "Have you ever had the flu? You're dizzy. You sit up and you get dizzy. You've got diarrhea. You're vomiting. You can't eat. You can't drink anything. You've got a fever. You're sweating. You're lying there in bed, just wishing you could die. How does that feel? The difference is the majority of them go on to stop breathing. When you have a real bad case of the flu, you almost wish that would happen. That's basically how I'm sure how those dogs feel."

We talked about how the disease robs them of their sense of smell and taste, their appetite and all the joys of being a dog.

"I'm sure in an acute case they wish they were dead. I'm sure the majority of them go on to die, but that's only because of organ failure. God, it affects every organ of the body practically. They're really sick. ... We're talking about the acute phase where you have fever, diarrhea, vomiting, gunked up nose, pneumonia. Your eyes are all full of mucous. You can't see. Are those dogs comfortable? No they're miserable. They're in severe pain and they don't like what's going on. They're hurting.

Now, if you go to the secondary phase, remember there are several depending on the age of the dog. You can have hardpad, which makes it almost impossible for the dog to walk. Consider somebody shaving off all the skin on the base of your foot and then ask you to walk across the room. You can't do it.

Think about the dog that gets bad teeth, loses all the enamel on their teeth, and then they have secondary problems there. Or the ones that lose their ability to make tears, so they can't even blink. These are all secondary problems that occur to the acute phase of the disease. Then you have the neurologic problem, which occurs, and it can occur within two weeks or it can occur within eight years after the infection. Now, that's a different ball game. Is there pain involved with that? That's a good question. I think some of those dogs look like they have headaches. Some of them don't. And how do you know a dog has a headache? If you look at a person with a headache, they have that look on their face with their eyes squinched down and they're kind of depressed. They're not looking at the world around them. They're just kind of squeezing in. Dogs do the same thing. If you've ever watched one of your children with a real bad headache, your dog looks exactly the same when it's got a bad headache. It's a matter of just observing. That's all."

I asked whether dogs feel anything during a seizure. "No, they're unconscious. Totally unconscious," he said. But I have heard from some owners who describe their dog as screaming or crying, something my distemper dogs did not do.

"I'm not sure whether that's pain or not," he said. "I can't answer that because I've never had a seizure, so I don't know. And you can't ask the dog because that's not possible. You'd have to ask somebody that's had a seizure whether there is pain associated with it. And I have not had the occasion to ask anybody that's had seizures that question." (In my non-expert opinion, there is probably something else going on, twisting and contraction of muscles, nerves and bone to cause pain like that. But again, a veterinary professional could explain it better.)

The ultimate value of Project Carrè came down to learning all the impracticalities of a non-scientist seeking to get published in a scientific journal. Just as there is a blood-brain barrier in the body, there is a scientist/non-scientist barrier. I am a molecule on the wrong side of the barrier and cannot cross to the other side. At least I would now understand these limits. But I have an adage I follow in my new pursuit as an inventor: You don't know whether something will work or not until you try.

So, I tried.

For me, the suffering of distemper dogs and their owners made the attempt worth it. Dr. Nancy Kay, a veterinarian and author, once estimated it could take no more than 4 minutes and 23 seconds to fall in love with a puppy.[82] "And four minutes and 22 seconds just isn't enough time to make sure all the necessary medical checkups have been performed – or if they have, to study the results!" she writes.

Since it can take up to two weeks for a dog exposed to distemper to show symptoms, that adds up to plenty of time to make a new dog a full-fledged member of the family. And a lot of grief as that family watches their new friend suffer and die.

Dr. Sears had come to accept the difficulties of getting other vets to accept that dogs do not have to die from distemper.

"You know what? I'm going to be long gone by the time that this is accepted by my profession," he said with a laugh. "I don't expect it to be accepted within the next 10 years, OK? I've been playing with this for 50 years, and I still can't get them interested. It boggles my mind."

When the first posting about Project Carré went up on the Kind Hearts In Action website in mid-June 2011, I sent the link to Dr. Sears. It laid out a plan to raise funds, make the NDV serum, collect lab reports to confirm diagnosis and document outcomes.

At this point, the project had no funding and no participating vet. The fundraising goal had been set at $5,000, a rough number I'd calculated from collecting examples of veterinary bills from dog owners around the country. That seemed a reasonable budget to ensure one vet could treat and document a small group of dogs.

"Very good start," replied Dr. Sears. "You are now where I was 35 years ago. How to get the profession to pay attention? The best way would be to set up a full test at a university … I wish you the very best in your efforts. Mine have been exhausted. Doc."

Agreed. A university study would be ideal. Even as the project began, I hoped that some university professor would take on this task instead, but since that didn't seem to be happening, I fell back on that motto made famous by Teddy Roosevelt: "Do what you can, with what you have, where you are."

The vet clinic would make the serum and treat the animals, and I'd collect the case files and lab reports and compile the article. Since the files need to be collected before they got swept back into the standard filing system for the office, I'd need to do this in person. However, since the vets using NDV at this time were in Florida, Texas and California, I didn't know how I could pay for so many airline flights.

After all, I still was not gainfully employed. Since leaving Ithaca College, I'd been writing, but not getting paid. I hadn't found my new direction. The canine distemper cause was never meant to be my career. My purpose was merely to put this information into the hands of the scientists and veterinarians in a format that might be accepted. Once safely in their hands, I planned to walk away. My needs for a career and professional fulfillment would come from elsewhere.

I studied submission guidelines and requirements for veterinary journals, read books about writing scientific papers and about other non-scientists who worked their way into the world of science. I wrote to book authors and others I'd known in the world of science who might have advice. I reconnected with Dr. Kim Hee-Young, who had returned to Korea to accept a professorship there, and then made contact with my cousin, Dr. Kathleen Triman, a biology professor at Franklin and Marshall.

I saw no direct stipulation forbidding a non-scientist from writing a journal article. But I also reasoned I would most likely encounter unexpected obstacles and make amateurish mistakes. In "The Cure" by Geeta Anand about the efforts of John Crowley to save his children from Pompe disease, I'd read how Crowley made such mistakes when he threw himself into the pharmaceutical industry in a bid to save their lives. In 1998, two of Crowley's children, Megan and Patrick, had been diagnosed with this severe neuromuscular disorder. A Harvard MBA, Crowley established a foundation and used his skills as a businessman to co-found a biotech company to find a cure. A chapter about his ill-advised involvement in an actual laboratory experiment burned into my mind.

Under tremendous pressure to show "proof of concept," Crowley brushed off the objections of his chief scientific officer and persuaded an undertrained employee to inject an experimental enzyme into laboratory mice. When they presented the data to their investing partner, the experts in the room tore them apart. For a while, Crowley's company came off looking like a fraud. A costly lesson, but one he learned from.

Another adage I learned years ago: "A smart man learns from his own mistakes. A wise man learns from the mistakes of others." What could I learn from Crowley's story? Even though the lives of his children were saved, Crowley's strengths lay in business, not science. Mine are in journalism.

Since we had different skills, got involved in a different profession which had different ways of operating and confronted a different disease, I expected to have different obstacles and dilemmas from Crowley. I couldn't know how to avoid these until they happened. There may be no rule in the book that says a dog can't play baseball, but that doesn't mean it's a good idea.

My sister Jane became a key adviser on setting up the fundraising for Project Carré. My best friend, Jeff Schnaufer, helped search for grants. At the end of July, we joined Microgiving, a crowd-funding website which helps people and groups meet financial goals by seeking lots of small donations. In August, we applied for a $5,000 grant from the ASPCA.

At the end of August, the Microgiving campaign launched with the headline "$5 will change the world for dogs." If a thousand people donated just $5 each, we'd reach the goal.

Building the project

Jane surprised me by posting a matching grant for any donations made in September from Eco Dog Care of Los Angeles, a dog-washing and doggy-day care business she and Karen had opened on Pico Boulevard. Even though Jane still lived in New Jersey, they'd started the business as cross-country partners.

The next day, the ASPCA responded with a form letter rejection on the grant application.

"Oh well," I wrote to Jane. "The faster you get through the 'No's', the faster you get to the 'Yes.' Other opportunities still on the horizon."

"Exactly," she replied. "In the end, hope is a choice."

By the end of September, we'd raised about $1,200 from Microgiving and from other donations that came in through Paypal, Google, Facebook and Network for Good. The Eco Dog match doubled these donations, which were typically $25 or so. But the grants search kept hitting a brick wall. The foundations willing to fund veterinary research insisted on only going through programs at universities. For others, the requirements were too difficult to meet because of the size of Kind Hearts In Action. After all, our entire organization consisted of Jane, Karen, myself and a handful of board members/volunteers. And Jane and Karen had to focus on their business. We weren't equipped to jump through a lot of bureaucratic hoops.

As I searched for traction on this new project, another venture had begun in a small town in the Blue Ridge Mountains of Virginia. The Mountain View Veterinary Clinic in Woodlawn had opened in October and was quickly overwhelmed with a distemper outbreak.

Dr. Amber Melton grew up on a small horse farm in nearby Hillsville. Her family had lived in Carroll County and this part of Virginia for at least a century. "When I was in kindergarten, you dress up as what you want to be, and I dressed up as a vet," she said. "I just knew. Always."

The horse farm inspired her interest in animals – cats as a close second to horses. Her parents, Kenny and Jane, helped Amber pursue her undergraduate education at Virginia Tech and at the Virginia-Maryland Veterinary School of Medicine, where she received her DVM in 2006.

"Well, I'm an only child too, and I'm really close to my parents," she said. "They've always been good to me. They paid my way through vet school, through undergrad. They've done everything for me. I can never repay them."

When the time came to set up her own veterinary practice, it was her parents and her husband Andy who made it happen. Kenny had found the building, which had once been a carpet and flooring business. It took only six weeks to convert the one-story building into a veterinary practice, adding the walls needed for exam rooms, surgery, kennels and a stall for larger animals. The floor plan included a room with access to the outside from the back of the building that could be used to isolate contagious cases.

Not long after opening, Mountain View got a call from a volunteer named Laurie who had been rescuing puppies from a local animal shelter for transport each month to a New York City area rescue group. She had at least a couple dozen puppies in a barn owned by another vet clinic, and they were being attacked by distemper.

"She could not find anybody to help her," said Samantha Jennings, the receptionist and veterinary assistant at Mountain View. "All the dogs were dying."

Samantha and Laurie searched the Internet for a solution and found the Kind Hearts In Action website.

"I actually found your website, right about the same time that she found it," Samantha told me later. "And we both called each other and said, 'Hey, guess what?' "

On Oct. 5, this email landed in my inbox:

"I am writing you from Mountain View Veterinary Clinic in Woodlawn Virginia. We have had a recent outbreak of distemper and are experiencing nearly 100% fatality rate. This is very disheartening and Dr. Amber Melton and the rest of us in the office are very interested in trying your serum. We have a couple of dogs that we can utilize in vaccinating and collecting the serum. We would like some more information or any advice you may be able to lend to help us. The death toll in the area is quickly climbing and our local animal shelter is closed temporarily until the problem is under control. I really appreciate your time and any information you can give us! Thank You, Samantha"

I responded with links to the protocols on the website, contact info for other vets and mailed them a copy of Dr. Sears' DVD. Dr. Melton and the staff called the vet clinics in Texas using NDV and were told what to expect.

"We were kinda desperate a little bit," Dr. Melton told me later. "We felt, Why not? Let's just try it. Most of the other vets around here wouldn't try it. Why not? They're gonna die. So, we're gonna try."

Without the time to make NDV serum, the clinic opted for the IV injections. Laurie ordered the NDV from a supplier. About 16 puppies died before they could be brought in for treatment, but on Tuesday, October 11, Laurie drove seven 16- to 17-week old puppies to the back door of the isolation room at Mountain View. The pups were mixed breed boxers, shepherds and Australian shepherds.

When Jen Roberts, the veterinary technician, injected the first one with Newcastle Disease Vaccine, the puppy collapsed.

"You are doing a protocol that's not nationally recognized," Jen said. "And you think you've just killed an animal because you've done something wrong. Then, it is very scary."

Frightened for the puppy, Samantha ran for the phone.

"I called the people in Texas and I'm like, 'This just happened,' " Samantha said. "And they're like, 'It's OK. Just slow it down.' "

The collapse lasted only seconds. As quickly as it had dropped, the pup was awake and up again. It had a reaction to the IV injection of NDV, something the vets in Texas encountered and had realized could be avoided by giving the injection slowly over the course of a few minutes.

The solution Mountain View decided on was to give each pup a sub-cutaneous injection of Benadryl. This stopped the reactions. All seven puppies in that first group improved by the next morning.

"Pretty cool," said Dr. Melton. However, one of those first seven did die of a respiratory infection a few weeks later.

"Distemper was a death sentence until this to me because I had seen these other little puppies suffer," Dr. Melton said. "They suffer very badly, and die. Your hands are pretty much tied. You see them come in, and you give them this vaccine and then the next day they're kinda like, 'Ok, I'm fine.' They're not 100 percent, but they look a lot better the next day. They eat and drink and everything. Even a couple of them were really, really bad and we gave them this vaccine. The next day they're eating."

The clinic still had their work cut out for them. Another 19 puppies and dogs came in over the next month from the Wythe County Humane Society.

"Jen, Samantha and I, we were all here till 10 or 11 at night sometimes," Dr. Melton said. "Treating these dogs. And they were pitiful. Some of them were really pitiful."

They didn't have enough cages in the isolation room for the dogs. Many just stayed in the crates they were delivered in.

"We kinda got hit fast," Dr. Melton said. "We had kennels everywhere. The poor distemper dogs were packed on top of each other because there were so many of them. We didn't really have enough room for them all coming here because they were all sick."

She gives much of the credit to Jen and Samantha. The dogs not only needed the NDV injections, but also the antibiotics, fluids and other supportive care for distemper dogs. "They're life savers," Dr. Melton said. "I couldn't do it without them because when you see how busy we are out here, they're fabulous."

They estimated they treated as many as 45 distemper dogs with the NDV injection in the next couple of months. Only five had died. Usually, the sick puppies were in the clinic for only a day or two before they recovered and could leave. The isolation room had a constant rotation of distemper dogs being treated, recovered and replaced.

"At one time, I think there were 13 or 15 dogs back there," Jen said. "We're not set up for that many. We had them all in crates. They just left them in their crates, but they were bringing them in by the van loads. As soon as these guys showed any symptoms, which usually was the sneeze or the runny nose, bring them in to get the NDV vaccine."

Seeing so many cases survive with just one addition to the accepted treatment made a compelling argument for Jen.

"It was amazing," Jen said. "We were like, 'Oh man, this is really gonna work.' We saw a lot of dogs. [Before] we had to sit and watch a lot of dogs on IV fluids and getting antibiotics die because we didn't know what else to do. Then whenever you see those and the only thing you change – always getting the same fluids, they had the same catheters, they had the same antibiotics – and the only thing you change was that vaccine and the next day they're almost 100 percent normal. It's amazing. Absolutely amazing."

Answering a question posed in Houston

Meanwhile on another front, something unusual had happened in another part of the world. I'd been waiting for a couple months to hear from Chantel van Rensburg from Sasolburg, South Africa. She had first written me at the beginning of September about her pit-bull puppy, Tjoppie, and I had been wondering whether he had survived.

When she first wrote me, he was 11 weeks old. He'd begun having kennel-cough symptoms at the end of July and later began twitching all over. The vets in Johannesburg diagnosed distemper. "That's when I was told that there is no cure or treatment," she said. "I couldn't leave it at that and couldn't believe that death is going to be my puppy's fate."

South Africa had been especially resistant to alternative treatments to distemper. Almost without exception, owners there would tell me the vets would not even consider the NDV protocols. However, in 2010, a vet in Darling on the west coast of South Africa had made the NDV serum.
Since Tjoppie had already reached the neurologic stage, it seemed too late to try the NDV serum. I sent Chantel the information on the protocols and contact information I had. Somehow a miscommunication happened, and the vet in Darling sent the NDV serum – not the straight vaccine – to a veterinary neurosurgeon in Bryanston, a suburb of Johannesburg, to use in a spinal tap. I learned this after the fact.

At the beginning of December, Chantel sent me an update:

"Today my pup is 6 months old and doing VERY WELL!!!!! 3 Days after the spinal tap he was a completely different puppy! His energy levels rose, his appetite grew, running around, being naughty and playful like a healthy puppy should be. Although he still has the twitching, but that is also improving as he is going for hydro therapy twice a week and he also gets a supplement called Muscle Dog to help build his muscle strength. His overall health is very good and haven't had any more problems thus far, he is improving every day, I can honestly say that he or any of the symptoms of distemper HAS NOT worsened at all!!!

She sent me before/after photos and video of Tjoppie, showing him wheezing and crying before the treatment and then up and playing five days later. She also sent a video of his hydrotherapy, in which he regained his strength by swimming in a pool while supported with a harness attached to a line overhead.[83]

So, by accident, a vet in South Africa had stumbled into possibly answering a question Dr. Sears had asked a couple of years earlier: Could the NDV serum be used in a spinal tap? They had just substituted one material for the other. No need for a catheter with continuous injections as Dr. Sears had thought. This variation in the protocol was something I would let other vets know about when the opportunity arose, and it was something I would hear second hand that others had tried. But since we had not yet demonstrated the effectiveness of either the serum in pre-neurologic cases or the straight vaccine in the NDV spinal tap, this didn't go out into the world as its own protocol.

Moving forward

As Mountain View kept writing to me about the distemper cases they were treating, I realized this could be the opportunity I needed. A nine-hour drive connects Horseheads to Woodlawn, Virginia, just straight down from Corning, via Route 15 to Interstate 81. For once, I was near to enough distemper cases to make a difference. On Dec. 19, I asked Samatha to see whether Dr. Melton would like to participate in Project Carré, which would mean they would make the actual NDV serum and let me document the outcomes.

Dr. Melton called me the next day, excited to join the project. They were going to look for the right kind of dog to use as a blood serum donor. As Amy and I work, we usually kept a window in iMessenger from AOL open to each other on our computers. I immediately shared the news.

"Hey, I got a call back from the vet in Virginia," I wrote. "We are moving forward on Project Carré! …They are so excited, and they were so grateful to find the treatment. They were overwhelmed with distemper dogs dying on them, and then they finally found this treatment.

Their serum donor dog walked in the door the next day.

"We have dogs that come in needing homes from time to time," Jen told me. When possible, Dr. Melton adopts these dogs herself. This time it was an unspayed 45-pound, 2-year-old dog named Jett.

"And as soon as she came in, we had just got off the phone with you, like the day before," Jen said. "So, we did a blood panel. We dewormed her. We did a fecal. We did a 4Dx test for Lyme and a heartworm disease and stuff like that to make sure everything was negative. Everything looked good. We dewormed her anyway even though we didn't see anything in the fecal."

To make sure the dog of the dog's health, they waited a few weeks before making the serum.

By the end of the year, we'd raised about $3,000 for the project. Another $220 had come from my in-laws, unexpectedly. At a Christmas party, the adults of the Clark family hold a $5 gift exchange. No present can be above that value, but the limit inspires a lot of creativity. Each family member donates $20 for charity to participate and blindly chooses a package, which could contain something funny, useful, completely useless or poignant. Or you could steal an already opened present from someone else, forcing that person to choose a new present. One of the packages contained an angel ornament, and whoever ended up with the angel got to choose which charity the pool of money went to. That Christmas, my niece Shannon Williams got the ornament and she picked Save Dogs From Distemper.

We were short of the $5,000 goal, but it was enough to get started. In my mind, I had earmarked some of our personal savings for the project if needed. But Project Carré had become a reality.

In January 2012, I updated the stats on cases treated for the website:

REPORTS FROM VETS

19 veterinarians treat
519 dogs with NDV

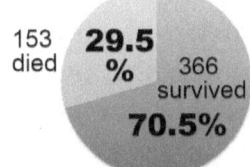

153
died   **29.5
%**   366
survived
70.5%

| 225 dogs treated with NDV serum | 157 dogs treated with NDV as IV | 137 treated with NDV spinal taps |

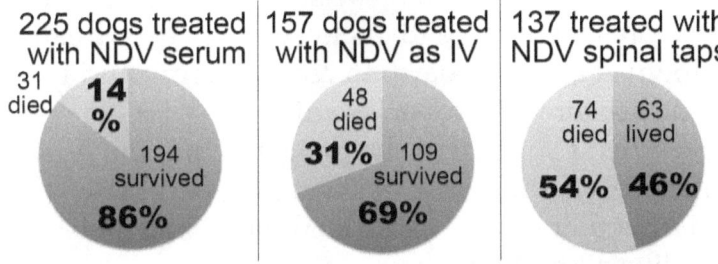

31
died   **14
%**
194
survived
86%

48
died
31%   109
survived
69%

74   63
died   lived
54%   46%

Kind Hearts In Action website
January 11, 2012

REPORTS FROM
DOG OWNERS/CAREGIVERS

724 dogs
467 treated   with distemper   257 not treated
with NDV   with NDV

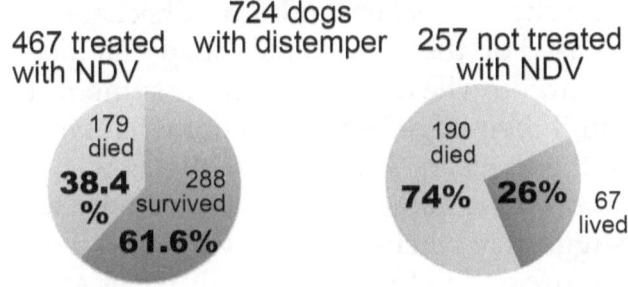

179
died
**38.4
%**   288
survived
61.6%

190
died
74%   26%   67
lived

| 195 dogs treated with NDV serum | 100 dogs treated with NDV as IV | 172 treated with NDV spinal taps |

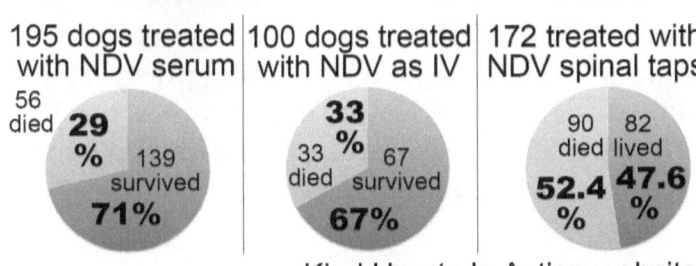

56
died   **29
%**   139
survived
71%

**33
%**
33   67
died   survived
67%

90   82
died   lived
**52.4
%**   **47.6
%**

Kind Hearts In Action website
January 11, 2012

2012 brought many surprises, some good but many unpleasant. The weather stayed mild through January, which allowed me to keep up my jogging. The foot braces still worked and the pounds had started coming off. Then about 15 minutes into one jog in mid-January, a sharp pain snapped across my left foot. The pain and location matched the injury inflicted by the L.A. Marathon back in 2000. I knew this would require surgery, but I put off going to the doctor for as long as I could. The foot pain would plague me all year.

A week after this came another twist in my life, a good one. The universe presented me with a new calling. In a dream, Amy and I sat down at checkerboard. In real life, Amy and I had never played checkers. However, we did play a lot of backgammon. So when I suggested she make the first move, she just looked at me oddly, as if to say, "I don't play checkers." Then she picked up a pair of dice and rolled them. She then moved a checker like a knight in chess.

"Very funny," I said. "But that's not how you play checkers."

But in a flash, I realized it could be. In the next moment, I realized I was dreaming and that I had invented a completely new game combining chess, checkers and dice. Checkers could make chess moves based on the roll of a pair of special dice. One die was a standard d6. The other die had the symbols for the 6 chess pieces. Roll them together to find out what kind of move to make with the checkers. I woke up with a new purpose. When I showed the game to my son, Jack, who was then 12, he made suggestions including a way for the king checker – whose capture ended the game – to flip over and go into hiding. We called that "stealth mode." The boys and I played the game all day, and I realized something pretty cool: "This is fun!" Game design would lead to a new career, but I kept my invention to myself at least until a provisional patent could be filed. That would take months.

A couple of days later, the Star-Gazette published a small story about Project Carré with the headline "Vet has distemper cure, area man believes." The story by my former colleague Jeff Murray included an old photo of me with Galen and Shadow. When the story ran in the Star-Gazette's sister paper, The Ithaca Journal, it prompted this letter to the editor from a vet student at Cornell University:

> "I was shocked by a glaring omission in the article about the dog supposedly 'cured' of canine distemper.
> An extremely effective vaccine has been available for this disease for about 60 years, and it is routinely administered to nearly every dog in the world who receives regular veterinary care -- or even sporadic veterinary care.
> The reason that distemper is rare in this part of the country is because the rate of vaccination is very high. Strangely, this basic preventative measure was not mentioned at all in the article.
> A roughly $15 shot at adoption could have saved each of this man's dogs, and it is a disservice to the public for the Ithaca Journal to fail to disclose this critical fact.
> Heather B.
> Cornell University
> College of Veterinary Medicine
> Class of 2012"[84]

Of course, Jeff's story didn't have the space to explain my puppies had been rescued from the streets after they had already been exposed to distemper. So, he wasn't able to get into the subtleties. Throughout the Save Dogs From Distemper campaign, we had emphasized the importance of vaccination. Better that a dog not get sick in the first place. But then, what do you do after they get sick? Just watch them die? We needed to prove the alternative to euthanasia. I needed to get down to Virginia, but I also had to find a schedule opening in my most important job: being a Dad.

As I had gotten deeper into this cause, I recognized the danger of becoming obsessed. Answering emails from all over the world, updating the websites, editing videos and posting to social media tended to suck me into the computer for hours at a time. Amy once had to call me to dinner table repeatedly as I messaged with someone from Honduras. This threatened to undermine the two key pieces of advice I'd heard when I became a dad for the first time: "Be there" and "Have duct tape" [because stuff breaks!].

So, I made sure canine distemper took a back seat to other priorities in my life: getting the boys to soccer practice or baseball games, Boy Scout trips and Cub Scout meetings and attending school concerts and plays. The emails still came in at all hours of the day and night, but I had to accept that they could not all be answered right away. Along with finding a new profession, I needed to sleep, eat, help maintain a house and be a dad and husband. Some replies would take longer than others, but after all, I was only one person and a volunteer at that.

A week after going to winter camp with Liam and his Cub Scout Pack in February 2012, I drove down to Woodlawn, Virginia. As I pulled off Interstate 81 after a 10-hour drive, the scene struck me as familiar – Horseheads, but in a different scale. Woodlawn was about a third the size of Horseheads, but instead of surrounding hills, they had mountains. The town sat deep in the Blue Ridge Mountains, part of the Appalachians. The foothills of the Appalachians stretch to my part of the Finger Lakes Region of Upstate New York, where the green hills don't get much higher than 1700 feet. The Blue Ridge Mountains top 6,000 feet.

After a night at a motel, I drove up to the Mountain View Vet Clinic on Industry Lane, which sat among a collection of commercial buildings including a dog spa.

Until now, I had not usually gone much farther into a vet clinic than the exam room. This trip gave me a look behind-the-scenes and all the people coming and going. Dr. Melton would explain that only about six were actual staff. The rest were volunteers who observe and sometimes help with the kennels. Morning appointments flowed straight into afternoon surgeries with no break for lunch. Friends from the local community often brought in food for the clinic, and they worked as they ate. When Dr. Melton finished with her duties at the clinic, she'd then go off on farm calls into the afternoon and evening.

In mid-afternoon, I got the chance to talk to Jen for a few minutes about how it went when they made the NDV serum with Jett, who had by now been adopted by a new owner and renamed Bella. They'd followed Dr. Sears' protocol line-by-line, she said. I asked if shock from blood loss was a problem.

"No, I watched her tongue," Jen said. "Once it started to fade to a paler pink, we quit. She was a young dog. She had already been a blood donor before. I think we got about 100 mls of blood out of her. So, once she started to fade in color, we stopped on how much blood we were pulling."

The 100 mls of whole blood spun down to create 20 or 30 mls of serum, which they stored in red-topped tubes in the refrigerator.

"She recovered fine," she said. "There were no issues. She actually went to her new home afterwards."

Samantha gave me the copies of the files on 29 of the distemper dogs treated with the intravenous injection of NDV in October and November. In the files, only four had been listed as having died after the NDV treatment. (One puppy died weeks later of a respiratory infection.) Another vet in the clinic talked to me about three other dogs they'd treated with NDV as IV that had been brought in by a private owner a couple of months before my visit. Two of the three were still alive.

"So, what do you think?" I asked. "Do you think we're onto something here?"

"It seems promising to me," she said. "With these three dogs in particular. None of them had been vaccinated in years. We know that one died from distemper. The other two obviously were exposed. They all stayed together. We don't have cause or diagnosis on either of the two that survived at this point. But I still think … I agree with the owner. We would have lost all three if we hadn't done something. My opinion is with a disease like distemper if they're going to die anyway and there is something we can try to do to help them, then we should try."

"But a lot of vets don't have this attitude," I said.

"I was gonna say, some people don't agree with that," she said. "And quite honestly, I don't understand. I don't understand not at least trying."

At her vet school, they didn't talk a lot about distemper. It was not considered a problem. "They basically said it'd been eliminated with vaccination," she said. "Well, it's not."

That reminded me of a story from my future brother-in-law, Alan, I told her. He'd recently been on a flight, sitting next to a veterinary professor from Colorado. "He was trying to tell him about what I was working on," I said. "His reaction was, 'Distemper? I didn't know that was still a problem.' "

Something occurred to me that had been lurking in the back of my brain.

"Check me on something here," I said. "When a dog dies of distemper, you don't report it to anybody."

"No."

"So, nobody is keeping track of the stats."

"It's not a reportable disease," she said. "It's not reportable, and when you think about which animals are most likely to be the problem to come in contact with it, to show signs, to die from it, most of the time it most likely is the shelter animals, the strays, the ones that a lot of times people don't have the resources to put towards testing. So, how much of it is going undiagnosed for years is part of the question that is in my mind too."

Dr. Melton explained distemper is not a reportable disease because it does not infect humans and the animals that suffer from distemper are not in the food chain for humans. "I think it's a bigger problem than anybody realizes," she said.

But making it a reportable disease would be difficult.

"I think it would be fabulous if there was some kind of way to report it," she said. "Because it would be nice to realize where it is hitting in these little outbreaks we are having. But trying to get them to report it would be hard. Because, like you said, people don't care because it doesn't affect humans."

I brought up the letter to the editor from the vet student chastising me for not getting my dogs vaccinated.

"That's the vet student attitude too," Dr. Melton said. "They're kind of in ivory towers."

They had not yet been out in the real world, treating cases.

"In a perfect world, everybody would vaccinate their dogs against distemper, and nobody would ever see the disease, but you get out here and people aren't going to do that. People don't vaccinate every single animal in the world," she said. "And vaccines are not 100 percent. No vaccine is 100 percent."

The letter had been bothering me, though. I told her it felt like "because I have a dog with distemper I must be a bad owner."

She shook her head.

"No? Ok. I'm taking it too seriously then."

"I don't think they have seen enough real life things to know," she said.

We talked about off-label treatments. Dr. Melton explained how off-label uses are common in veterinary clinics, especially with cattle and horses.

"As long as you have a patient-client relationship, you can do that," she said. "We use things off-label a lot in the veterinary world. It should not be a problem."

I spent a couple of days at Mountain View, and each was hectic for the clinic. Mostly, I observed, asked questions, relayed their questions via email to Dr. Sears and Chuck Whitt and made sure they had all the materials they needed. Hopefully, I did not get in their way too badly.

Having collected the records and notes and seeing that they had the serum at the ready, I got on the road for Horseheads, with plans to return in a couple of months or so.

On March 4, Brittany R. of Lexington, Kentucky, emailed:

> "... I am in need of help for my dog Abbey. We adopted 2 10 week old pups 11 days ago and they both became very ill within 24 hours. We took them to the animal hospital in Lexington Ky. They tested positive for parvo and both were hospitalized. In addition to parvo symptoms, both developed pneumonia. After several days, one pup died after a grand mal seizure. Two of their other litter mates were taken to another vet and died. Autopsies confirmed BOTH parvo and distemper. We have one pup left who is completely recovered from parvo (her cbcs white blood cell counts are normal and no more vomiting, diarrhea, etc.). She was just about to be released from the hospital when the neurological signs appeared- at first just mild chewing gum fits. They subsided for 2 days with phenobarbital but are back now for the past 36hrs becoming more frequent.

> "There hasn't been any grand mal type convulsions but she is generally disoriented and uncoordinated, facial and head seizures. They have stopped the phenobarbital and given her muscle relaxers. We want to try this procedure. Where can I get the Newcastle Vaccine and if these vets won't do the spinal tap procedure, then do you know the closest vet that will?"

When we started the project, I explained to Mountain View that Kind Hearts In Action would not be paying for any NDV spinal taps. That was because I needed to focus the effort on treating dogs in the pre-neurologic stage with the NDV serum. We could treat and document more dogs that way. If we paid for spinal taps, too, that would wipe out our budget quickly on a procedure that at best had only a 50-50 chance of success. However, Dr. Melton was still willing to perform the spinal taps if the owners were willing to pay.

So, I sent Brittany the contact info for Mountain View. But Abbey died that next morning after suffering from unbearable seizures. It seemed the end of another sad story. "OK, I am so sorry," I wrote. "That's such a tough thing to go through. I lost two pups to this disease years ago, so I've been there."

But the next day, Brittany sent an email about Pax, another puppy from the same litter co-owned with her partner Mary B.[85] "I just wanted to tell you that we are taking the last puppy from the litter to the vet in Virginia. She is not showing neurological signs, just a cough and runny nose. She will start treatment tomorrow. I will keep u posted. Thank you."

On the way down, Brittany noticed the puppy's face twitched as she slept. "Not sure if she was dreaming or if it's the first neuro signs," she wrote to me later. But the staff at Mountain View did not see the neurologic symptoms. In my humble opinion, I don't think you can diagnose a dog with neurological problems until you also see what happens when the dog is awake and unable to stop the movement.

As part of Project Carré, Kind Hearts In Action gave Mountain View a small digital video camera to help document the cases. Jen Roberts held up the puppy to the camera on March 6:

"This is Pax, presented to us for distemper," she says. The camera zooms in to show her crusty nose. She holds up her right paw. "There's her paw pads because they've got a little bit of stuff on those too."

She pats Pax reassuringly severely times and places her in a cage. Pax takes a couple of bites from a bowl of wet dog food. In the notes for Pax's case file, she is described as having "nasal and ocular discharge, hardened paw pads."

On March 9, the staff picked up the video camera again. Pax stood on top of her cage while being comforted by Samatha. Dr. Melton stroked under the puppy's snout and petted her back as she discussed the case [But accidentally refers to her as male]:

"This is Pax, a 12-week old cocker spaniel-mix puppy. Four of his littermates have died of distemper... This dog came from Lexington, Kentucky, for the NDV treatment." According to the case file, Pax received 2.5 ml of NDV serum at 9 p.m. March 6, then again at 9 a.m. and 9 p.m. March 7. At the 9 p.m. injection, the notes read "Very BAR," which stands for "Bright and Alert."

Dr. Melton continues in the video: "This is the condition now. I think he has improved some. He does still have pneumonia ..."

At this, Pax coughs a few times.

"... as you can see from the cough. He is eating and drinking well. And he is going home today. He's going home on Orbax, amoxicillin and cough tabs as well. He's going back to Lexington, Kentucky."

Pax continues to cough as Samatha picks her up. They hold up her paw pads. "Which I feel have improved," Samatha says.

"The paw pads are soft now," says Dr. Melton. "He's still crusty around the nose, but there is minimal discharge from the eyes. Ocular discharge and nasal discharge are minimal. He has not had any seizures, or focal or the fly-biting seizures. Neither of those."

The clinic had sent a sample for PCR testing to Abaxis Veterinary Reference Laboratories at Kansas State University. The lab would confirm Pax had distemper in a report dated March 14.

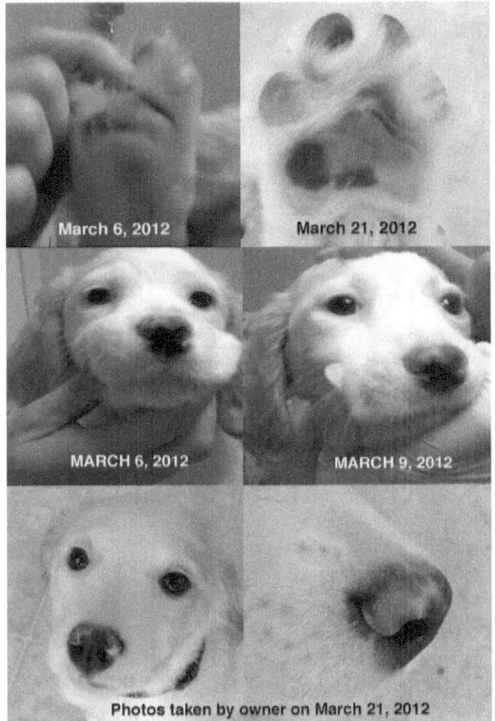

March 6, 2012

March 21, 2012

MARCH 6, 2012

MARCH 9, 2012

Photos taken by owner on March 21, 2012

Meanwhile, Brittany kept me up to date on her recovery and sent more photos and a video on March 21 in which Pax playfully chews, chases and wrestles with her toys on the living room floor. She grrrs happily as she bounces.

"She has been to the local vet a couple times and her pneumonia is getting better," Brittany wrote when she sent the photos and video. "She still coughs some but is otherwise very active and playful and a bit destructive (HAHA)- just like a puppy her age should be. She is now 14 weeks old and has gained weight and grown quite a bit since we got her."

Life gets in the way of a return trip

At the end of May, Amy's sister Beth fell ill. Then, after a weekend golfing with his son Bill and grandsons, Amy's dad Howie came down with pneumonia.

This double crisis stressed the whole family. In the hospital, Howie's pneumonia led to one problem after the other and he died on June 19. In the meantime, J.D. Ward had sent me an email on June 1 that Bruce Parker, who had helped with the DVD filming in Houston, died of cancer at age 37. "Mother and father were holding his hands when he took last breath," she wrote.

All this happened just as I cleared a major hurdle in getting the patent on my game. Over the next month, I had to focus on working with the lawyers on the application for the full patent.

On June 15, Brittany sent me a new photo of Pax, (see below) at 7 months. "She is in perfect health, she was spayed last month and even has a new playmate. She's a great dog! Thanks again. :-) oh, and her nose is completely normal now."

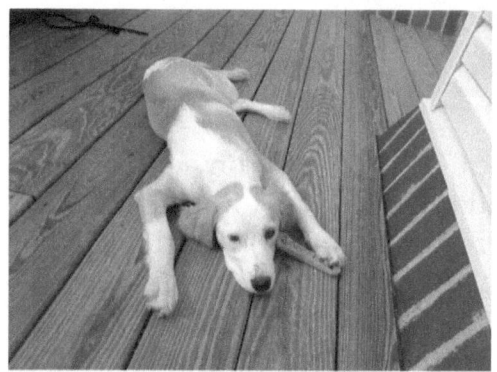

I forwarded the photo to Mountain View, but I would not get back down to Woodlawn until the end of July. When I did, I came back with a handful of records of dogs treated with NDV serum, diagnosed with distemper via lab tests. Six dogs were treated with NDV serum, 4 lived and 2 died. They also gave me the records on three dogs treated with the NDV spinal tap. One lived, one died and in one case the outcome was unknown. Only one of those cases was confirmed by lab test. I also received records of three additional NDV as IV cases, one died and two survived.

The plan had been to return to Woodlawn later on to collect more cases. But a series of events prevented that.

The patent on the game was filed on July 25, with Jack listed as co-inventor. With that obstacle cleared, I needed to move forward on my business. Project Carré was important to me, but this game was a chance to bring income into the family and to pursue an original idea that I loved. I hired a computer coder to work with me to develop an app for iOS systems so that people could download and play the game on iPhones or iPads. The computer coder, Harold Serrano, and I had decided we'd aim to be finished within a month. That seemed like a reasonable amount of time to put Project Carré on the back burner.

But a month proved to be way too optimistic a projection. The game needed a name, a logo and artwork. We found a logo by running an online competition among artists, and then I did the rest of the art myself. So, I had to teach myself more skills in Photoshop and Illustrator. Each version of the program had to be tested over and over, trying to ensure each variation of the game worked. Then, with each version, the game had to be tested on every iOS platform – iPhone, iPad and iPod. Each version, each platform, each option on the game could have their own unique bugs. Jack and I play tested constantly. Harold stayed cool through all of this and just kept working as one month stretched into two, stretched into three.

Finally, in mid-October, Stealth Checkers launched for iOS devices.[86] But getting the game up on the Apple store was not enough. I had to promote it if it was to get noticed among the million other apps available.

Still, the files of distemper cases waited next to my desk. How do I turn this into some sort of scientific article? This was not my kind of writing. The task stumped me.

As I pondered the records, a storm system formed south of Jamaica. It became Superstorm Sandy.

By coincidence, my sister Jane and her fiancé Alan, had planned a vacation to the Caribbean at the end of October, and she asked me to spend that weekend with our mom. Mom lived alone in the house we grew up in two blocks from the beach on the Jersey Shore. She was 85 years old and semi-independent. Jane would visit weekly to check on her and the elderly all-white husky-mix dog, Katie, who had once been hers.

Saturday night, Oct. 27, I answered an automated phone call at Mom's house. In a recording, an official of the Borough of Avon-by-the-Sea informed us they could not guarantee the safety of any resident who remained in town on Monday, when the storm was expected to make landfall. The next day, I took Mom to church, then to breakfast at a local Greek restaurant. Then we packed up my car and evacuated with Katie to Jane and Alan's home in Flemington.

My childhood had been punctuated with hurricanes and major storms, which would sweep in over the beaches and snap the boardwalks like bed sheets. But they always lost impact once they moved inland. Surely, we would be fine in Flemington, more than 70 miles away in the woods of western New Jersey.

Their three-story house sits up a hill at the end of a cul de sac surrounded by hundreds of trees. Because it sits on a hill, the main entrance is on the second floor with the living room and kitchen. A tenant lives in the bottom floor, and the top floor has an office for Alan and a guest room.

Their two dogs, Abby and Charlie, plus multiple cats greeted us. A sitter had been visiting the pets each day while they were away. Jane had given Katie to Mom because Abby had been attacking her, so we had to take precautions to keep them apart. Otherwise, Mom and I settled in fine. I went shopping and on Monday we mostly watched the TV news about the movement of the storm. As usual, I answered distemper emails from my laptop. Jane and I stayed in touch. She suggested a couple of things to secure in case the winds got too strong.

Early that evening, I helped Mom get to bed in the guest room on the top floor. Then I went back downstairs to watch TV with two of Jane's cats on my lap: Katrina and Sandy. Superstorm Sandy did not break up at the shore. Parts of western New Jersey recorded winds above 80 miles an hour. The power went out around 7:30, and trees crashed all around us. Would one smash through the roof?

I moved mom downstairs to Jane and Alan's bedroom.

The tenant, Radek, had been a tank commander in Poland and now worked in construction to support his family back home. Radek and I stood in the dark in the living room for a while and watched as more trees fell around us. Eventually, he went back to his room while I stayed on the main floor.

I spent the night camped outside of the main bedroom, huddled in a swivel chair with my back to the large bay windows of the living room. News reports of the flooding, fires, power outages and high winds hitting New York City played on a battery-powered radio. When a tree crashed in the driveway, it made an odd thud, I texted Amy that I think it hit my car.

"Don't go out there," Amy texted.

I had no plans to.

Meanwhile, at Mom's house in Avon, the power outage knocked out the sump pump in the basement. For years, that pump had kept the house dry from a tiny underground creek that flowed under the property. Water now attacked the house from at least three directions: from the beach, two blocks away; from Shark River Inlet, one block away; and from the creek under the house, which filled up the basement.

In Belmar, the town immediately south of Avon, the storm surge swept in and erased Silver Lake, the site of my high school cross-country meets. The ocean water kept going and flooded St. Rose High School, where the Bonds had all gone to school. When school officials eventually got back to the property, they found more than 700 pounds of dead fish and live sea turtles swimming through the hallways.

In the morning, the storm subsided in Flemington. Warm tropical air still blew through the trees, but more gently now. Radek and I found several large trees had fallen across the long driveway to Jane's house, and yes, one had landed across the second row of seats of my Toyota Rav4. But none had hit the house. If I had to pick anything to get hit that night, I would rather have it be my car than their house. Later, Jane and Alan would discover a tree could have hit the house, but as it began to fall, the branches of another tree had caught it.

Without power, this house would not be a comfortable place for my 85-year-old mother. Mom and I needed to leave, but two of the trees on the driveway looked to be more than half as thick as a man is tall. I didn't see how we could clear the driveway without help. However, Radek remained undaunted. He started a fire in the kitchen fireplace for Mom. Then he brought out two chainsaws from the garage.

I had little chainsaw experience, so I helped with the small stuff closer to the house. Radek took care of the large trees. A neighbor had come over to ask for help, and when I realized we were going to be able to get out after all, I walked through the woods to help with their driveway. By the end of the day, I'd become a chainsaw veteran.

By mid-afternoon, the driveway had been cleared. I took Jane's car from the garage, loaded Mom and Katie into it, and drove off through the back roads of western New Jersey, heading for Horseheads.

Along the roads, rows of telephone poles had been snapped at their bases, but the poles had not fallen over. They dangled, suspended in mid air from their wires because just enough other poles had remained intact. We would not find a restaurant with the power on until we reached the Poconos that evening.

Compared to many, many others, the storm had given our lives a glancing blow. After Jane and Alan returned from their trip and the power came back on, she came up to Horseheads to pick up mom. From then on, Mom would live with Jane but then come to live with us a couple of times a year. Jane took on the bulk of the challenges in trying to rebuild the house in Avon. The water had flowed into the first floor, and the repairs needed went all the way to the roof.

So, this is a long way to say that not much work on Project Carré got done in November. I kept going through the files, and it began to dawn on me that I needed "professional help."

As to December, I had another small matter I had been putting off all year. I'd finally met with an orthopedic surgeon, who scheduled surgery on my foot on Dec. 3. That morning, Amy and I walked into Arnot Ogden Medical Center in Elmira. I remember thinking I would be walking in on two feet, but would have to be rolled out in a wheelchair when this was over. With every step, I felt pain. I'd gotten used to that pain over the years, but the time had come to do something about it.

As I lay on the pre-op bed, the surgeon did something I appreciated as a former copy editor. She asked which foot they were operating on.

"My left foot," I said.

She drew a smiley face on my left shin with a ball-point pen. Always double-check your facts.

She had already explained the plan. The marathon in 2000 had pulled a tendon in the arch of my foot. It had lost its elasticity, like a rubber band that had over-stretched and would not return to its proper shape. She would replace the bad tendon with one from my toes. Then, because the position of my heel made me susceptible to this kind of injury, she would break it and reposition it.

"How are you going to break my heel?" I asked.

"With a saw," she said.

Then a large screw would be drilled up into the middle of the heel to hold it in the new position.

So, I spent the rest of December in a recliner with a cast attached to an ice cooler. The cooler pumped cold water across my foot to keep the swelling down. The hospital sent me home with some good drugs, at least. I could use my laptop to answer emails about canine distemper, promote my game online and play with the art for the next version of the game.

But the drugs made me too loopy and getting around the house on crutches became too treacherous for me to venture down the steps into my office to work on Project Carré. I also had not been directly in touch with Mountain View since July.

Professional advice

Another pursuit of mine had been writing children's books. In the past year, I had joined a children's book writing group in Ithaca and gotten to know its leader, a fellow named Jim Radke. Jim is a Ph.D., a trained scientist and medical writer who'd been working on a project to use comics to educate children about their illnesses and injuries. I had learned not to burden new friends with the whole spiel about canine distemper when we first meet. So, I had held off on that for a while.

A few days after the surgery, I fired off a drug-addled email to Jim:

> "I have a non-children's book question to ask you. It has to do with you being a medical writer. The non-profit I am working for may have the need for a medical writer. We have been working with vets to document the effectiveness of a treatment for canine distemper. We want to help them to compile this information into the proper format to submit it as an article in a veterinary journal."

Jim was very frank and open to explaining what it would take, and I told him I would send more info when I got back on my feet. That evening, I managed to do an hour-long phone interview about distemper with a web-based radio program. Mostly, I spent the month writing silly Tweets about moments in history where Stealth Checkers had nearly been invented. [87]

As if to punctuate the frustration and difficulties of the year, Amy's sister Beth died just two days before Christmas. As Amy puts it, 2012 had been the year of hell.

On January 8, 2013, Jim wrote me:

> "I looked over your website last night and I am very impressed with the amount of work you have put into this and you have done a great job trying to be enthusiastic about the treatment while at the same time being honest with the expectations. That is a difficult thing to balance. Did some research on the subject last night and would like to talk to you more about what I think your options are moving forward. To be blunt, I do not think your study will be accepted by a peer reviewed journal such as JAAHA. ... The fact that you are not part of an academic institute or major vet clinic will be a major detriment to getting published. It sounds [like] bias but from the journal's perspective, those larger institutes have rules set in place that filter out unconventional methods so that the science and methodology of any procedure have already been reviewed by administrators at the clinic or university before they reached the journal. The equivalent would be sending a manuscript to a major publisher before you have let an editor look it over and make corrections. Most publishers would not even read it and odds are JAAHA would not as well."

I appreciated his honesty, and over the next few weeks and months, we kept talking about ways to move forward. He reviewed the copies of the files I had so far and he explained the issues in emails and phone calls of what he saw as the main problems.

These included:

- "The fact that there is no 'dose' for the treatment is a major stumbling block that most of journals at the JAAHA level are going to be sticklers about. I could be wrong on that but that is my interpretation." This confused me. Of course, there is a dosage. The protocols stipulate how much NDV serum to use. But the problem was that we don't actually know what is in that vial of serum. If it was interferon – and it isn't – we could say how much interferon is in each treatment and what the effect is. Since we don't know, that creates a hole in our presentation that will be hard to address. The scientific explanation for how NDV works is unknown.
- We need the reports to be more consistently detailed, with more specifics. The dog's weight and temperatures should be recorded when they come in and when they leave. More details would help the credibility. Jim said our files "do not have consistent post NDV symptom check other than they lived/discharged or they died."

Placebo – A material without a therapeutic benefit used to help establish controls in scientific studies.

As we talked, it became clearer to me as to why Dr. Sears' submissions to the veterinary journals had been rejected. Jim also explained even in animal studies, a journal article had to account for the **placebo** effect, where a subject gets better just because they believe the drug being used will help them or the extra care that went along with the treatment was responsible for the observed improvement instead of the treatment itself.

Jim offered me some suggestions, which included:

- Going to an open source journal. These have looser restrictions, and usually the author pays for publication. However, open source journals are controversial because of their lack of peer review and a reputation for allowing hoax papers to be published. "They tend to cost money to publish and they are not read by many people nor do they usually look very professional," Jim said. "However, it will give you a published article that you can show people."

- Have the vet make a presentation at a conference. "Making a poster or slide presentation of the data is a good way to get a feel for the story the data is giving you. It also allows the vet to get 1) feedback from other vets 2) something published (an abstract at least) 3) the data in front of academic vets who can take this to the next level. That last point is very important. No matter what happens, your data needs to reach the right academic vet who can do well planned studies. That is the only way this procedure is ever to gain acceptance. Wish that were not the case but it is."

- Create a for-profit enterprise. Perhaps a business could be developed around these treatments to promote the protocols. He told me I could be missing out on a big opportunity.

The business idea did not appeal to me. Frankly, that resurrected the old "snake oil" comment from that vet back in 2009. That memory stung, and I had resolved to not do anything that could be seen as taking advantage of people desperate to save the lives of their dogs. "Money always talks," Jim said. "When you do it as a business instead of a nonprofit, you get more done." This had been John Crowley's approach. I understood what Jim was saying, but I had little interest in going down that road. I did not intend for canine distemper to be the business of my life. I wanted to get this into the right hands and somehow in the right format and walk away.

I would keep the open source journal idea in the back of my mind. The conference presentation sounded like a good idea, but that was not what I had asked Dr. Melton to do. She had not signed up for that.

It would require facing a room full of colleagues most of whom would meet this with derision. Jim's reasoning was that if the presentation was made to 1,000 vets, probably 900 are not even going to listen. Of the 100 who do listen, maybe only 10 would take an active interest. Of those 10, maybe only a handful would want to do something about it. But of the handful, the question could be asked. "OK, you've found this so far. What can we do with it next?"

It could also go badly as it did when Dr. Sears tried to present his discovery in Las Vegas in the 1970s. I told Jim about the encounter Dr. Sears had with Dr. Ott. "He did everything wrong," Jim said. Perhaps if we had a time machine, Jim could have helped Dr. Sears put together a slide show or charts with all the details of the protocol and documented results of cases he'd treated. Then, maybe request a slot to give a mini presentation at the convention. Hindsight, as they say.

Since nothing could be done about the Las Vegas convention in the 1970s, what could be done now in the spring of 2013? I emailed a summary of the issues and the options Jim raised to Mountain View but received no reply. My calls to Dr. Melton were not returned. "I'm very sorry we lost contact," Dr. Melton wrote in a note to me later. "I had some medical issues myself during that time."

Without a reply from Mountain View, I decided to wait a bit, step back and think things through. Before, I had approached them with a clear-cut plan, but now that plan careened sideways. Better to not push this any further until the project goals and plan had been squared away.

I had not yet completely given up on the idea of submitting to a veterinary journal. Jim and I continued to talk about what would be needed. He guessed that hiring a medical writer – either himself or someone else – would cost up to $5,000. Non-profits would get a discount, but since the information they provide would be not as well organized, the hours on the job would be longer. So, the price would probably be about the same.

To move forward, we would need to either salvage additional information on the cases we already had and/or fully document at least another 15 dogs. Could we just start over? Was that too much to ask of the vet clinic? I'd also need to raise more money. I seemed to have gone from walking a tightrope without a net to walking a tightrope without a tightrope.

Later I would learn White Angel Animal Hospital in Austin, Texas, ran into about the same obstacles I had. Tal Shohamy, the manager of the clinic, found that despite their optimism they were not able to compile enough data and submit a paper about the NDV spinal tap.

The problems they ran into included:

- Getting all the lab tests conducted consistently. Not all owners were able to afford them. "We were trying to be affordable and work with people," Tal said.
- Getting consistent data on outcomes. "Because not everybody got back to us," Tal said.

- They also had the challenges of running a full-time clinic and Dr. Zilkha giving birth to a baby girl. They just did not have the time.

"It's impossible to write something that meets the standards of Big Pharma," Tal said. The contact at Texas A&M had not reconnected after the treatment of the corgi. I imagine the issues Tal and I faced were very similar to what the vet clinic in Houston encountered when they treated the 150 dogs with the NDV serum.

The heaviness

For me, the daunting problems also fueled another issue I had been grappling with. At this point, I walked with cane and my foot in either a cast or a special boot. I had not regularly exercised since the injury in January 2012. Looking back at spring of 2013, I've come to realize I also had an undiagnosed injury: clinical depression.

This book is supposed to be about canine distemper, but the depression does play a small role in the story. Since I believe that stigmas about mental health issues need to be dispelled, I'll try to talk about it briefly and without being ... depressing.

Compared with many others, my experience with depression created only a temporary setback. My case is more like receiving a sharp injury that took a while to recover. More like that injury to my foot in the marathon.

That foot injury had plagued me for years. By continually using my foot, the tendon could not recover. The point of the surgery was to repair the damage so that the foot could heal and get stronger. The mental injury also needed to be repaired so recovery could happen.

The mental injury happened in the spring of 2010 when both my journalism and teaching careers had ended. In my brain, I had shrugged at this turn of events. "I'll find something else." After all, this was possibly a chance to pursue my fiction writing. I was also glad to have the time to devote to a cause I cared about.

But even though my brain shrugged, my emotions had their own reaction. Letting go of both of those careers had been a big blow to my identity. For 25 years, I had either been a journalist or a journalism teacher.

Simply put, I was sad. This did not surprise me. No big deal. People have sad things happen to them all the time, and much worse than what I had. For example, Amy lost her dad and her sister within six months. So, my career setbacks do not come close to what she went through. However, a counselor later explained to me that after about two years, the sadness I still felt could change the chemistry in my brain. This makes it difficult to attempt tasks.

For anyone who just says depression is "all in your head," they are right. It is. But that doesn't mean it is not real or that you can just "get over it." Back in the 1980s, Rodney Dangerfield had a bit in his comedy routine where he talked about "The Heaviness." He would say, "The heaviness is always there." Now, I understand what he was talking about. Tasks and goals now came with an extra weight. I could feel them grow heavier as I approached them, as if slogging through a tar pit. Anxiety and self-esteem problems also go along with depression. It took great effort to make phone calls, and receiving phone calls from people I didn't know or expect sent me into a tail-spin.

Makes it difficult to be an advocate for a cause. I had fallen a long way from what I had been at the L.A. Times.

As I write this, my feet are stronger than they had ever been. I can walk barefoot without pain. I can run or walk for an hour or more. I just played a game of badminton on my brother-in-law's front lawn IN MY BARE FEET! And just as my feet could be fixed, so could my brain. The damage to my brain chemistry has been adjusted, and the heaviness has gone away. But diagnosis always comes first, and in spring of 2013, diagnosis remained more than two years away.

Project Carré remained at an impasse. Perhaps someday, I might get the data from the project privately published, such as in a book. [88] As this was going on, a parallel story had unfolded which I haven't had a chance to tell you about yet. So, I'm going to have to roll back the clock a little bit and cover some of the same ground from a different angle. This other story began in South Dakota in May 2012.

Nilla

.

As a puppy, Nilla had been such a timid border collie.

"I just didn't dare scold her because she was so sensitive," said Clark Audiss, a pastor/farmer in Colome, South Dakota. "Even if you just changed the volume in your voice. I was afraid she wasn't going to turn out to be anything, she was just so timid."

The mostly black border collie with white paws, chest, nose and black freckles, had been given to Clark's teen-age son, Nathan, after the family began raising sheep in 2010. His friends had talked Clark into adding sheep to their horse farm to prepare him for his ministry.

"Everybody told me that if you're going to be a shepherd, you need to learn about sheep," said Clark, who had been an insurance agent before becoming a minister. "I've learned that when Jesus was telling us we're all like sheep, he wasn't paying us a compliment. Sheep are pretty stupid. They're about the dumbest animals on the face of the Earth. They can't do anything without their shepherd. So, they're totally lost."

Clark grew up on a farm about 10 miles south of Dallas, SD, a town of about 100 people. His wife, Jennifer, grew up in a suburb of Lexington, Kentucky, and they had met as students at Trinity Bible College in Ellendale, North Dakota, in the early '90s. They eventually married and left Bible college.

Clark had always planned to get back to the calling of ministry, and in the meantime, God had blessed them with a 40-acre farm and two children. Their daughter Rachael is two years younger than Nathan. When the family battled canine distemper in 2012, Nathan and Rachael were 19 and 17 years old.

The entire family puts a priority on service to God and others with Sunday school teaching and missionary work. "God's got a hold of us, and it's a good thing," Clark said. "It's a good place to be."

A couple of years earlier, the family bought 41 ewes and 50 lambs, a trailer-load full. The investment could help pay for Nathan to attend Bible college. But a friend knew that a farm with sheep would need a border collie, and he offered Nathan a 3-month old fluff ball that the teen named Nilla.

The family already had two dogs, an aging German shorthair named Millie and a miniature pinscher named Bosley. But border collies were bred especially to herd sheep. The name of the breed derives from their probable origin along the Anglo-Scottish border, and they are renown for their high energy, intelligence and obedience.

The sheep investment paid off financially, and the new dog had a deeper impact on their lives. But Nilla's first encounters with sheep did not go well.

"The lambs were about as big as she was," Clark said. As a puppy, Nilla would hang out and play with the lambs.

"Pretty soon, them ewes started getting after her and chasing her and knocking her over a couple of times," Clark said. "And I was afraid she was going to have a bad experience and be ruined. So, I pulled her out of the sheep."

Meanwhile, Clark's daughter Rachael had been raising about 20 ducks.

"Nilla took a keen interest in those ducks," Clark said. As it turned out, it was with the ducks that Nilla developed her skills as a border collie.

"She'd just go stalk them and go around them," Clark said. "The border collie is a mustering dog. So, her natural point was some place on the other side of the critter from me, to bring it back to me. Well, she got so good at bringing those ducks back to me. She wouldn't just bring them back in my general vicinity. I'd stand there and tell her to go get them up. And she'd go down the hill, underneath the apple trees and she'd bring them ducks up the hill. She'd bring them right up to my leg. So, they'd be crowding around my leg, and I could just reach down and grab a duck. That's how close she'd herd them to my legs.

"I could just walk off across the yard, and she'd make them ducks follow me wherever I went. I'd take off across the yard, and she'd just make them ducks follow me. It was the craziest thing. So, then, I began to work with her and teach her commands for left and right, which was 'come by' and 'away.' I taught her 'down.' At her peak here, she learned about 15 different commands that she was real good with. Just a phenomenal dog."

When the friend who had given them Nilla saw what she could do, he said, "I'll give you $400 for that dog right now."

Clark said, "It ain't gonna happen."

By then, the whole family had fallen in love with Nilla. When Millie, the German Shorthair, had to be put down at age 15, Nilla helped fill the void. "The more time I spent with her, the more I loved her," Clark said. "Nathan and I had to have fights over whose dog she was."

Nilla loved to jump and to ride things.

"If you go out the door and you're going to jump on the 4-wheeler, she'll meet you on the 4-wheeler," Clark said. Nathan also trained Nilla to ride a horse.

"He'd be on the saddle on the stallion, and he'd say 'Up,' and she'd jump up on his foot and springboard onto the back of the horse."

Bosley, who liked to run off and hunt rats, would sometimes draw Nilla off into trouble.

"My dad always told me that if you have one dog, you actually have a dog," Clark said. "But if you have two dogs, you only got half a dog. And if you got three dogs, you ain't got any dog at all because they get in trouble together."

Distemper strikes

One day, the family came home and each dog had a face full of porcupine quills. Another day in the spring of 2012, they came home to find Bosley looking like he'd been in a fight with something.

"He got all tore up," Clark said. "It looks like he got a coon. His neck was all swelled up. It had cuts in it. He was like oozing, like blood and pus. He just looked terrible. He looked like he got drug through a rat hole. He just looked terrible. We took him to the vet, and they treated him with antibiotics and stuff. But he never got sick."

While Bosley had been vaccinated as a puppy 8 years earlier, Nilla had not. They would later wonder if somehow this raccoon encounter led to Nilla getting distemper. As Clark described it, most people in his area vaccinated livestock, but not their dogs.

"If they vaccinate for anything, they usually vaccinate for rabies," Clark said. "I've talked to numerous people since this around the area and they are like, 'No, we don't vaccinate our dogs.'"

A couple of weeks after Bosley's run-in with the possible raccoon, Nilla showed signs of being in heat. They decided to breed her, and Clark knew of a red-and-white male border collie owned by a man who ran a sheep feedlot. They dropped her off there, with the hope this encounter would produce puppies.

"He was glad to see her cause he had 8,000 sheep in the feedlot. He needed an extra dog anyways," Clark said.

But something went wrong.

"After about a week or 10 days, he called me," Clark said. "He's says, 'I think you oughta come and get her because she's not acting right. She's acting homesick.'"

When Clark picked her up, she had her head down, acting depressed. He worried she was mad because she'd been left with a stranger. But it didn't take long to realize she had a fever. The local vet diagnosed her as having a tick-borne illness such as Rocky Mountain spotted fever and treated her with antibiotics and steroids.

Nilla's health seemed to bounce back. About this time, Clark had retired from his job as an insurance agent and was hired as a part-time associate pastor at their local Assembly of God Church starting on May 1. That year, they had also sold off their mares but kept the stallion. But in the meantime, Nilla's health went downhill again.

"We started noticing things like her balance was off," Clark said. "All of a sudden, she started walking sideways. She started stumbling. Things like that. Her head started bobbing. So, we knew something was drastically wrong."

Nathan, home from Bible college, went with Clark to the vet, who was now 98 percent convinced of distemper. He sent a test off to a lab to check.

"This is a death sentence," they were told. "There's no cure for it."

The news hit them both hard. Nilla stayed overnight in a horse stall in the back of the vet clinic. By the next morning, she could not stand at all. The vet told them, "Take her home over the weekend. Love up on her. Bring her back on Monday and we'll put her down."

Devastated, they took Nilla home. "So, I was praying for Nilla and arguing with God," Clark told me. "I wasn't getting no answer. But I just felt like I needed to get on the Internet, and I did. I got on the Internet. And the first thing I did was I pulled up Google. And I typed 'distemper cure.' And I'm telling you, I just feel that God led me to do this. The first thing that happened was I pulled up your website. Your website was the first thing that came up in the search engine."

He'd found one of my videos, which gave him a glimmer of hope. On Saturday, May 5, 2012, his first email came in through one of my old secondary Yahoo! accounts, which I had set up to forward to the main Gmail address:

> "Help me please! The vet says our 2 year old border collie Nilla has distemper. She is already experiencing neurology from it and loss of control of her muscles. Call me at … if you can help in any way!
> Thanks,
> Clark Audiss"

Clark kept searching and found my other email addresses. He sent a message to my personal Facebook account, but I may not have seen that since we were not already "friended." This one came directly into my distemper Gmail account a little later:

> "Hello,
> Saw your video on You Tube about distemper cure. Our dog Nilla is a 2 year old border collie and has been diagnosed with distemper. She initially presented with weakness, lethargy and depression then we realized she had a big fever. The vet gave her antibiotics, IV and

steroids. Then for a week and told us it was
probably one of 3 tick born
illnesses. She responded very fast to that first
round of antibiotics, which told the vet they were
on the right track. After the 1 week of treatment
she began to deteriorate neurologically and now
cannot stand. Her balance is way off and she
cannot track very far with her eyes. The vet now
says he is almost sure that this is distemper,
however blood tests are pending.
Help!"

My reply:

"You didn't let me know where you are.
Please, let me know.
In the meantime, here is some general information
for you…"

The answer:

"Hi Ed,
This is the wife, Jennifer…. we live in South
Dakota.
Nilla is our son's dog. And I just to give you a
little more background…. We also have an 8 year
old MinPin that is not showing any signs of illness
at all. He was attacked by something, we think a
coon, about 3 to 4 weeks ago. Our vet has done
some research and found that coons are one of the
biggest carriers of distemper and since Bosley was
vaccinated against it he may have just become a
carrier, although he also says we are not "out of
the woods yet" with him….

"Thank you so much for getting back to us right away. I will pass along the other sites to Clark as well. This has been very hard for my husband and kids. A little over a year ago we had to put down our German shorthair.... she was 15. Nilla filled the "void" of Millie. She helped the kids and especially my husband heal...Millie was his dog. She also helped me through some tough times of my own.... I lost my mother and 2 brothers within the first 6 months of 2011. She would lie on my lap and let me cry...

I know you understand how animals can be more than pets. They become part of the family. Thank you for all of your help.

Sincerely,

Jennifer"

I groaned when I realized where they were. Three facts stood out:

- Their dog had already hit the neurologic stage.
- The closest vet willing to perform the NDV spinal tap was 1,000 miles away.
- It was the weekend, which makes it difficult to get anything done.

I replied with a copy of the full protocols and the list of available vets at that time, which were in Texas, Florida, California and Virginia.

"I kept remembering I was frustrated with you at first because I wanted you to call me," Clark said with a laugh. "That's what I wanted you to do. But you wouldn't call me. So, I was dealing with you by email."

At about that time, I'd also been replying to emails from the Aegean Coast of Turkey, The Philippines, Canada, North Carolina and Florida. I had long-since decided to primarily respond only via email. If I called back everyone who emailed, I'd never get off the phone. Also, I worried that I'd make a mistake by trying to verbally explain everything. I could get complete information into the hands of the owners quickly and accurately through email.

For those reasons – plus the anxiety I felt every time I got on the phone – I only called on very rare occasions when it seemed that was the only way the dog owner could understand the information.

Clark understood very quickly that if he ordered the NDV online, it would not get to him until Tuesday or Wednesday, which would be too late. Somehow, he would have to find a source of NDV and a vet to perform the spinal tap before the weekend was over.

"So, I just decided, well, I've got to find this now," he said. "I can't wait to order this. And besides, if I have to go somewhere, where do I have this shipped? Do I have it shipped to my address or somewhere else? I don't even know where I'm going. It was just this big scramble and so I knew I needed to find the vaccine now."

The big scramble

With doggedness, Clark pursued every angle he could find. Since NDV was a bird vaccine, he called a local pheasant farmer he knew. That led to a poultry business. He tracked down three phone numbers at the poultry business and got an answer from someone cleaning the office.

"He didn't speak a lick of English," Clark said. "But I got enough information in his ears that he gave me a number."

He called that number and was told, "I'm the egg guy. You need the chicken guy."

But the chicken guy was unreachable because of the weekend. That sent Clark to another poultry business and the numbers for their three managers. He tried all three. On the third number, the woman on the other end told him he needed the manager on the first number.

"And I said, 'Well, I tried him' And she said, 'Send him a text message. He'll respond to that.' "

Clark sent a text: "Help. My dog's dying."

The confused manager called back, and Clark explained the situation.

"Give me some time. I need to think about this," he said.

Clark hung up the phone and prayed.

"I can tell you exactly the prayer that I prayed," Clark said. "I prayed, 'God, give me an open door.' I said, 'If you just give me an open door, I'll walk through it. I won't even ask any questions.' "

The manager called him back. "I don't have the chicken vaccine Clark, but I've got a number for you to call."

That was the state poultry inspector for South Dakota. He didn't have the vaccine either, but he gave the number for the state poultry inspector for Iowa. He also didn't have the vaccine, but he also had a number to call.

"So, I called it, and it was the largest producer for Iowa," Clark said. He reached him late Saturday afternoon. "He says, 'Clark, I've got 5 million doses of this sitting on my shelf. When can you come over here to Spirit Lake, Iowa, and pick it up?'

"And I was like, 'Thank you, God. Thank you for an open door.' "

Meanwhile, he'd also been trying to find a vet to perform the spinal tap. His local vet could not do it, and he also called a friend who was a veterinarian. He couldn't do it either.

"Well look, I need someone to do this," Clark told his friend. "I'm willing to take a chance if you'll try it."

His friend offered advice: "Clark, I would love to help you. But don't just let somebody try the spinal tap. You need to find somebody that does these. That knows how to do these. You're going to have to go to a specialty hospital that has a surgical team or a veterinary teaching hospital. So, those are your options."

That sent Clark off on another round of phone calls. Finally, he connected with a clinic in Sioux Falls; they referred him to a veterinary hospital in Omaha. The hospital in Omaha said the vet who did spinal taps no longer worked there. They referred him to another specialty clinic in Omaha. That clinic was closed for the weekend and would be open at 8 a.m. Monday, but according to their website they did perform spinal taps.

"So, my plan was to go get the vaccine and head for Omaha and be on their doorstep Monday morning," Clark said. "That was my plan."

Clark wrote to me about the plan. "This trip may be a big fail because I haven't actually talked with the clinic but I'm willing to take the risk that they can help. She doesn't seem to be in any respiratory distress, she pants a little and I think she's still running a fever. She can lift her head and pick up her ears but her vision is going and she bobs her head quite a bit. She's still eating and drinking, which I would think would be a good sign."

I had my doubts.

"I must warn you that showing up at a clinic unannounced with a distemper dog and NDV is not a recipe for success," I wrote. "That is mainly because these treatments have not been published, so they are not widely accepted and understood. ... The NDV spinal tap is the treatment needed for a neuro distemper dog, and it needs to happen ASAP, but it may take a while to find a vet local to you who is willing to do this. But it may happen. It is usually motivated, committed owners like you who find ways to open doors that ordinarily would not have opened. I hope you succeed."

"I understand that I may be chasing my tail on this one showing up unannounced," Clark wrote back the next day. "We are getting ready to head out this morning to go get the vaccine."

Meanwhile, Clark had been calling veterinary hospitals at Colorado State, Kansas State, Iowa State and the University of Minnesota. They each asked for him to send the protocols, but said although emergency hospitals were open, they would not be getting back to him with a decision until Monday.

Sunday morning, Nathan and Clark loaded Nilla onto blankets in the back of Nathan's 2004 Saab and headed out on the 4-hour drive east to Spirit Lake, Iowa.

A glimmer of hope

About 3 hours into the trip, Clark got a phone call from a small animal internal medicine resident[89] at Kansas State University. She told him she had shown the protocol to Dr. Ken Harkin, Head, Section of Medicine, at the veterinary hospital.

Clark was told: "He has looked at it, and he doesn't see any reason why it would work, any scientific reason why it would work. But he said that we would do the treatment if the dog has distemper and you want to proceed. We'll do the treatment."

However, they had to first confirm the distemper. Clark asked how much the spinal tap would cost. "She told me it was going to be $1800."

This took Clark aback. He'd heard from me the range of prices from other vets: $500 to $1500, and he'd been hoping for it to be closer to $500. He could buy a really good border collie for $1800.

"I was thinking, 'Wow,'" Clark said. "Cause, you know, as much as I loved the dog, I was raised on a farm and I was raised that you cut your losses when they get too high. No. 1, we had just gone into ministry, and I'm on a part-time pastor's salary and we really didn't have $1800."

He asked to think about it. In the meantime, they pursued the original plan to go to Spirit Lake and then Omaha. He hoped that maybe the clinic there would charge closer to the $500.

The NDV supplier waited for them in his pickup truck in front of a general store in Spirit Lake. They drove up to him.

"And I rolled down the window. And he rolled down his window and I looked at him and I said, 'Is this where we get the drug deal?' He laughed, and he said, 'Yeah, this was the place.'"

He had a bottle of dry vaccine powder in a cooler with ice packs. He explained how the powder is reconstituted with the liquid diluent and how it was used on chickens. He asked for only about $10.

"I knew that he had driven a ways to get there," Clark said. "Can I pay you for gas?"

"No," he said as he reached into the window and petted Nilla. "No, I'm a dog lover too. You just take this and you save your little girl."

They turned south and drove another three hours to Omaha, Nebraska, and found the clinic, which would be closed until the next morning. But Clark and Nathan went into an emergency animal hospital next door to see if they could get her stabilized until the next day. They left Nilla in the car with the air conditioning running.

"They just kinda looked at us like we were nuts," Clark said.

Finally, they got to talk to a vet and explained the situation. The vet made a call and found out that the doctor who could do the spinal tap would not even be in until Tuesday and his schedule was booked solid. They could not treat Nilla.

Clark sent me an update on their situation and asked if there was a fund available to pay for doing Nilla's spinal tap at Kansas State.

I had to think this through.

Kind Hearts in Action had money earmarked for Project Carré. The whole purpose of the project was to get the NDV protocols published in a veterinary journal, and my plan had been to demonstrate this through the use of the NDV-induced serum. I had specifically told Mountain View that we would not use the Project Carré funds for NDV spinal taps.

A couple of reasons had led to that decision: 1) The NDV spinal taps showed a lesser survival rate, only about half of those dogs survived. 2) The NDV-serum treatment cost less. More dogs could be treated with the serum while in the pre-neurologic stage. Only three or four spinal taps could wipe out our budget, and with much less a chance of success.

As Nilla fought for her life, I was in between my two trips to Mountain View. I wanted to make sure that we had enough funds to keep that project going. But how could I say "yes" to a spinal tap in South Dakota and "no" to a spinal tap in Virginia? If I said, "yes" now, would I need to say, "yes" to every other spinal tap case?

Clark and Nathan got back into their car.

"Nathan, what does God say to you?" Clark asked his son. "Is God speaking to you about this?"

Nathan said, "Dad, I just need to pray."

They parked at an apartment complex in Omaha with trees and shade and grass.
"We laid her out under the grass and trees and tried to water her," Clark said. "By that time, we were trying to water her with a syringe because she couldn't drink. She had too much head bounce to on her own. She couldn't drink. So, I left Nathan alone with her. I went to the car and I began to pray."

After praying, Clark came back to Nathan.

"Dad, I just feel peace," Nathan said. "I feel like we need to take her to Kansas State. They've opened the door for us there. Nobody else has opened the door, and we need to take her there. I know we don't have eighteen hundred bucks, but we need to go."
"OK," Clark said.

They loaded Nilla back into the car and headed for Kansas State University. They hadn't even gotten out of Omaha when Clark's phone rang.

I called and offered to pay half of the hospital bill.

"And that was another answer to a prayer, Ed," Clark said with a laugh. "When you called me."

What changed my mind was the purpose of Project Carré. The entire goal of our social media campaign and the project was to get the NDV treatments into the hands of the veterinary experts so they could see the possibilities for themselves. Clark had opened the door, and we could not afford to miss this chance. I only hoped Nilla's case would fall among the nearly 50 percent who lived and improved after the procedure.

I also wrote Dr. Sears to let him know what was going on and that they may need to consult with him.

Kansas State

They drove another three hours from Omaha to Manhattan, Kansas, and checked into a Super 8 motel that evening. As Nathan tried to get Nilla to stand, with his hands under her ribs and stomach, Clark filmed a video. Every time Nathan let go, Nilla toppled over. Her eyes rolled back and forth, unable to track herself or objects. Her head still bobbed.

"She had a little bit more energy when we actually got to the hotel," Clark said. "She'd been riding the whole trip. Hadn't moved a muscle. She couldn't do much, but she showed more activity like she was going to live the night anyways."

They'd find out later that Super 8 would waive the pet charge for dogs being treated at Kansas State.

The next day, they drove to Mosier Hall, the veterinary medical teaching hospital at Kansas State. Because she was contagious, Clark and Nathan had to leave Nilla in the car while they went in and filled out paperwork. A senior veterinary student took down the medical history. He went out to the car with a quarantine cart to pick up Nilla. "Oh my God, she's gorgeous," Clark remembers him saying. They placed her in a quarantine kennel and ran tests on her.

Some of the notes from the case file on Nilla's admittance:

- Recumbent and non-ambulatory
- Stiff right limbs, but decreased withdrawal reflexes
- Head tilt to the left
- Head turn and torticollis [twisted neck] to the right
- Positional vertical nystagmus [involuntary eye movement indicating loss of vision] after
- Inducible ventral strabismus [lack of alignment] of the right eye
- Absent menace reflex bilaterally [eyes not blinking in response to approach of object, another sign of vision loss]
- Bradycardia (heart rate 52 beats per minute)
- Urine soaked coat

Clark and Nathan went back to the hotel. Clark texted me the news that if Kansas State did perform the NDV spinal tap, they would document the results and send me copies of the file. The next morning, they came back with some boned chicken for Nilla. They couldn't see her, but the staff fed it to her. She still had an appetite.

They found a local Assembly of God Church and went in to pray. While there, they met the youth pastor. He invited them to lunch at Pizza Hut to hear their story. He asked Nathan to come speak to their youth group the next night.

At lunch, Clark's phone rang. The veterinary resident at the hospital called to report the tests confirmed distemper. The PCR tests were positive on conjunctiva scrape and in the cerebrospinal fluid. "Do you still want to proceed with this treatment?" he was asked.

"And I said, 'Yes. Absolutely.' "

They went back to the hospital to sign some papers, including a liability waiver. But as they sat in the waiting room for the papers to come out, Clark's phone rang again.

"It was Colorado State University," Clark said. They'd reviewed the protocol. "His words were, 'This is quackery.' He says, 'Clark, this isn't good medicine. This is quackery. There's no reason this would work.' He says, 'We are a state-funded facility. We're a state-funded hospital. And if we were to try this, we could put our funding in jeopardy. I'm afraid you're not going to find anybody to do this procedure for you.' "

Clark thanked him for his time and hung up.

"I just didn't have the heart to tell the guy that we were sitting in Kansas State, ready to go in and do the procedure," Clark said.

But according to Clark, even the veterinary resident had her misgivings. She told him the dog should just be put down so her misery could end. Between Sunday night and Tuesday afternoon, Nilla had gone completely blind. She was almost completely paralyzed.

"We love Nilla," Clark told her. "We're just trying to do the best thing for her. If this doesn't work, we will be the first ones to say, 'Let's put her down.' "

Clark looked at her and said, "Now, who's going to be doing the procedure?"

"I am."

"Have you ever done this before?"

"Yeah, I did one this morning."

"Then you're exactly the person that I want to do this for Nilla," he said. "I trust you because we're just trying to help our dog."

Some questions needed to be answered first. They needed to double-check on how the NDV should be reconstituted into a fluid for the injection. They also needed to clarify some questions on the procedure itself.

I ran errands around Horseheads when I got texts from Clark that they needed to connect with Dr. Sears. However, I had not had a reply from him since my email on Sunday. This probably meant he was travelling and unable to respond. Often he was helping one of his four grandchildren celebrate a landmark such as a graduation. Also, I did not have a smartphone at this time, so I could not instantly check my email. I replied by saying they should contact the vets in Texas and California who had already performed the NDV spinal tap.

Luckily, when I got home, I found an email from Dr. Sears.

"Wow! At last, 40 years after Dr. Adams and I did this in the basement of UCLA," he replied. "I would be thrilled to be part of this in any way."

"I'm sending them your phone number, so you might get a call. They just gave the go-ahead to perform the procedure. The distemper has been confirmed in the patient."

Dr. Sears talked to Clark and the veterinary resident. According to Clark, the phone call with Dr. Sears helped turn the corner. The staff at Kansas State may also have thought the NDV spinal tap nothing but quackery, but since the distemper had been confirmed and the dog would likely die anyway, they were at least willing to try.

Clark remembers the resident saying before the procedure began, "Don't worry. If my hands are not steady, Dr. Harkin is right there to take over for me."

They went outside Mosier Hall, and Nathan filmed a video update of Clark. "We're hopeful this procedure will work. We'll keep you updated," he said to the camera. "We're hoping for the best."

Nathan and Clark went back to the hotel during the procedure. They got a call from the resident later on to say Nilla had come through the operation and was groggy and in recovery.

Meanwhile, I waited for news on the outcome too.

The father of Amy's karate teacher had died that week. Wednesday morning, Amy and I drove up to Cortland to attend the funeral. After the service, I stepped outside onto the grass in front of the church and turned on my cell phone.

The text from Clark:

> "Nilla is awake and she was able to sit up in the night and change sides she was laying on. She ate and drank this morning and is wagging her tail. They're calling her the miracle dog in ICU this morning! No seizure activity and no facial pain is evident yet. Since the optic neuritis should be one of the first things to clear they are checking her vision every hour."

A wave of relief swept over me. "Thank God," I thought.

But she still had the chorea, the head bouncing, blindness and paralysis. Wednesday night, Nathan preached at the church youth group where he had been invited.

"He preached a sermon on the potter and the clay," Clark said. "He said that the potter has the right over the clay, and God is the master potter. He talked about that God has a plan for your life. God wants to use you. ... He told them the story of Nilla, 'If God's got a plan for Nilla, then God's got a plan for you.' "

On Thursday morning, they got to see her, at first only through a little window. She moved her head slightly when they called her name. She might have reacted with a reflexive action when the staff tested her vision earlier. But they were not sure and could not repeat it. So, they concluded she was still completely blind. The latest she could stay without any further charges was 11 a.m. So, Clark and Nathan checked her out.

But Clark became insistent about something.

"I wanted to see Dr. Harkin," Clark said. "They're like, well, you know, he's busy. Finally, they just went and told him 'Look, this guy is not going to leave until you come down here and shake his hand.' "

Clark chuckles lightly as he tells his story.

"He come down, you know, and I thanked him for doing what he did, and opening up the hospital to us and agreeing to do this treatment. I was just amazed that he did. It seemed to me it was a miracle that he was willing to do it. Everybody else turned us away, and here's this one guy who is evidently quite well respected in his field and well known, that he would open himself up and open the hospital up like this and the school to this. I was just struck by that and I wanted to thank him."

They shook hands as Clark thanked him.

But Dr. Harkin had to be straight. He said, "Now, Clark, I need you to understand we don't think this is going to work. You need to go home and prepare to put her down."

He was told to check in with his local veterinarian. If Nilla got any worse, she would need to be taken to him right away and put down.

"He was pretty unemotional about it," Clark said.

Items listed under "Diagnostics and Findings" on the discharge papers included:

- Conjunctival scrape for PCR: positive for distemper …
- Cerebrospinal Fluid Analysis: Marked lymphocytic pleocytosis with possible intramacrophagic distemper inclusion bodies…
- CSF Distemper Titer: pending
- CSF Distemper PCR: pending

From the "Assessment" on the discharge:

"Based on PCR and CSF analysis, Nilla has been diagnosed with distemper infection in her brain. The prognosis for neurologic distemper is very poor and no known treatments have been shown to be effective in the veterinary literature. ... At your request, we have performed an intrathecal (into the cerebrospinal fluid) injection of Newcastle virus vaccine according to the Sears protocol. As we have previously discussed, we do not know what side effects may occur with this injection. However, thus far we have not seen any adverse events related to the injection – Nilla's neurologic status is unchanged and she shows no abnormalities on her bloodwork post-injection."

They packed her in the back seat of Nathan's car. Before getting on the road, Nathan filmed Clark.

"Nilla is here in the back seat, she's pretty comfortable."

Her head rises up at her name, rotates and goes back down.

"She's just chilling. She's responding to stimulus. She definitely has not deteriorated during her stay here at Kansas State. But she hasn't really improved much either. There seems to be some discussion about her vision, about whether that is returning or not. We're going to continue to test her. They've given us protocols. We're going to go to a park right now and let her smell the grass and relax. We'll keep you informed as we go. Thanks for your prayers."

About 70 miles out of Manhattan, not very far from I-80, they stopped at a roadside cemetery. They laid her on the grass under a big tree and fed her turkey slices from a deli. They gave her a drink of water with a syringe.

"I noticed that she started watching my hand," Clark said. "That when I moved my hand, she was moving. It wasn't just a smell. She wasn't just smelling the turkey in my hand. She was watching my hand movements."

The realization dawned on them.

"Oh my God, Nathan, look at this."

"Dad, she can see!"

Nathan took out his Android smartphone and shot a video of Nilla tracking Clark's hand.

Clark called the vet student who had checked Nilla in, saying: "We're about 70 miles away from you. We just stopped, and I just want you to know this dog can see."

"You're kidding," came the reply.

"I said, 'I'm not kidding you. I'm as serious as a heart attack. We just took a video of her. We're going to send it you, email. You take a look at it. We're going to stay right here until you call me back.' "

He called back to tell him to keep a daily log of Nilla's progress. They stopped a few more times. "Her vision just kept getting better and better," Clark said.

He emailed me that night:

"Just made it home with Nilla and her vision is improving rapidly. She is increasing with alertness and energy also, sitting up frequently. We will keep you posted. I would love to hear some of your ideas and be a sounding board and help you any way I could."

On her first night home, Nilla crawled around but could not control her bowel movements. The family found a mess the next morning, marking where she had crawled. Clark gave her a bath, during which she lifted up her leg and licked it. After the bath, she groomed herself, licking her fur.

"Not long after that, she sat up," Clark said. "Then her vision really started coming back in leaps and bounds. We just knew that we had a miracle in our house."

On May 11th, I wrote a very enthusiastic email to Dr. Harkin explaining what our group had been working on and the possibilities of treating dogs with distemper before they reached the neurologic stage. I asked if there could be some sort of collaboration. Very politely, he let me know I was getting ahead of myself:

"Thank you for the email. My first reaction to the NDV protocol when it was forwarded to me was one of extreme skepticism ... Still, given that both viruses are in the subfamily Paramyxoviridae and Nilla seemed to have almost 0% of survival with her form of distemper, I decided it was worth the risk of looking ridiculous.

As we still don't know Nilla's outcome, I am reluctant to jump into any sort of commitment for collaboration at this time. If, however, Nilla defies the odds and goes on to apparently recover (I suspect that I will ask Mr. Audiss for a follow-up visit with Nilla if she does show solid evidence of recovery), I agree that a full-scale investigation into this treatment option is warranted and I will spearhead the hunt for grants to pursue this doggedly.

"At this time I would prefer to keep the details of our using this experimental treatment quiet. When the time comes for us to pursue this fervently, I will most definitely seek your help for collaboration."

So, we had done what we could do for now. The next steps were up to Nilla.

Literally.

The Big Picture

"Get'im up!" Clark commands.

"Get'im up!"

"Get'im up!"

Nilla's head stretches for the lamb, which they had been bottle feeding. Clark holds the lamb just out of her reach. As she lies on the ground, her front claws grip the grass and pull. Her back feet tuck under her prone body as she propels herself forward. She relies on her front legs, which are more functional than the back.

Briefly, Bosley gets between Nilla and the lamb.

"No Bosley! Bosley get out of here."

Clark shoos the black Mini Pinscher away so Nilla can get back to the job.

"Oh good girl!"

She flops on her side. Her front paws reach for the lamb as the back legs kick in unison.

"Oh good girl!"

Nilla's tail wags. She looks around proudly.

"One more try? Move them legs! Move them back legs!"

She's got a system down. Her front legs work the ground, getting traction on the grass. The back legs kick off to one side, the edges of her toes and legs adding just enough forward momentum. Her teeth reach the lamb's back legs, just enough to nibble.

"Oh yes!" says Clark as he rubs Nilla on the head. "Good girl!"

Clark looks up into the camera.

"Sheep Therapy 101."

Three weeks earlier, Nilla had been injected with NDV into spinal canal via the foramen magnum at Kansas State. By appealing to her herding instincts, the Audiss family had found a way to inspire their border collie during her rehabilitation. They sent me videos or posted them on YouTube from the end of May through August 2012.[90]

Each video showed some kind of improvement. Two days later, they started with the lamb several yards away from Nilla. Rachael held the lamb between her legs and guided it in front of Nilla as Clark urged her on. "Get the sheep! Get the sheep!"

Nilla began crawling as she had the other day, but then got her back legs under her. This gave her enough momentum to get up on her front legs and dive for the sheep, just missing it.

"Good girl!" calls Clark.

Nilla collapsed back on the ground, wagging her tail.

Rachael brought the sheep back. This time, Clark held it as Nilla aggressively crawled after the sheep, just barely nipping at its shoulder.

"Oh good girl!" he said, patting her side. "That'll do! That'll do!"

Some of the other milestones:

• They tried a doggy wheelchair, but Nilla kept falling headfirst into the ground. The doggy wheelchair never appeared again.

• Nilla stretched and crawled after a Frisbee, which is tossed further and further away on each attempt.

• To climb a hill towards the house, Nilla at first moved only her front legs, dragging her back legs. Then she pulled herself up onto her front legs and lurched forward. She brought her back legs under her, hopped a couple of steps and then fell. She pulled herself back up again, got her back legs under her again and fell forward. Eventually, she propelled herself forward by using her back feet in a unified hopping motion.

• While chasing a squeaky ring toy, Nilla crawled, then pulls herself up on all fours and for a second or two all four legs support her fully as she walks.

• She briefly chased Bosley and played tug with her toy.

• Nilla followed Rachael and Bosley out into the pasture, walking in a straight line for several seconds. Later, she climbed to the top of a hay pile.

• With Rachael's encouragement, Nilla climbed up and down the steps to a deck. When Rachael opens the door to the house, Nilla just barely got around it and slid onto the floor inside.

• On June 20, Clark gave the squeaky toy a strong toss across the yard. Nilla ran after it for a solid 8 seconds, only dropping to the ground as she reached the toy. She promptly chewed on it.

• On July 4th, Nilla chased a pillow thrown across a platform, going up one side and off the other. Clark used the pillow to get her to chase him. She ran normally until she reached the deck. The front legs leapt onto the deck fine, and she let her back legs slide onto it.

• Three weeks later, they filmed Nilla climbing into the passenger seat of their pickup truck. The same day, Nathan filmed Nilla running some sheep back into their enclosure.

Nathan reaches down from the top of the 4-wheel ATV and pets her after finishing the job.

"That'll do! That'll do!"

But would it do for Dr. Harkin at Kansas State?

What I had been learning

By now, I had seen dogs survive canine distemper for 15 years. I'd seen this in the life of my own dog and in the emails, photos and videos I'd received from all over the world. However, I knew all too well my anecdotal info, my numbers, videos and all the website posts and social media sharing didn't mean much in the scientific world. Saving the life of one dog – in this case, Nilla – also did not prove a treatment to be the Holy Grail.

I also knew dogs in neurologic distemper that received the NDV spinal tap had a 50 percent survival rate at best. This was the riskiest procedure on which to prove the effectiveness of NDV. My hope was that Nilla might open a door at Kansas State that might lead to a study of the NDV serum or NDV as IV treatments for dogs in the pre-neurologic stage of canine distemper.

Even if it didn't, the videos from South Dakota cheered me. In June 2012, our family went into crisis mode as Howie Clark died and the health of Amy's sister Beth deteriorated. At the same time, I wrestled with government bureaucracy and legal requirements to get my patent filed. The videos of Nilla wagging her tail as she regained more and more ability brightened those days.

In the meantime, I'd also been busy doing some research about viruses and NDV. I'll try to explain what I've learned. Brace yourselves. I'm about to get back into some nitty gritty science for a few pages. While doing this, I hope to not get too far out on a limb and make misleading conclusions.

Virotherapy – Genetic reprogramming of viruses so they might be used to treat disease.

Dr. Sears had said for years he did not know how his serum worked. But we knew there were some unusual properties to NDV. The recently emerging field of **virotherapy** has found some intriguing ways viruses could be used as tools against disease. The three branches of this field are: oncolytic virotherapy – viruses as a weapon against cancer; viral gene therapy, using viruses to deliver genes to cells; and viral immunotherapy, using viruses to introduce specific antigens to an immune system.

For decades, Newcastle Disease Vaccine had been known to be an inducer to create interferon. As a virus that attacks bird cells, NDV has proteins that counteract the bird's immune response. This makes it more effective in making a bird sick. However, the same proteins that help make the bird sick are quickly flagged by the immune response of a mammal, which results in interferon. (Zamarin and Palese 2012)[91]

As mentioned earlier, NDV also has a reputation for attacking cancer, but it seems to be able to do more than just destroy cells. Laboratory and animal studies have shown NDV can stimulate other indirect immune responses. These include the activation of natural killer cells, which are white blood cells that can attack tumors. Also, NDV can affect changes to the surfaces of tumor cells, making them more likely to be flagged for attack. (Zamarin and Palese 2012)[92]

Could the mechanism saving dogs from distemper be one of these? Or is there some other mechanism of NDV inside the biology of the dog that has not been discovered by science? After all, biology is also a science of discovery and nature continues to surprise scientists.

For example, scientists in 2008 discovered a tiny virus called Sputnik inside a mimivirus, which is one of the largest known viruses. This was the first and so far only example found of a virus directly attacking and infecting another virus.[93] More recently, there have been studies in HIV research on using non-lethal viruses to block or lessen the impact of lethal viruses. (Paff at al., 2016)[94]

Walking on a new continent

Dr. Sears and I had found tantalizing hints that the answers he needs might be found by someone smarter and better funded.

> **RNA interference** – When an RNA strand binds with another RNA strand and blocks the genetic message.

In November 2010, Dr. Sears came across the research on **RNA interference**, which had earned the Nobel Prize in 2006 for Craig Mello of the University of Massachusetts and Andrew Fire of Stanford University.[95]

"At last I have lived long enough for the science of what I discovered has come to light," he wrote in an email. "Problem with the universal brain is you need to be smart enough to ask it the right questions. Answers are there."

He sent me the materials on RNA interference along with his original notes on the book, and we talked about it a few months later.

In the cell, DNA determines how a cell grows and functions. This is a complex, double-stranded molecule wound into a helix shape like a twisted ladder. Most DNA is in the cell nucleus, and it sends RNA out into the cell to carry its messages and commands.

RNA is another form of genetic material, which usually exists as a single strand – just one side of the ladder, not as long as a full DNA strand and a slightly different chemical composition. Also, many viruses are just strands of RNA encased in an envelope of proteins. Some viruses are DNA.

An experiment on petunias in the 1990s had led to the discovery of RNA interference. Molecular biologists had been confused in an attempt to intensify the red color of the flowers by adding more of the RNA for red pigment. Instead of the result they expected, the gene for red had been blocked completely, resulting in a white flower. Fire and Mello found the answer to this puzzle while working on muscle proteins of worms.

Fire and Mello discovered in their worm experiments that two single stranded RNA molecules of opposite type could bind to each other, form a double-stranded RNA molecule that would block the signal for the genetic message from the DNA.

That's RNA interference, and this effect has also been cited as a defensive mechanism against viruses. An attacking viral RNA strand can bind to a type of RNA molecule from the defending cell called a Dicer, which destroys the attacking virus. [96]

"But is it everything?" Dr. Sears said in during one of our phone calls in 2011. "No, it's only what they've discovered so far. It's like walking into a continent and starting on the East Coast. What have you got in the rest of the country?"

Ultimately, it may not be that the mechanism of RNA interference explains how Dr. Sears' NDV serum might work, but it is an example of how difficult it may be to unlock all the interactions between cells, viruses and the compounds that affect them.

A deep mystery remains. In a normal attack, the distemper virus attaches itself to the cell membrane, passes inside and uses the mechanisms of the cell to make thousands of copies of itself. While some viruses do this by invading and taking over the nucleus, paramyxoviruses replicate in the **cytoplasm** of the cell. Eventually, so many copies are made that the cell may explode and spread new virus throughout the body.

If NDV cannot infect a dog's cell, where in this process could the addition of NDV block the distemper virus? How could NDV boost the standard immune reactions to seemingly shut off a distemper attack within a day or two? What exactly is happening?

"I don't know," Dr. Sears said. "I don't have an answer for that."

Cytoplasm – The material within a cell that is not the nucleus.

Antibiotic – A material that can destroy or inhibit bacteria.

Although the dots might be coming together, we can't really draw a picture from them. The inability to explain this NDV reaction sits at the core of the skepticism. But in this way, Dr. Sears inhabits a similar position as Carré when he made his discovery in 1905 but could not show his virus to the world. In his time, Jenner could not really explain how cowpox could prevent small pox. Before Sept. 28, 1928, Alexander Fleming could not have imagined how mold could be used to kill bacteria. All the same, he discovered the first **antibiotic** by a fortunate accident of science when his petri dishes were contaminated by fungus.

The early astronomers calculated the orbits of the six planets visible to the naked eye and could see how they interacted with each other. But the math did not add up. Some hidden force beyond the known universe pulled on Saturn and Jupiter. It led astronomers to search the skies further and to eventually find Uranus and Neptune. More recently, astronomers have been baffled to discover the universe has more material and energy than thought. They cannot see this matter or energy, have no idea what it is, and simply call it "Dark Matter" and "Dark Energy." But the effects are real. The universe has evolved the way it has and is expanding as it does because of these unknown factors.

That's what we have here: an uncomfortable possibility that science may not have all the answers. New worlds remain to be discovered.

To figure out what is happening with NDV, it would take a microbiologist, someone a lot smarter and with a lot more resources than Dr. Sears or myself. But Dr. Sears remains convinced this NDV effect cannot be replicated in a test tube, it is something that occurs within the living body. As he said in Houston in 2009, "This is a material that stirs up the immune system and manufactures by a variety of different kinds of cells, antiviral products which work in concert to knock viruses out."

But viruses are still pathogens. They can cause disease and trigger tumors. So, researchers still have a lot of issues to resolve on the safety of viruses as a tool against disease. On one website of a veterinary clinic which refused to try the NDV treatment, the dangers of combining viruses were raised. Because of the frequent changes in versions of influenza – the flu – in birds and other animals, the clinic did not want to take a risk by giving a bird vaccine to a dog.

This would put a scary question into my head.

Could I kill Gweneth Paltrow?

In the 2011 movie "Contagion" starring Matt Damon and Gweneth Paltrow[97], a new and highly dangerous virus threatens humanity after the wrong bat met the wrong pig. Paltrow's character is infected by this new virus on her visit to Hong Kong and she brings the disease back to the U.S., passing the virus off to nearly everyone she meets before it kills her.

The film eerily portrayed events similar to how the COVID-19 crisis unfolded in 2020. The novel coronavirus or SARS-CoV-2 is believed to have emerged from bats and somehow jumped to the human population, possibly in markets where wild animals were sold as meat in Wuhan, China. [98] The ensemble movie was ahead of its time in educating the viewer about the dangers of viruses and how they are spread. The villain of the movie – a former journalist using a website to declare he had a cure for the disease – left me simultaneously uncomfortable and outraged. This opportunist, Alan Krumwiede, as played by Jude Law, took advantage of the panic to make millions off his fake cure although he was eventually exposed as a fraud and arrested at the end.

So aside from having a character who portrayed everything I did not want to be seen as, the film raised a very big question for me. Could using NDV against canine distemper create a dangerous new virus?

I asked Dr. Sears about this in an email.

"Yes, combination genus viruses from different infected host species can combine," he wrote. "That is how flu virus transforms. However, getting two different viral genuses to combine – extremely rare. Do not think this is common."

Later on, he added, "If it were going to happen it would have decades ago as the NDV has been in farm yards for eons and the cross over to dogs with distemper would have occurred. Seems many species have distemper but no mammals have NDV and as far as I know no birds have distemper."

That made sense, but I was not completely reassured about Gweneth Paltrow's chances. I turned to my cousin, Dr. Kathleen Triman, the biology professor at Franklin and Marshall, to get her opinion. As I wrote her in mid-December, I realized it was the middle of final exams. She might be too busy. Luckily, my timing was favorable. She answered within a couple of hours:

> "Dear Ed,
> I am proctoring my final exam today, so I have time to respond!
> … Recombination is also an extremely rare event. However, I do want to assure you that these very rare events can THEORETICALLY occur. They are not IMPOSSIBLE. You have touched on a major problem...we do not know enough about viruses or about transmission of genetic information from one species to another.
> Please remember that medical opinion (including veterinary medical opinion) is just that and can only be based on the (current) training of the person expressing that opinion....
> Best wishes for a happy holiday.
> Kathleen"

So, anything is possible. But to better understand the chances for Gweneth Paltrow and the rest of the human race, let's discuss three ways new viruses emerge:

1) **Reassortment**: When the genes of a virus exist as segments and the gene segments of one virus swap with the gene segments of another virus. This usually happens as both viruses infect the same host cell.
2) **Recombination**: The swapping of a gene within a single segment to form a new virus.
3) Single point mutation: A change in the amino acids somewhere along the chain of the gene strand, resulting in a new virus. For

example, when measles evolved into canine distemper in 18th Century South America.

"Viruses can modify their behavior and increase their virulence as they evolve through changes in their genetic material. Such genetic evolution can occur through reassorting of viral genes, recombination of a viral gene or mutation within a viral gene. Reassorting occurs when a virus has multiple gene segments and swaps one or more of its segments with those from a different virus to form a new virus ... For humans, swapping of an influenza gene from birds or pigs with an influenza gene of a man resulted in a new form of influenza virus that wreaked havoc on a human population." [99]

Viruses can combine with each other to create new viruses the way a baker may combine ingredients to make a new cake batter. To make it happen, you need a mixing bowl.

For influenza, the pig is one of the better known examples of a "mixing vessel." Both bird and human strains of influenza virus can simultaneously infect it. (Ma et al. 2009)[100]

Again, viruses are inert outside of a cell. They can do nothing without the energy and materials provided by the host. But a pig cell can play host to the two different strains of virus.

It is as these influenza viruses replicate that the segments of their genetic code can separate and then reassemble. If another influenza virus is also replicating, the genetic segments can swap and create a new virus. But it is important to understand the strains of influenza (flu) virus – for bird, pig, human, etc. – are in the Orthomyxoviridae family.

The Orthomyxoviruses are described as having genes in 8 strands of RNA. So, influenza viruses readily swap their gene segments with other influenza viruses – reassortment.

But the Paramyxoviruses – distemper, measles, Newcastle disease – have a single strand of RNA, not in segments. (see my graphic on next page) These viruses are more antigenically stable, (Pringle 1991)[101] which is cited among researchers discussing the safety of using NDV. Without segmentation of its RNA, these viruses cannot undergo reassortment. This created an obstacle for researchers trying to understand the molecules of the virus because they were not as easy to breakdown and identify the individual components.

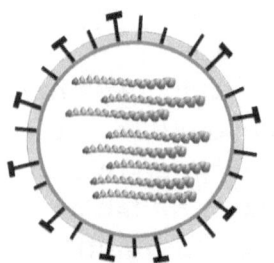 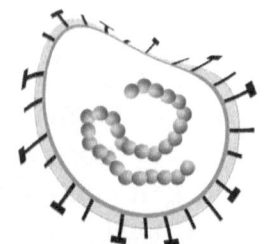

Orthomyxoviruses | **Paramyxoviruses**
Influenza A, B, and C | Distemper, Measles, NDV

"Previously, genetic manipulation of paramyxoviruses was not possible because the genome is not infectious alone and RNA recombination is essentially non-existent. This posed an obstacle to the molecular and biologic characterization of these viruses." (Samal 2011)[102]

Single-point mutation has been the most common way paramyxoviruses have changed. This is how canine distemper evolved from measles. Somewhere along that single chain of RNA, a change happened and created a new virus. If that new virus is able to keep infecting hosts, it survives. In the creation of distemper, the mutated virus could now infect dogs instead of humans. But the overall structure remained similar, and single-point mutations are not happening because of an interaction with other viruses.

In a study of 13 strains of NDV isolated over a period of 50 years, "It was concluded that the different strains appeared to have evolved by accumulation of point mutations and that no gene exchange by recombination had occurred in generations of the three lineages." (Pringle 1991)[103]

It was not until reverse genetics techniques developed in the 1990s that researchers have been able to better understand the function of the proteins and genes in paramyxoviruses. To do this, they needed to employ a form of cloning so they could break down and identify the molecules.

When concerns were raised about an increase in recombination events reported in NDV, a study in China investigated and attributed the trend to errors and artificial alterations of the virus by researchers. "It appears that the recombination of NDV is not as common as has been reported." (Song et al. 2011)[104]

Note the phrasing: "essentially non-existent" and "not as common." Paramyxoviruses are "characterized by low rates of recombination." In that single chain of RNA, recombination is rare, but not impossible. For example, recombination of distemper was documented in a giant panda in China in 2008. The two parent strains of distemper apparently came from a lesser panda and a fox. So, this created a new strain of distemper. Again, this was possible because two strains of the same virus were able to simultaneously infect a common host cell. (Han et al. 2008)[105] But I have not found any published papers about a recombination between distemper and NDV. In March 2012, I summarized my thoughts in another email to my cousin, asking, "Can you tell me if my logic is on track?":

- Pigs are an ideal mixing vessel for influenza virus because they can be infected by multiple strains simultaneously.
- As of that time, I had not found any example of a dog becoming a mixing vessel for a virus. [106]
- For a dog to become a "mixing vessel" for both distemper and Newcastle Disease, both viruses would need to be able to connect to the cell receptors of the dog. This might be possible if there was a mutation of Newcastle Disease. But for now, dogs do not get Newcastle's Disease. Chickens do.
- The vaccine used in the NDV-induced serum is LaSota strain and is off-the-shelf. No special reverse engineering is used. A mutation that would make NDV infectious to dogs seems unlikely.
- Still, we can't completely rule out the possibility because we are still learning what viruses are capable of. However, the use of the NDV-induced serum – created by injecting a healthy dog with NDV – rather than straight injections of NDV into dogs that are sick with distemper – limits the risk further.

- Since NDV does not infect the cells of the dog, the disease-fighting reaction apparently happens elsewhere in the dog, possibly floating in the blood serum, where the immune system creates this unknown material as a response to the virus that can save a dog from distemper.

"I do not detect a flaw in your logic, but I am no expert!" she replied.

I appreciated that reply because over the years I'd run across people who would claim to be experts who clearly were not. So, I found it interesting that my much-better educated and experienced cousin would not call herself an expert on this subject. It takes a level of understanding to know what you know and don't know.

I review all of this research as a tourist. I do not possess the education and experience to make conclusions. I simply pull together information that seems to be relevant and hope to make these issues clearer to the average reader. But I could never claim to be an expert, no matter how many web posts I write or journal articles I read. I had admonished my followers about this on the Kind Hearts In Action site in this post:

> "You should be careful when someone claims to have a cure for canine distemper. You should be skeptical. You should ask questions. Look for red flags. If someone says they are an expert, check it out. By the way, I do not claim to be a veterinary expert. Those are called vets, and I am not one. I can answer questions about the NDV treatments as they have been explained to me by Dr. Sears, but when the questions get too technical I will refer you to him or to another vet."
> Nov. 25, 2010

As I read about the risks of viral therapies, the somber realities of promoting an unpublished treatment came into focus. For any scientist, researcher or veterinarian to pick up, study or use such a treatment, there is a judgment call to be made that is far above my pay scale. So, I can only be grateful to those who had picked up these treatments and gave them a fair chance.

Going old school

Most of the recent NDV and cellular research can be easily found online (although sometimes expensively for a non-scientist like me – often $35 for one article). But I had some more questions, which required old-fashioned hard-copy research.

In February 2012, Liam, Amy and I went up to Cornell Vet School for an annual celebration of cats. Liam, then 7, loves cats above all other animals and was always up for anything cat-related. The Feline Follies, held each year at Cornell, offer educational programs about cats, competitions for longest tail, most toes or best trick, as well as other cat activities.

The Follies were held in the veterinary school's main lobby, and I promised Amy I would behave myself. So, I refrained from leaving copies of Dr. Sears' protocols and DVD around the school or pestering faculty with his wild ideas. I admire and respect Cornell Vet School, but I had already made my attempt at knocking on their front door with Dr. Sears' protocols. My approach had not been compelling enough to warrant a response, and I still had not improved my position enough to make another try.

Instead, I slipped away from the festivities to use the veterinary library upstairs.

I needed to settle an issue with the timing of Dr. Sears' discovery. Whenever I had asked him when he made his discovery, his answer ranged between the late 1960s and early 1970s. His 40 years of veterinary practice had blended together in his mind. So, at the veterinary library, I flipped through the *Journal of the American Animal Hospital Association* from the mid-1960s to early 1970s.

In the July/August 1972 issue, I found an abstract titled "Interferon Response in Cats" about an experiment on creating interferon in cats using NDV as described by Bruce McCollough at Ohio State University. I made a copy of this and other articles and sent them to Dr. Sears. However, he insisted this was not the same article that had inspired him to try to make interferon in dogs. As he remembered it, he read about the procedure in a special handout or flyer put out by JAAHA, and it was by a different researcher and a few years earlier.

"I have never been able to find the original article," he wrote to me. "Nor have my friends at [U.C.] Davis been able to find it in the library."

A letter I wrote to JAAHA asking about the existence of a special handout or flyer on the subject went unanswered.

The full paper by McCollough had been published in the *Journal of Infectious Diseases* in February 1972. In the opening paragraph, it reads, "Although the interferon response has been investigated in several animal species, no reports on the interferon response of the cat have been published." The article had been originally submitted for publication in March 1971 and resubmitted in August 1971. (McCollough 1972)[107]

It also reported "the interferon levels in serum were found to be markedly elevated in **specific-pathogen-free** cats within 6 hr after iv stimulation by NDV."

Despite the confusion, it seemed reasonable to me Dr. Sears read about this area of research sometime around 1972 and decided to make interferon in dogs using NDV then. To me, the inability to produce the actual article as he remembers it does not take away from his discovery. It may still exist, but it has not yet been found.

But then, I asked another question. Why hadn't anybody else thought of making interferon in dogs? I went back to the library.

Specific-pathogen-free (SPF) – Laboratory
animals established to be free of particular
pathogens to ensure they do not affect
the outcome of tests.

In the March 1979 issue of the *American Journal of Veterinary Research*, I found an article titled "Interferon Induction in Dogs" and co-authored by Max Appel of Cornell University. The article described using inactivated Newcastle disease virus, B-1 strain in 3 to 7 month old Beagles and found "Serum interferon concentrations usually reached a peak by 8 hours after inoculation, rapidly declined thereafter and were nondetectable in most instances at 24 hours." (Tsai and Appel 1979)[108]

It went on to report "Blood samples were taken from jugular veins before inoculation and at 2-hour intervals from 2 to 12 hours and then at 24 and 48 hours after inoculation for interferon assay [testing]."

As Dr. Sears had done, they withdrew the dogs' blood serum at 12 hours after the NDV injection. The material in that particular sample was presumably identical to the one Dr. Sears had sent to Cornell in 1972. But they had only tested for interferon and found it lacking. And the test for interferon is in vitro – in glass tubes. They had not used that material on a dog sick with distemper.

Then again, why would they?

Without any published information about an NDV serum being used against distemper, there was no reason to try it. Dr. Sears' apparent mistake in the timing – withdrawing at 11½ to 12 hours – and in using his serum directly on a sick distemper dog seemed to have sent him off onto a tangent others in veterinary research did not follow even though they were within reach of it.

My research on distemper, measles, interferon and multiple sclerosis continued at the library and in online articles, mostly through PubMed. But again, I reviewed all of this as a tourist, not a scientist who lived with this material and mode of thinking daily.

The hope remained for someone on the research side of things to look at this and have the light bulb switch on. Would that light switch on with Dr. Harkin?

Returning to Kansas State

Clark Audiss stood in front of several round hay bales and a tall pile of loose hay. He addressed the camera:

"All right, today is August 12th 2012, and on May 8th Nilla had a treatment to cure distemper. It was experimental, but by golly it sure worked. We're just a few weeks out from going out and seeing Kansas State University. They've asked us to come back. We have an appointment with them on Sept. 10th. They're gonna take a look at Nilla and find out why she's cured. So, we want to show you how good she's doing."

The camera pans to Nilla, who stands on all four legs and pants expectantly.

"Here Nilla. Here Nilla. We're going to show you on this bale."

Clark tosses a stick for Nilla about two-thirds of the way up to the top of a big pile of hay. "Go get it. Go get it." She easily walks up the pile and picks up the stick in her mouth.

"She can climb now. Doing pretty good. Tearing it up."

She brings the stick back to Clark,

"Good girl. Good girl."

He tosses it again, this time over the top to the other side of the pile. She runs over the pile, tossing hay dust left and right.

"Boy she can tear it up," Clark said as Nilla climbed down the back side of the pile. "Hind legs are working great. She's got a little bit of bounce. C'mon dirty face! C'mon. Drop it."

She's now dusted with specs of hay.

"I'm gonna show you her running away."

He threw the stick down a dirt road. She runs for it with no problem. When she brings it back, he gives the command "Down," and Nilla lay on the ground.

"You ready? You ready? OK, go get it."

He throws the stick over the top of the pile. She pops up and runs after it, churning up another trail of hay dust.

"I don't care what you say," Clark said. "That's pretty darn good."

With two quick whistles, he calls her back. She returns, tongue panting happily, tail wagging. She shakes her head to throw off the hay.

Later I asked Clark whether Nilla could jump like she could before. She used to be able to spring up onto a horse or the four-wheeler.

"No, she doesn't have that ability," he said. "She's recovered, but she's still not 100 percent. Because of this spinal cord damage or this bounce that she has in her hind legs, it's really taken her confidence out of her to jump."

On September 9, Clark and his daughter Rachael drove to Manhattan for Nilla's appointment the next day. The intern who checked them in was someone they had not met before. They were taken into a treatment room and placed Nilla on a stainless steel exam table. As the intern asked questions to enter into her file, Dr. Harkin walked into the room.

"Where he had been unemotional before, he was clearly emotional now," Clark said with a laugh. "He grabbed her and started petting her like she was his dog. He just kept saying, 'Nilla, Oh my gosh! This is incredible.' He kept saying, 'This is amazing. This is amazing.' He was looking in her eyes and looking at her nose, looking at her paws. He opened her mouth and pressed on her gums, and he just kept saying, 'This is incredible.' "

They sat Nilla on the floor.

"And she run around a little bit," Clark said. "He got to watch her, and he says, 'Well, she still has a little bit of that leg bounce. I don't know if she'll ever come out of that.' And I said, 'Well and her vision isn't 100 percent.' And he looked at me and said, 'Yeah, but she should be dead.' "

They needed to take her away for more tests. The intern took her out into the hallway on a leash. Clark realized something unusual was happening as they walked into the busy hallway with staff veterinarians, students and other animal patients.

"They walk her down the hallway and these vets just kind of step off to the side and they are watching her go," Clark said. "It's like everybody just stopped what they were doing and watched her walk down the hallway."

Everyone stopped talking. Pin drop silence. They all knew about Nilla's case, Clark said.

Later, Dr. Harkin informed Clark the tests showed Nilla's cerebrospinal fluid – which earlier had been full of occlusions and indications of distemper – was now clear. The PCR testing of the CSF was negative for distemper. However, the conjunctiva scrape was still positive for the virus.

Again, Clark made sure to talk to Dr. Harkin before they left Kansas State.

"I said, 'Dr. Harkin, is this a good thing?' He said, 'Yes, Clark, this is a very good thing.'

"I said, 'Is this going to go somewhere or is this going to die here?'

"He said, 'I can guarantee you, Clark. This is not going to die here.'

"He said, 'We're going to do something with this.'

"I said, 'What is your next course of action?'

"He says, 'We need to study this further, and we need to evaluate it, we need to write about it, we need to get funding and things like that.'

"I said, 'I know for a fact that Ed Bond has got distemper cases, right now, that he's getting calls about. And Dr. Sears is getting calls about distemper cases all the time. Do you want these cases? Can they start sending these people to you?'

"And he says, 'Yeah. Yeah.' He said that what they wanted was about eight cases, is what he told me. If they could get this treated with eight cases, then they'd have enough to write a paper or publish it or something. And that would generate enough interest he thought, that they could get funding."

The entire adventure with Nilla became a source of inspiration for the Audiss family and their faith.

"I'm starting my pastoral career," Clark told me. "This has been one of my greatest sermons is this story about Nilla and the journey. And it's been very inspiring to people that God has a plan for their life. It's been pretty cool. Our family, we're very humbled that this had happened."

I asked him what he uses as the closer to wrap up his main sermon about Nilla.

"We only see the little picture," he said. "We see with tunnel vision. And when I started this process, you understand that all I could see was my dog. All I could see was how can I make my dog well. And God had a whole different plan. He not only wanted to make my dog well. But he wanted to touch a young man's life in a youth group. He wanted to confound the wisdom of the doctors. He wanted to use the foolish things of the world to confound the wise. Do you see what I'm saying?

"He wanted to increase the faith of my son and I and my whole family. And God worked this on multiple levels. That's how God works because he sees the big picture. He not only sees the big picture for the dog. He sees the big picture for you and me, you know, in our life. There's a big picture, and we have a tendency to only look two-dimensional and God is like six dimensional. You know what I mean. He's like all these different levels he hits things on because he's got the big picture."

Working My Way
Out Of A Job

"I'm dipping my toe into the water, not diving into the deep end," Dr. Harkin told me when we talked on the phone. I'd been hoping Nilla's recovery could lead to a broader study of the NDV serum or NDV as IV, but Dr. Harkin had no interest. He'd read the research that some dogs who get distemper can clear the disease on their own without going into the neurologic stage.

To prove a pre-neurologic treatment was making a difference, he said, it would take hundreds of dogs treated in a **double-blind study** to tell whether the serum was useful. The recovery of a dog not in neurologic stage was not interesting to him. Instead, he just wanted to treat 8 to 12 dogs in the neurologic stage of distemper with the NDV spinal tap so he could submit a paper.

Double-blind study – When neither the researcher nor the subject knows which type of treatment has been received until after clinical trial is over.

C-peptides – A material that aids in the formation of insulin.

Again, I had been getting ahead of myself.

But then he told me about three other initials: BCG.

In August 2012, a study on the use of the BCG vaccine against diabetes had been published. (Faustman et al. 2012)[109] The bacillus Calmette–Guérin vaccine – from a bacteria – is used against tuberculosis, mostly outside of the U.S. Ten years earlier, researchers at Harvard Medical School and Massachusetts General Hospital had shown the BCG vaccine helped diabetic mice by blocking the immune responses that cause diabetes.

The 2012 study had been conducted on adult humans in a double-blind, placebo controlled trial of adults with long-term type 1 diabetes, a good example of the steps needed to establish proper controls. It also is an example of the kinds of measures that would be needed to demonstrate the effectiveness of NDV against distemper.

In the study, six insulin-dependent adults received either two doses of BCG or two fake vaccinations. The two groups were compared to one another, also to 57 diabetes patients, and to 16 people without diabetes. The study found that autoimmune cells responsible for the disease died in subjects treated with BCG. This also allowed a regeneration of the pancreas and a boost in the **C-peptides**, which indicate levels of insulin.

Oddly enough, even one of the placebo subjects – the control group that were not treated with BCG – showed improvement. The researchers realized this was because the patient had been infected with mononucleosis after entering the study. Mononucleosis –also called the Epstein-Barr virus – is also known to be an immune inducer.

As a treatment, BCG would require diabetes patients to receive lifetime injections, but the researchers concluded the patients could withstand such injections. The study also offered another example of using a pathogen to treat a disease.

While I was disappointed Dr. Harkin had no interest in a broader study on the NDV serum, I couldn't deny the logic of a small study on just the NDV spinal tap. To this day, I still hear of vets who aren't sure they have a distemper case until the neurologic stage begins. The response from many vets who hear of dogs treated before the neurological stage is often "Well, that wasn't distemper." That's a criticism Dr. Sears heard throughout his career. There also seems to be debate and questions about the reliability of diagnosis through lab results.

With a study of 8 to 12 dogs in the neurological stage of the disease, Dr. Harkin could focus on indisputable facts. Tests of the cerebrospinal fluid might show whether NDV had an effect or not in cases where the distemper diagnosis is not disputed.

I emailed Dr. Sears about Dr. Harkin's plan.

"Interesting," he replied. "Why would they not be interested in acute distemper? Lots more cases, and many more dogs dying. Oh well, I shall take what I can get. Any little bit helps."

This could help him tremendously. If Dr. Harkin had a successful study, that would at least put Dr. Sears on the map. Other researchers might take a closer look at NDV and distemper. Perhaps it might allow me – or someone else – to give a tap on the shoulder at another vet school. Or perhaps Kansas State might want to keep pursuing the possibilities?

Yet again, I keep getting ahead of myself ... crossing bridges before I get there ... counting chickens before they hatch ... insert your favorite adage about expectations and how they don't usually work out ... here.

I'm also putting all my eggs into one basket.

Dr. Harkin needed to follow the science as he saw best. That had been the hope all along, that someone on the research side of things would look at these protocols and evaluate them on their own terms. Still, I had the same worry I did when Nilla was being treated. Not all dogs improve after the NDV spinal tap. From my informal stats, at least half still die.

For now, we just had to get more dogs to Kansas State. The rest was up to Dr. Harkin.

That conversation with Dr. Harkin happened in September 2012. In the next few months, I would also be launching an iOS app, evacuating my mom from Hurricane Sandy, replacing a smashed car and undergoing surgery. Fortunately, I had become efficient at answering a lot of email about distemper in my spare time.

Unfortunately, we had a problem of geography. While distemper cases can happen anywhere, the disease spreads more readily in warm climates. This makes sense, as dogs are more likely to roam and interact with strays or canid wildlife in warm weather.

So, in the continental United States, most cases happen in the south and west – Florida, Texas and California. Less often, I hear about cases in the Northeast and Northwest. Emails also came in from Canada now and then. However, the vets who were willing to give NDV a try also were in these warmer climates. My thinking is they were the ones being overwhelmed with a lot of cases, had grown tired of euthanasia and were willing to try anything to prevent the death of a dog.

This was why the story of Nilla had been so amazing to me: a dog already in neurologic distemper in South Dakota – on a weekend – and more than a thousand miles from the closest vet willing to use the NDV spinal tap. Clark Audiss performed a minor miracle in finding an open door at Kansas State, but now that open door was more than a thousand miles from the highest concentrations of distemper cases.

In mid-January 2013, I checked in with Dr. Harkin again:

"In the past few months since we talked, I have had a couple dozen owners of dogs with neuro distemper contact me who were within a day's drive of Kansas State. These have ranged from Kansas/Missouri area to Colorado, New Mexico, Oklahoma, northern Texas. I think a couple were as far away as Arizona and Michigan. Have any shown up at your door?"

His reply: "I haven't had a single one show up. I've talked to 4, but none ended up making the trip."

The next day, Clark Audiss gave me a call. Nilla had a seizure.

It was her first seizure. All I could recommend was to contact his local vet and update Dr. Harkin. They might need to put her on an anti-seizure medication. Many post-NDV spinal tap dogs are prescribed with phenobarbital. But for now, this appeared to be a one-time event.

California investigates

A week later, a crisis erupted in California. Through my contacts on Facebook, I heard from a dog rescuer that the only vet using NDV in California was being investigated by the state of California. He now had to drop the NDV treatments too.

His license and career hung in the balance.

"Is there anything I can do to help?" I wrote to him. "I can have owners of dogs who you've helped write letters of support."

I also told him about the potential for research at Kansas State.

"Thanks for reaching out," he replied. "I meant to contact you and let you know. I'm still waiting to hear back from the state board. I think it will be ok, but the state vet had never heard of NDV."

He told me a former employee had filed a claim with the state, alleging the NDV spinal tap amounted to torturing dogs and doing experiments on animals just to make money.

"I would love if you could have some clients write letters on my behalf," he said. "I will get you the investigator's number and if you could call him that would be great. Also if Kansas state could call them that would help too. I will get you his number. Thanks again for checking in. Oh and until this clears I have decided not to do the treatment. Unfortunately I just don't want to risk my license. I will keep you posted."

When he sent me the name and phone number of the investigator with the California Department of Consumer Affairs, I decided to wait a day to gather my thoughts.

The next morning, Amy drove me to the doctor's office to get the cast taken off my foot. This was not the liberating experience I expected. The ligaments had stiffened from lack of use. Every time I moved, I felt winded, tired, sore and disoriented.

"I don't think I will represent the cause well on the phone today," I wrote to the vet. "But I feel confident I will feel better by Monday and will take care of this then."

When I called Monday, the investigator had gone on vacation. So, in the meantime, I sent the vet copies of NDV research I had found and contacted former clients to write letters of support.

"At no time was I ever a witness to any cruel or unusual treatment of any of the animals..." Pamela Nabors of Santa Cruz wrote to the investigator about the vet's treatment of her Border Collie, Mojave in July 2011. "In fact, I was very reassured by the love, gentle treatment, and caring attitudes towards all of the pets in [his] care. I was even allowed to spend time with Mojave during his recovery phase and again observed the wonderful and patient care given to every pet. ... I now have, at almost two years post treatment, a very healthy, active, and distemper free Border Collie thanks to [him] and his team of excellent caregivers."

By the time I reached the investigator on the phone on Feb. 12, he had already received a stack of info and research papers from me – including the papers by Dr. Adams at UCLA – 7 or 8 letters of support had been sent from clients, and I gave him Dr. Harkin's phone number at Kansas State. We had a reasonable and pleasant conversation about the history of NDV. Mostly, he was grateful to have someone explain this procedure he had not heard of before, and he told me he would pass along the information to the state Veterinary Review Board.

Despite the good mood of the investigator when I called, this did not mean all would turn out well. As I wrote to Dr. Sears a couple days later, "Sometimes when people are happy to see you, it isn't good news for you, but simply good news for them in that you made their jobs easier."

Seeing a vet under threat for using the treatment was nothing new to Dr. Sears. This is why many just stay with the standard protocols. "The euthanol is always close and available and ethical," he said.

The crisis had been dealt with as much as possible for now. But it would loom over our heads, and the NDV treatments had yet again lost the only willing vet in California. We would not know the outcome of the investigation for more than three years.

Unexpected progress

So far, Dr. Harkin still had not had any takers show up at his door. Between mid-January and mid-March, I had sent his information to about 20 owners of dogs in neurologic distemper who had written to me from around the country. I was not publicly posting this option on the websites or social media. For now, we were keeping this treatment opportunity quiet. It was only as a private referral via email to owners of dogs in neurologic distemper who might benefit from the NDV spinal tap. Some sought treatment closer to home when they could find it; others sought other options, and some just never replied.

The cost and the travel expenses were probably a factor. Any of these owners who would opt for the treatment would have to pay for the entire procedure out of pocket. Kind Hearts In Action had about $2,000 in the bank, and at this time I was still holding onto the hope of getting the Mountain View data published. But Jim Radke had explained how steep that climb would be. I needed to be conservative with the money.

Ideally, I'd reply to everyone who contacted me with the same help I gave Clark Audiss. Something like: "Kind Hearts In Action will pay travel expenses and half of the veterinary services for every dog treated with the NDV spinal tap at Kansas State." But that would zero out our account within a handful of cases. Indecision handcuffed the cause as I pondered what to do.

Part of the reason I helped Clark was because he specifically asked for help, because he had the obvious willingness to get to Kansas State and the money was the only obstacle. With money as the only obstacle, I was glad to help.

On Tuesday, March 19, as my physical therapist evaluated my foot, my phone's text alert went off from inside my jacket. When I dug out the phone later, I found a message from Clark Audiss:

"Nilla jumped into a tall feedbunk 2x today!"

Once again, the South Dakota border collie made my day. My phone did not save my reply of congratulations. But a few minutes later, he followed up:

"Yeah, she got her confidence back and that was all it took!"

Nilla's progress reminded me the successes from the past will sometimes return to help you. Sometimes, in ways you never would have suspected.

The physical therapy slowly brought back flexibility and strength to my foot. The pain lessened somewhat, and they transitioned me to regular exercise equipment and recommended I join a local gym.

On May 13, I checked my email before heading out to the Planet Fitness in Horseheads, and found a slightly cryptic message from Elizabeth Nelson of San Antonio, Texas.

> "Hi Ed,
>
> "How are you???? I've missed corresponding with you but I'm sure you agree that it's good that we haven't needed to talk about dogs with distemper for a while. ... I emailed Dr. Sears at ... Is this still his email? My number is ... and I'd really like to talk with him about a study of the serum that I've been following. I'm hoping you have his phone number and you could give him a call and ask him to call me. Thanks Ed, Elizabeth"

Elizabeth had first written to me in April 2011 about her Chihuahua mix, Bella, who came down with distemper but survived after being treated with the NDV serum and the NDV spinal tap. We posted a story and video of Bella on the Kind Hearts In Action website, and Elizabeth had a hand in coordinating treatment for a few other cases in Texas. She is a passionate animal lover who has been one of my trusted advisers. We'd also discussed strategies to get acceptance for the NDV protocols.

So, her use of the word "study" caught my eye.

My reply: "I'm fine. As always, answering e-mails from all over the world. I believe the best e-mail for Dr. Sears now is ... Who is doing this study of the serum?"

Her reply:

> "Thanks Ed. I just emailed Dr. Sears. Not trying to hide anything but I'm very excited and thought Dr. Sears should be the first to know. I also assume he'll call or email you right away about this. If I'm wrong let me know. I haven't told anyone about this because I didn't want to have a big disappointment to report. It's been so hard to wait and I know you will want to help any way you can now that it's going forward. I just think Dr. Sears deserves to be the person to tell you about it. Does he read his emails often?"

I told her that sometimes it takes a while to reply if he is traveling. Then I left for my workout at Planet Fitness. It made sense to let Dr. Sears be the first to hear the news, whatever it was. But I could think of nothing else as my legs pumped away at the elliptical machine.

That evening, Dr. Sears sent me a copy of Elizabeth's email. "I also mentioned to you that I was very serious in pursuing a clinical trial for the serum," she wrote to him. "Well, it's been a long road but I didn't give up."

During her battle to save Bella, Elizabeth had spoken to Dr. Sears about what was needed to get his treatment accepted. He had told her about the need for researchers to put the serum to the test and publish the results. She had mentioned this to a friend, who had a friend at Texas A&M, who knew of a veterinary professor at a Midwestern university who researched canine distemper.

"I've waited a long time to be able to happily tell you that he has used the serum successfully in this clinical trial," Elizabeth wrote. "I just found out today and thought you should be the first to know. The problem is that the treated dogs continue to test positive for the virus (one in particular for 9 months) even though they are healthy. So the study is ongoing and has great potential. My number is … Once again I congratulate you on your discovery and your tireless work in helping dogs with distemper. Thank you Dr. Sears, Elizabeth Nelson"

The next day, I received an email from Dr. Sears:

"Ed, got a chance to talk with Dr. […] [110] Very interesting man. Has already used the serum successfully. Is working on more data. Just what we need. A professor of Vet med. He would like to talk with you. So, at your convenience give him a call."

I called and emailed and received a reply.

"Sorry I missed your call. I was out of town giving a seminar. Thank you also for your email. I will be gone all next week but would like to talk to you about some of the information you have on treatment of CDV and some of the studies we have done recently and those we plan to do. I will call you during the week of May 27."

This professor was studying the NDV serum in pre-neurologic cases. The academic world was now looking at both sides of Dr. Sears' protocols.

My mind kept playing a scene from the end of "Return of the Jedi." The rebels are losing, but Admiral Akbar orders a concentrated attack on the Superstar Destroyer. The attack succeeds and the disabled ship loses control and crashes onto the surface of the Death Star. As it explodes, the entire rebel fleet cheers!

But, the battle was still not over. Oddly, I never got the call back from that professor. None of my emails or phone calls to him were returned after that day.

I checked in on Dr. Harkin to ask about his progress.

"I had one recently from our area," he replied. "I also had 3 from Alabama ~6-8 weeks ago. That's it, though. I just submitted a research grant for a pilot study, so we'll see if that gets funded. It will provide for a small incentive."

That would solve a major problem. If the grant funded the cost of treatments, then the only obstacle would be the costs of travel for someone coming from far away.

Then, there was a question about what to do about the Mountain View data. I gave Jim Radke a call to update him on the situation with Kansas State and the new study on the NDV serum. We agreed my Project Carré efforts were now unnecessary. Best to leave it in the hands of the professionals. Later, I sent an email to Mountain View to thank them for all their help and let them know the project was being shelved. I packed the records into a box next to my desk.

The remainder of the Project Carré funds could be used to help dog owners get to Kansas State. But that would be on a case-by-case basis if they expressed a need, showed they were otherwise willing to get there and the money was the only thing holding them back. It also depended on Dr. Harkin getting funding for his study approved.

In July, I dropped an email to Elizabeth Nelson to thank her and let her know I still had not had any reply from her professor. We agreed that sometimes it is just difficult to get in touch and stay in touch with vets and researchers. All we could do was wait for news.

This would take time, and I had to learn to be patient. "You can't turn the ship of medicine that quickly," Dr. Sears had said once.

"You've helped me have patience and given me hope on many occasions," Elizabeth Nelson wrote to me. "Please don't drop your efforts completely – I, like you, have to sit and wait to see what happens."

"No, I won't be dropping this entirely any time soon," I told her. "My plan is to hold firm with what I've been doing – answering every email as quickly as possible and networking in whatever way becomes available – up until the day it is published. After it is published, the strategy will switch to a straight-out public information campaign, which I will be pushing for at least a year afterwards. But at the same time, I think a lot of bigger groups will be willing to step in and take over the load, and I won't be needed for much longer. And that is my long-term plan – to basically work my way out of a job!"

I waited until September to contact Dr. Harkin again. His reply:

"No, I haven't seen any in quite a while. Had a few calls, but none of them ever turned into visits. ... Although the research committee was interested, in the end they decided not to fund a clinical study. I have decided to evaluate a few more cases and obtain more clinical data (if we ever see any) before re-submitting a proposal to a different granting agency. Also, I wish you would present this differently to people that call you. When they call here they all think we have a study on-going, which makes them think they are going to get something for free. That's not the case. I've agreed to do the NDV treatment on dogs with ODE, but it's not a study per se."

Nuts. Nuts. Nuts. Obviously, I'd done a poor job of explaining things. I made a note to clarify the situation to the dog owners. As always, people needed to have the proper information going into these treatments. Anything less is just a waste of time. I mulled over the situation some more over the next couple of weeks and came up with another suggestion for Dr. Harkin:

"I was thinking about the grant you applied for, and I had a thought. Would it be OK or appropriate if I pursued my own contacts within the non-profit world to help get you the funding you need for a study? This would by no means be any kind of public campaign, but really just some quiet networking to find the people who can help push this over the finish line. I once was a college professor and a chair for a journalism department, so I have some experience in dealing with bureaucracies, applying for grants and dealing with complex applications.

"I just can't help thinking that there must be
someone out there who will see the value in this
and help bring all the elements together.
Let me know if that makes sense to you."

His reply:

"Sure, I'd be happy to get targeted donations
which could then be used specifically for this type
of research. That certainly would help drive some
of the preliminary studies that need to be done. A
shelter near Wichita had a big CDV outbreak a
couple of weeks ago. I didn't find out until all of
the dogs were put down (I think a problem was
that they were looking for something exotic and
didn't even consider distemper until the
necropsies were done). Still, if we had funding for
a project that was known within the college, at
least when the first of those dogs were being
submitted it might have prompted a pathologist to
contact me before all the dogs were put down."

He estimated about $50,000 would be enough to launch a
pilot study. I began searching for a source. It only took me a
couple of weeks because I'd laid the groundwork a couple of
years earlier. Back in August of 2011, when I'd been searching
for funding for Project Carré, I had made contact with a handful
of foundations that politely informed me they would only work
with proposals from university veterinary programs. One of
these had been Maddie's Fund, a family foundation, which
strives to help dogs by funding veterinary research. They began
with a $300 million endowment and had disbursed $118 million
so far. According to their website:

"Dave and Cheryl Duffield founded Maddie's Fund to honor their sweet yet feisty and spirited dog. It's the fulfillment of a promise made to Maddie while playing together on the living room rug, that if they ever had any money, they would give back to her and her kind, so that other families could experience the immense joy they have with her. And the rest, as they say, is history."[111]

So in October 2013, I reconnected with them to let them know about the possible Kansas State study. This time, my email was met with more interest but I was told again that the application would have to come from the professor himself. I passed along the information to Dr. Harkin so he could act on it as he saw fit.

I forwarded this news to my sister, Jane with the words, "Making progress ... I feel like I earned my pay today. I hope it works out."

Of course, that's a low bar. My canine distemper work pays nothing.

"Really terrific," she replied. "Wonderful to connect these dots!"

Distemper around the world and in my backyard

The marketing and communications director for the USA Bobsled and Skeleton team emailed me in March 2014 about a 2-month old puppy she had rescued at the Sochi Olympics in Russia. Amanda Bird of Nashville, Tennessee, rescued the shepherd-mix pup just before the Russian authorities carried out a massive extermination of the street dogs of Sochi.

A news producer flew the puppy back to the U.S. for her, but the puppy fell ill and was diagnosed with parvovirus. Then as Sochi, the puppy, recovered during its mandated quarantine in Los Angeles, he was diagnosed with distemper. "I am sobbing as a write this," Amanda wrote. "This dog, our dog, doesn't know enough about love yet. He doesn't know what home feels like. He just has to make it through this, too!"

She had found the Kind Hearts In Action website through the Jason Debus Heigl Foundation, which had been paying for Sochi's treatment. With their help, the vets caring for Sochi agreed to use the NDV treatment and Sochi recovered. I later heard the vets treating Sochi were not convinced the NDV saved his life, but he successfully completed his quarantine in L.A. and finally joined Amanda in Nashville.

As I looked at the pattern of distemper cases occurring around the world, one thought kept coming up. The odds were that eventually I'd hear about a case right here in my backyard, in my part of Upstate New York. What would happen then? Would I be able to help? Would it open another door for us?

The chance came in early April with an email from a senior at Cornell University who is from China. "Lizzy"[112] wrote on a Sunday night:

> "I'm [Lizzy], currently a senior student from Cornell University and I reside in Ithaca, New York, US. My dog, Ranger, has been diagnosed as having distemper three days ago. He is a 4-month old Siberian husky, very cute and smart, so I'm doing anything I can to help him fight this disease. Unfortunately, by the time he is diagnosed, he had developed neurological signs such as twitches and unsteady walk ... My boyfriend and I are very upset to find out that Ranger has distemper, but we strongly believe he will be able to recover from this disease. Time is so precious at this stage for Ranger. So if you see my email, would you please contact me as soon as possible?"

I emailed her all the information on the protocols and contacts I had. Then I called them. Just as with Clark Audiss, Lizzy and her boyfriend faced an uphill battle. They would have to knock on doors to find a vet or facility willing and able to perform the NDV spinal tap. I told them that if it became possible for Cornell Vet School to perform the procedure, Kind Hearts In Action would help with the expenses.

When they contacted me, Ranger was a patient at a private vet clinic in Ithaca. Cornell Vet School had seen Ranger 10 days earlier, but the distemper test then was negative. But later on, a test from a lab at Michigan State declared him positive for distemper. The next day, they asked the local vet clinic to perform the NDV spinal tap.

At first, the clinic refused their request. The practice manager would not approve of an unpublished treatment. Again, malpractice worries loomed over their decision.

Then, a small surprise. The practice manager called me to ask how to get the NDV. We talked briefly, and it seemed like they might change their mind. But then ultimately they decided not to perform the procedure. They referred the case to Cornell.

While Lizzy and her boyfriend took Ranger to Cornell, I couldn't really do much else for them. The owners are the ones with authority to make decisions about the care of their animal. But the reporter in me wanted to try any options. However, I found that as a matter of policy the switchboard operator at Cornell Vet School would not allow me to connect with the vet they were seeing. An email I sent was not answered. Again, I have no standing within the veterinary community.

Not surprisingly, the vet they saw at Cornell would not perform the unpublished treatment. Instead, the vet offered to perform a published treatment: Botox injections.

According to the paper published in JAAHA a year earlier:

"A 13 mo old spayed female mixed-breed dog presented in a nonambulatory state that was attributed to severe **myoclonus** secondary to distemper. The authors hypothesized that mitigating the myoclonus would help the dog become ambulatory and expedite convalescence. They injected the severely affected muscles with botulinum toxin on two separate occasions over a period of 18 days. Those injections reduced the myoclonus, helping the dog become ambulatory and attaining a comfortable, functional state." (Schubert et al. 2013)[113]

Myoclonus—A sudden, involuntary jerking of a muscle or a group of muscles

But it would cost up to $4,000 to hospitalize and treat Ranger under that plan.

Instead, they took Ranger down to Mountain View for the NDV spinal tap. They got to Woodlawn on Wednesday. Lizzy texted a photo of Ranger, saying, "Sending Ranger's greeting to you!"

I replied: "Hey Ranger! Hang in there buddy!"

On Friday, I heard from Lizzy: "Morning. :D he's still in the hospital and recovering from that. He walked out of his cage by himself yesterday and ate a little bit."

The next day, I drove up to Ithaca for a Saturday morning meeting about getting the book published. Afterwards, I sat down to a lunch in a courtyard of the Ithaca Commons when I got a text from Lizzy that Mountain View called. Ranger was eating and drinking and walking a lot more. "They think the result is amazing!" she wrote.

This put an image in my head: Lizzy and her boyfriend take Ranger back to their vet in Ithaca for a follow-up visit. They let the vets there see the dramatic recovery. Perhaps nothing would even need to be said, but the word would get back to Cornell that Ranger had recovered after treatment with the NDV spinal tap.

But then on Monday, I learned Ranger died.

When Nilla was about to be treated, my hope had been she'd be a survivor in this 50-50 coin flip. With Ranger, the coin had landed the other way. As I often tell dog owners, distemper is a terrible, nasty disease that does not play fair.

Mountain View buried Ranger for them. Kind Hearts In Action paid the vet bill of more than $600 and helped with the travel expenses. They had not opened the door to Cornell Vet School, but they had enough faith in the cause to try. I was grateful to them.

"Although Ranger did not make it, I still appreciate your help," Lizzy texted me a few days later.

A seismic shift

At about the same time Lizzy and her boyfriend fought to save Ranger's life and Sochi struggled through his quarantine in Los Angeles, I learned about cracks opening in the veterinary doctrine that distemper dogs could not be saved. This shift did not mean the NDV treatments were openly accepted, but they were beginning to be treated fairly. More importantly, experts came forward to publicly assert dogs did not have to die from distemper and shelters did not have to "depopulate" – kill every dog in a facility – when an outbreak occurred.

In a webinar from March 13, 2014 – posted to YouTube on April 9 – Maddie's Institute posted a lecture by Dr. Cynda Crawford, DVM, Ph.D., of the Maddie's Shelter Medicine Program at the University of Florida: "Everything Shelters Need to Know About Canine Distemper." [114]

Her webinar explained how to use testing to distinguish between vaccine-induced and active levels of distemper titers, how to prevent transmission of the disease throughout a shelter, how to save shelter dogs from distemper without euthanizing the entire shelter and how long after a distemper attack a dog could be expected to shed a virus and be infectious.

Dr. Crawford answered many of the questions and issues I knew rescue groups and dog owners all over the world worry about. Her lecture clarified a lot of areas of confusion, and I would encourage everyone to go watch it online. She said:

> "We have heard for many years distemper is a death sentence. What we've heard is that there is no way no way dogs can survive this without some heroic effort, and even with the heroic effort they are still likely to die. So don't try to save them. But thanks to some pioneering shelter vets ... we now know dogs can survive distemper infection and become a normal pet, doing all the things that pets do in life. These pioneers have shown us that it is possible to treat and save distemper dogs. Our program has had the good fortune to help shelters, rescues groups and community veterinarians treat and save hundreds of infected dogs taken from out of shelter outbreaks. You see, I was one of those who believed that distemper in a dog means death, but after working with distemper outbreaks, using intervention strategies, listening to the pioneers who know that you can treat and save dogs, I have really had my eyes opened to what can be accomplished with time and supportive treatment ... We should change our outlook about distemper and look for treatment options either within the shelter or out in the community including foster homes, rescue groups and community practices to save more of these dogs. In other words, we should start thinking about what we can do for each dog during a distemper outbreak instead of focusing entirely on what to do at the population level."

Dr. Crawford went into much detail about how dogs can survive distemper and the biosecurity measures to keep the virus from transmitting through the shelter. But the simplest answer would be to send the sick dogs to a foster home where they could be cared for without endangering other dogs. She also went into detail about which testing kits shelters could use on site to get immediate results on viral infections. I would also encourage everyone interested to go to the The Maddie's Fund website, which holds a wealth of information about saving the lives of shelter animals. [115]

In the Question and Answer section at the end of Dr. Crawford's lecture, someone in the audience asked her opinion about the NDV treatments. This paralleled the encounter Dr. Sears had with Dr. Ott in the early 1970s. I listened to her reply through my computer, bracing myself, head in my hands:

> "I am very well informed about this Newcastle disease vaccine practice for the treatment of distemper infected dogs. The Newcastle virus is a virus that infects chickens not dogs, but the chicken virus is very closely related to the dog distemper virus. They are in the same virus family. I don't really understand the rationale for injecting distemper infected dogs either with the Newcastle chicken vaccine itself or serum from dogs that have received this chicken vaccine. The thought is that there are antiviral factors in either the serum from the vaccinated dogs transferred to the infected dogs that can kill the virus or the chicken vaccine that is injected into the infected dogs induces the formation of antiviral factors within hours that effectively kill the virus. There are no controlled studies to demonstrate the efficacy of this approach. So, we don't have any evidence one way or the other that it works or does not work.

> "I know that there are veterinarians that use this
> method and they feel it has been successful in
> their hands. So, I personally have not used it. So,
> it's hard for me to make a comment whether it's
> good or whether it's baloney."

I looked up, took a breath, relieved. Her answer had been fair and rational. She didn't declare it impossible, just that it had not been proven. I also had hope that very soon data from academic studies of the NDV treatments might come forward. Either way, the tide of the battle to save the lives of distemper dogs appeared to be turning. Distemper was no longer universally viewed as a death sentence.[116]

In another video I found, posted by Maddie's Institute from a Shelter Medicine Conference at the University of Florida in October 2012, Dr. Ellen Jefferson explained in detail how dogs can be saved from distemper. Dr. Jefferson is the executive director of Austin Pets Alive in Texas and she explained their approach to get a distemper dog through the disease by addressing each symptom as it arises, even into the neurologic stage.

The vet and owner/rescue does not give up so long as the dog is eating, breathing, able to move and without overwhelming seizures. It also depended on how well the foster owner of the dog handles the stress of caring for the dog. Recovery may take a couple of months or more, and euthanasia would be used only in rare cases. "Where there is life, there's hope," she said. Again, I would encourage everyone to look up the video.[117]

Of interest to me, she told the audience they did treat distemper dogs with NDV. She did not believe the NDV helpful, but all the same, they were willing to give it a try mostly because the dog owners and rescuers kept finding the information on the Internet:

"There's zero really good evidence to prove that it's helpful in any way, shape or form. We started using it because we felt like when we were having the outbreak and we had so many people invested in these animals, so many fosters invested in each individual. They always find it on the Internet. So we were just like, all right fine, if you get some we'll try it because we don't know what our success rate on saving these dogs is anyway, why not try it? And what we found is that it's not dangerous, we've had zero side effects from it. I don't think it helps, but interestingly the 24 hours after we give it IV they seem to be better. And I don't know if it's just the stimulation of coming to the vet clinic and getting a shot, or if it's truly related to the Newcastle, but it definitely doesn't have any long lasting effects that I can tell. Of course, some of these animals made it, and it could be because of the Newcastle, but I don't think so. We do the IV and then we have not … we've done the serum I think on a couple of dogs but not since then. And there is somebody in Austin [White Angel] that does the spinal injection and we sent five dogs there, they were all funded through Chipins, and three of them survived. Again, I don't know if it was related to that."

At the end of the talk, she presented a case study of Reba, a dog who had been rescued in March 2010. Reba had been hit by a car and did not get vaccinated because of a fractured leg. She developed a fever and sniffles. After surgery for her leg, she became weak and wobbly and paranoid. Her back legs became paralyzed, and she had seizures.

They suspected distemper and began a treatment that included Newcastle vaccine, antibiotics and anti-seizure medication. A month after the neurologic problems began, the foster owner noticed movement in one of the rear legs. They began physical therapy. Dr. Jefferson played a video of Reba at physical therapy – walking on an underwater treadmill in a tank of water. Her motor function on the rear legs slowly came back.

"And we kept going, but you know, the question is – why did we keep going?" Dr. Jefferson said. "And again, every day, this dog would eat. And you're like, when she gets to the point – the foster and I would talk – when she gets to the point that she doesn't feel like eating, then that's when we need to call it. And she kept eating. Every day, she kept eating."

Eventually, Reba regained the ability to walk on all four legs. Dr. Jefferson played another video from 2011 as Reba trots down a hill to a small body of water.

"It's the outcome you hope for when you go through so much pain and suffering and they go through so much pain and suffering," she said.

Reba wades into the shallow water, panting and happily wagging her tail.

"She's not normal, but she's pretty close," she said.

The audience applauds as the video ends. I applaud too. I am always happy to see a dog survive this disease.

Good news for Dr. Sears

In May 2014, I heard through J.D. Ward that Dr. Sears had a heart episode. He emailed me later to say his doctors had implanted a heart stent. "It has been a week," he wrote. "Seems to be doing well. Doc says I dodged a bullet. Problem is all the blood thinners I'm taking have me bruising like a prize fighter. Drop in blood pressure is dramatic. Down about 30 points. However, no pain. If Doc correct then I'm good for another couple of years. Here is hoping. Still getting lots of inquires. Sending all to you. Thanks for the help. People are slowly learning there are cures for the incurable. Doc.'

Had he not dodged that bullet, I would not have been able to share with him the some good news, which came in June. I received this email from Dr. Harkin:

> "Just wanted you to know that the Maddie's Fund decided to fully fund the study evaluating changes in blood and CSF cytokines in dogs with canine distemper encephalitis following treatment with the Newcastle Virus vaccine. Funds should be available in the next 2-3 weeks, after which I'll begin recruiting cases. I have funding to completely support the treatment of 10 dogs, so long as the pet owner agrees to return for the follow-up testing, otherwise they are responsible for all costs incurred up to that point. I'm going to try and recruit from local practices, which should be sufficient, but if you hear from anyone that lives relatively close that wants to pursue therapy, please direct them my way.
> I anticipate that if recruitment goes well I should be able to finish this study within 8-12 months and hope to present this at the ACVIM [American College of Veterinary Internal Medicine] meeting prior to publication. I'll let Dr. Sears know, too."

Not long after this, I received this email from Dr. Sears:

> "Ed, finally someone of stature is taking a longer look at my procedure. Thought you might like to see this. ... Dr. Harkin with a note this AM and suddenly things are looking up. All of this might yet possibly be adopted by the Vet profession at some time. And then, my sincere hope is that the Medical profession will pick up on it for the treatment of Measles and MS in humans. Keep the faith. Doc"

The emails kept coming in from around the world. Even though I could not help many of those in the most exotic locations, the messages taught me a lot about geography. Dog owners had written me from wherever they could make an Internet connection: Mongolia, China – mainland, Hong Kong and Taiwan – Nigeria, Nepal, Thailand, Malaysia, Cambodia, Vietnam, Sri Lanka, Mauritius (an island in the Indian Ocean), Peru, Brazil, Colombia, Venezuela, etc.

My system had gotten faster and more efficient over the years. Blocks of text had been saved to my email so that if, say, someone emailed from the Philippines with a dog in the pre-neurologic stage of the disease, I could quickly copy/paste the key information with contact information and protocols. But the Philippines are made up of more than 7,000 islands (at low tide), and options were limited on many of the remote islands far from the capital, Manila.

Occasionally, someone would write and assume I was a vet or tried to get me to diagnose their dog. I always knocked that down in my replies. Sometimes people also reposted my reply on the Internet, causing trouble because that included private information and identified the vets using NDV who did not want to be known publicly. So, the signature on my outgoing Gmail messages became quite lengthy:

> "I am not a veterinarian or a doctor. The information I've sent is based on the discoveries of Dr. Alson Sears, but my e-mail is not meant to replace the care, evaluation and diagnosis of your pet by a qualified vet. These websites are a resource on Dr. Sears' discoveries, which can be used by other vets to save the lives of dogs. I can help explain the theories behind these discoveries, but when matters get too technical, I will refer you to a vet or another resource. More about Ed Bond: **http://kindheartsinaction.com/archives/870**

Please do not post this e-mail elsewhere on the
Internet. If you would like to help spread the
word about these treatments, please circulate my
e-mail address and the URL for Kind Hearts In
Action: **http://www.kindheartsinaction.com/**or
any of the Web pages on the site. Thanks!
How effective is NDV? Read our report
here: **http://kindheartsinaction.com/2011/03/24/re
port-on-effectiveness-of-ndv-treatments/**…"

Batman and Robin

Sometimes, a quick email would result in an unexpected
ally, even if we weren't able to save their dog. In June 2014,
Adriana Robles of Chihuahua, Mexico, emailed about her 10-
month-old pug in the neurologic stage of distemper. Two weeks
later, she wrote to say she had to put the put her dog to sleep,
but she was now trying to help a friend in Ecuador.

That led to an exchange about my limited vet contacts
throughout Latin America and the need for a Spanish-language
translation for the website. She offered to translate the pages of
the website. I asked if she could also help answer the emails I
was getting in Spanish. I'd been relying on Google translate to
answer these messages, but I knew it would be better if a native
speaker could explain the treatments to other dog owners.

"I work all day, but I would not mind to be responding
emails," she wrote. "I feel useful helping people and you are a
big inspiration."

By the end of July, she'd sent me 30 pages of translations,
and they kept coming. She was inspiring. Because of her, we
were able to post the entire website "en español." She also
translated the complete protocols and the transcript of Dr.
Sears' lecture in Houston (which I intended to add as captions
to the YouTube video, but I got overwhelmed.)

"I feel like we're batman and robin jajajaja!" she wrote when the Spanish section went up.[118] We also launched a Spanish language distemper page "Salve a los perros del moquillo" on Facebook, which I later handed off to a vet in Mexico.

In the meantime, I had heard little news about the study that Elizabeth Nelson had used her connections to get rolling. Aside from that one email at the beginning, I never got any reply to my emails or phone calls to the professor. By now, I had given up trying. Then I got an email from Elizabeth in July 2014:

> "I just spoke for a long time with Dr. ... I finally understand that he is a very busy man. I also think that this is not the priority for him that it is for us. That isn't a criticism. It's just a circumstance that we'll have to understand and hope that he will eventually get to this. I asked when he would be able to publish and he wasn't able to give me a timeline. ... So I wanted you to know what my latest communication was with him. I will continue to stay in touch with him and do everything I can to keep this going. He said he would get these things done ... just wasn't able to give me a time. Please let Dr. Sears know what's happening and that I'll never stop trying to get this done. Take care, Elizabeth."

By now, I had plenty to work on anyway. Over the past few months, I'd also been developing a non-fiction book proposal to send to a publisher. With the progress we'd been making lately, it had seemed possible this book could hit the mainstream publishing industry rather than just be a self-published affair.

From the beginning of my conversations with Dr. Sears, we had discussed either self-publishing or publishing as an E-book. But getting this story accepted by a mainstream publisher would be the brass ring. It would give not only a big jumpstart on spreading the message on the distemper treatments, but it could also prompt a larger discussion on what further research and education was needed.

Despite the videos from Maddie's Institute, I worried the overall state of treatment of distemper dogs around the world remained Medieval. While shelter vets in the U.S. may have been undergoing a shift in thinking, too many other vets still shrugged at a possible distemper case, waited for neurologic problems and euthanized. The message that it was so necessary and possible to treat these dogs was not being heard.

About this time, the story of Boko Haram's massive kidnapping of Nigerian girls had dominated the news. What impressed me was the power of Twitter to generate and maintain interest in a story. Posts of photos with #bringbackourdaughters were everywhere. This eventually gave me an idea I shared with Elizabeth Nelson in July:

> "We need one big public push to demonstrate that this is a priority for dog owners. I have a plan, but I am about to go camping with my son and the Cub Scouts for five days. … It's very simple. If you remember the #bringbackourdaughters campaign on Twitter, I want to do something like that. All I am going to do is have a picture taken of me in my backyard, holding up a sign that says, "I loved my distemper dogs."
> "It will have pictures of my distemper dogs with the hashtag – #savedistemperdogs along with the URL for Kind Hearts In Action. I will post that to Facebook and Twitter and ask that everyone who follows me to do the same thing … If their dog is alive, pose with the dog rather than the picture. I think that could make a big bump in awareness."

She liked the idea, but I opted to wait. It would be a good campaign to launch in conjunction with publication of the book. In mid-August, Dr. Harkin emailed to say he'd received his funding and the study could formally launch. Over the next few months, I continued to wrestle with a book proposal for publishers. Ultimately, I realized I could only go so far with it because I still did not know how this story would end.

"This is not going to go the way that you think!"
- Luke Skywalker

'Not always as we expect'

In October 2014, the first dog to be treated as part of the study arrived at Kansas State from Colorado Springs. However, after coming out of the anesthesia following the procedure, the dog died from complications related to pneumonia. The owners sent me a note about how compassionate Dr. Harkin and his staff had been.

My best friend, Jeff Schnaufer, came to visit from California in November. When he landed at the Elmira-Corning Regional Airport, he had booked a room at a local hotel so that we could catch up, drink beer and be loud without keeping the rest of my family awake.

I woke up in the hotel room at 6 a.m. and lay in my bed worrying about the book, the studies, the cause and a host of other things.

"Ed, you awake?"

"Yeah, how'd you know?"

He knew because he'd listened to my breathing as I slept. He recognized the patterns and knew what they meant. He'd been recently diagnosed with sleep apnea, and he realized I probably had it too. When you have apnea, it prevents you from getting enough oxygen as you sleep. You keep waking up – or nearly wake up – throughout the night. This keeps you from getting enough REM sleep, and you feel exhausted every day.

That was the first of a series of issues Jeff helped me recognize on that visit.

We went out to breakfast at a Cracker Barrel, and I caught him up on things that had been going on with my family and other friends.

At one joke, we busted out laughing. Hysterically. Thank God the restaurant was mostly empty. The laughter brought an unexpected and welcome relief. For the rest of the visit, we hit microbrews and bars throughout the area. Wherever we went, we brought the board game I'd invented – now called MetaCheckers. I only had the one real-world prototype of it, but wherever we went it drew attention. Whenever a bartender, waitress, customer or other passerby got excited about the game, it filled me with joy.

By the end of his visit, I realized I was happy. From that, I finally understood I'd been depressed for a long time, probably since the end of my journalism and teaching careers. To be honest, the thousands of emails I'd received about canine distemper also deepened the depression. More dogs were saved than lost, but many were lost. In the past five years or so, I'd received photos and videos of sick, dying and dead dogs from all over the world.

Even though I always explained up front to people that I am not a vet or a doctor and could not possibly diagnose their dogs for them [something that cannot happen over email] I still got copies of lab reports and close-up photos of dry paw pads, dry eyes, poop, diarrhea and rashes. Sometimes owners would send me videos of operations, dogs in seizures, dogs spasming, shaking and scared. Photos of dead dogs on blankets, pillows and next to shallow graves landed in my Inbox.

These owners needed to send these videos and photos because they were scared or grieving. They needed to express what they were going through and know that someone else understood without judging or blaming them. When our puppy Selkie died back in 1996, the vet who euthanized her admonished us afterwards, saying that we should make sure to get our next puppy vaccinated. That still pisses off Amy, the assumption being we had done something wrong to kill our puppy. We'd taken Selkie to our vet immediately for a checkup and vaccinations after adoption, but she had already been exposed.

When a dog gets distemper that is not the time to admonish the owner. A distemper case does not always mean vaccination was neglected. The veterinarian and staff should remember that vaccinations do not always work, especially if the dog is somehow immune compromised. They should at least ask about the dog's vaccination history before leaping to a conclusion.

For whatever reason the dog got infected, it happened. It's a fact that must now be handled. Do what you can to protect other dogs from infection. Most importantly, what you do have is a patient sick with a disease. What can be done now? The best time for the vaccination lesson is before (or at least when) the dog is adopted. If it is clear the owner of a distemper dog did miss the lesson on vaccination, you might find a compassionate way to let them know before they get away. But while I have your attention right now: Always get your dogs vaccinated!

When someone writes to tell me their dog died, I sometimes tell them I still remember what it was like to have puppies die of distemper. Sometimes I skip that part because not everyone feels the loss the same way. So, it's arrogant to assume you know what they are going through, how long the pain will last or whether a new pet will make things better. In my replies to these emails, I usually say some variation of "I'm so sorry for your loss. Distemper is a nasty disease that does not play fair. It is a terrible way to lose a good friend and family member. My hope for you is a future with happy, healthy dogs."

When I write these condolences, I remind myself of the joy of the dogs who have lived and the hope that someday perhaps dogs will no longer have to die of this disease. That's what kept me going.

The other weight that added to the depression was the unremitting silence. The unanswered phone calls and emails. The vets and scientists who refuse to even consider that distemper is a problem worth solving or that a solution is possible. I am aware of the dismissive criticisms online. I have no standing within the veterinary or scientific community, so I understand. Were I in your position I might say the same. But the universe gave me a choice: Do nothing and dogs would certainly die. Do something and perhaps some could be saved. Do something, and maybe canine distemper would stop being such a deadly disease.

So in December 2008, I chose to do something. I chose to try. I made that choice because I don't like dogs dying when they don't have to.

Recognizing the depression broke the hold it had over me. I quickly realized the anxiety and self-esteem issues that came with it and began to deal with those. When I felt dread as I approached a task, I recognized what was going on and fought to overcome it. In the next few months, I gradually got better but I would eventually decide I did not have the power to completely defeat the depression on my own. I'd need a little help.

Meanwhile, another issue came to a head. Up until this point, I had been pursuing the book as a co-authorship with Dr. Sears. I maintained his status as co-author despite advice that I should take over sole authorship to make a book deal simpler. However, I did not want to push Dr. Sears off his own book.

"Ed, that's very gracious," Al said when I told him and Ruth this in early December 2014. But then, they explained I did need to take over completely. Ruth told me Al did not have the mental focus to continue. "This is your book," she said.

On Dec. 21, I received an email from Debby Simms of Huntington, West Virginia, about a dachshund/Basset hound mix named Coal she was fostering from a local shelter. "He tested positive for distemper on Dec 15," she wrote in an email copied to her friend Barbara Bias. "He is still eating and eliminating. He was first diagnosed with kennel cough and then began losing weight. The return visit and testing gave the result of distemper. I have been researching on Internet and found you. If you know of a vet near West Virginia please let me know."

They took Coal to Ohio State a couple days later, but that only confirmed the dog had neurologic distemper. The school refused to consider the unpublished NDV spinal tap treatment, so I encouraged them to contact Dr. Harkin and get into his study.

"Coal has had the treatment!" Debby wrote on Jan. 2. "We were so impressed with Dr. Harkin and the med student … We will let you know as he improves. We can not thank you enough!!"

With the university studies now under way, the stats I kept became less important. Every few months or so, I had been sending out follow-up emails to any one who had contacted me, but by now additional anecdotal cases would not add anything further to the argument. So, I stopped the follow-up emails. When someone did offer an update, I would post that to the websites and social media as well as add to my tallies.

REPORTS FROM VETS

22 veterinarians treat
571 dogs with NDV

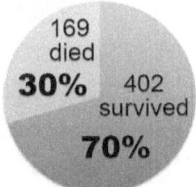

169
died
30% 402
survived
70%

265 dogs treated
with NDV serum

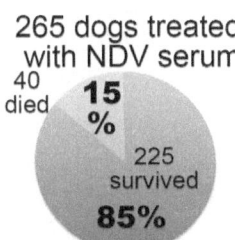

40
died **15
%**
225
survived
85%

162 dogs treated
with NDV as IV

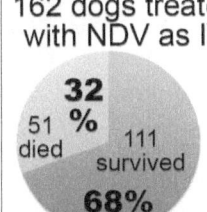

**32
%**
51
died 111
survived
68%

144 treated with
NDV spinal taps

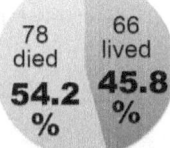

78
died 66
lived
**54.2
%** **45.8
%**

Kind Hearts In Action website
January 7, 2015

REPORTS FROM
DOG OWNERS/CAREGIVERS

941 dogs
with distemper

647 treated with NDV

294 not treated
with NDV

223
died 424
survived
**34.5
%** **65.5
%**

225
died
**76.5
%** **23.5
%** 69
lived

268 dogs treated
with NDV serum

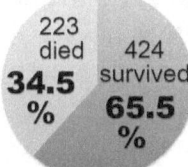

65
died **24
%** 203
survived
76%

160 dogs treated
with NDV as IV

**23
%**
37
died 123
survived
77%

219 treated with
NDV spinal taps

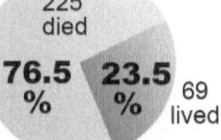

121
died 98
lived
55% **45%**

Kind Hearts In Action website
January 7, 2015

The countries where vets reported outcomes now included India, Israel, Hungary, Italy and Mexico among others. But these were not always solid, long-term commitments. I had learned a vet in India who had been using the NDV spinal tap later dropped it. Making connections in Israel became difficult. A vet in Canada who had been supportive dropped the treatments. So had vets in Florida. In many places, finding a willing vet was still hit or miss. The most reliable place was in Texas, which had a handful of willing vets. The other was the Philippines, which also had a few possibilities and I usually heard from there at least once a day.

Getting updated on the study

All we really could do was wait to see whether the academic research produced any fruit. In mid-January 2015, Dr. Harkin sent me an update on his research:

> "Thanks for the referrals of the distemper dogs for our study. The veterinarians in KS have not been very helpful about identifying and referring cases. My experiences so far (5 cases) have been less than encouraging, but I can make a few general comments. One, dogs with myoclonus (chorea) as their primary problem (especially whole body chorea) do not do well. My presumption is that those dogs have a significant polioencephalitis [a viral infection of the brain] and not just the leukoencephalitis [inflammation of the white matter of the brain]. This may also be a viral strain issue, but I can't confirm that at this time. I'm also surprised how many of these dogs turn out to have severe viral pneumonia at necropsy despite having normal thoracic radiographs. So, for now I'm encouraged with the dogs that have **ataxia**, weakness, paralysis, blindness, cerebellar signs, but not encouraged by those dogs that have chorea. Basically, 3/3 dogs with demyelination have done well (study and pre-study dogs) and 0/5 dogs with chorea (study and

pre-study dogs) have survived."

Ataxia – Loss of muscle control and balance.

In a follow-up email, he reported that dogs with chorea did not show distemper antibody titers in their cerebrospinal fluid. They also do not improve after the NDV spinal tap. But dogs with other versions of neurologic problems did show distemper antibody titers in the cerebrospinal fluid – CSF. But he added the distemper titers in CSF are not enough to confirm distemper.

I forwarded this information to Dr. Sears. His reply: "Wow! Great information. I wonder if this is why we only got 50% success when tried. Sounds like a reasonable assumption."

New beginnings and endings

Since I really had nothing else to do but wait – and answer emails – my focus began to shift more into my new career, game design. I began to teach myself software coding in an attempt to build a new app for my game under the new trademark MetaCheckers. After some experimenting with woods, stains and inks to make the special checkers and dice, Jack and I took 10 copies of a real world version of the game to our first gaming convention, Running GAGG in Geneseo, N.Y.

But as this new part of my life moved forward, others came to an end.

"FYI, Katie is not doing well," I wrote to Jane in mid-January about Mom's 15-year-old dog, Katie – who had been living with us since Hurricane Sandy. "She is in discomfort. She started singular barks about half-hour after we went to bed, which was unusual. I got up and let her out, and when she came back in she had a lot of trouble settling down, as if in pain. I don't think she slept at all. This morning she was just lying there with her eyes open and not able to get up."

When the vet evaluated her, she was not responsive. Since she had originally been Jane's dog, I checked with her and we agreed it was time to let her go. We were now down to two cats and one dog, Romeo.

About a month later, mom died comfortably in the recliner in Jane's guest room with an old cat named Panda on her lap. She was 87 years old. Although none of us want to go, I think that was about the best way any could hope for.

According to a post she submitted to the website for the Herald-Dispatch in Huntington, WV, Barbara Bias took Coal back to Kansas State for a follow-up evaluation on April 17, 2015, and had been told he was disease-free.[119] "Coal's new life began Jan. 2, 2015, and now a year later he is celebrating his New Year as a very active and happy 2-year-old doggie," Barbara wrote in the post.

Going public with the study

My next update on the study from Dr. Harkin came in August 2015:

> "I just treated a dog from Texas last week. He has done OK — at least he's still alive and no worse. The dogs with myoclonus seem to take a long time to recover (the myoclonus continues even though the CNS inflammation goes away). So, despite the first 4 dogs doing very poorly, the last 3 have gone quite well. I would like to have this moving quicker with patients, and as it stands I still have money to do more than the original 10 that was allotted (mostly because I built in enough cost to make sure we'd get 10 to follow-up). Thanks for sending the clients my way."

Since he was now interested in getting more dogs sooner, I broached the subject of publicly advertising the project on the website. At first, I was going to describe the project as being at a "Midwestern university," but then he allowed me to name Kansas State in the post so that people willing to drive would know how far they'd have to go. The blog post about the study went up on Sept. 22, 2015.[120]

Meanwhile, I'd received a Portuguese translation of the protocols for the website from Carmen Adorno of Sao Paulo, Brazil.[121] She wrote me in August 2015 while trying to get the NDV spinal tap performed on her 4-month old border collie, Blue. During our email conversations, we had shared a lot about the power of imagination sparked by dreaming. The awareness of dreaming – such as when I invent a board game or a sci-fi story – is called dream yoga in Buddhism, she said. Although Blue seemed to be turning a corner after the procedure, he died nearly three months later. Blue "was a brave warrior!" she wrote. "Now he is not suffering anymore. He rested."

"You certainly deserved to win this one because of all you did," I replied. "Also, I must say that you have been very supportive and inspirational to me, and that's usually my job."

"We had put a fight against distemper, and we lost!" Carmen wrote. "All animals deserve to be saved from distemper and from all kinds of suffering. I hoped Blue could make it because he would be a pioneer in Brazil and would give hope to other dog owners. Life is not always as we expect it will be. We have to accept that and move on ... I believe Blue had purified lots of karma, he helped me to develop patience and compassion and that he will come back soon in a human precious body. I am sure I will see him again in this life! Big hug."

We did not publicize this, but when a dog owner did express a willingness to get to Kansas State and travel expenses were the only obstacle, I did send them money. About $600 went towards those trips in 2015. By the end of the year, Kind Hearts In Action had only a couple hundred dollars in the bank. The costs of maintaining the websites and keeping the campaign going had also been whittling us down. I would add a few hundred dollars from my own pocket to give it a boost.

In November 2015, Clark Audiss called me with a problem. The family had to move, and Nilla couldn't go with them. As he wrote for a post to the website I made the next day:

> "I enjoyed visiting with you yesterday and catching up on the progress made in studying the NDV treatment. As I mentioned, we have accepted a new position as pastor of a small church and it appears we will be in a rent situation. Because it is a small town, rent opportunities are very limited and all we have seen currently say 'no pets'. Nilla's amazing story has touched so many people and we cannot just let her go without knowing she is in a loving home and being well cared for. I am tearing up as I type these words..., 'She is family'! Thank you for all you have done for Nilla and thank you for offering to help find her a good home. Jen and I are praying for the day when all the studies and all the research verify what we already know ... there is hope and there is a cure!"

His post circulated on the social media accounts. A month later, they found a solution. "Good morning Ed, We have found a home for Nilla! She will be staying here in SD with a friend of my wife's sister. Thanks for all your help (:"

A blog post on another website changed my life for the better. Wil Wheaton, who played Wesley Crusher on "Star Trek: The Next Generation," had posted a video online describing a panic attack he'd had at an airport. In that moment, his wife helped him realize he had a mental health issue. In his video, he explained how those with depression, anxiety and other issues could get help.

He helped me realize that although I had come a long way to climb out of the depression, I couldn't quite get all the way out of the hole without a little help. So, I went to counseling. The counselor had me get a prescription from my doctor. With the medication, counseling, much longer walks with Romeo at night and the music of Brandi Carlile, I began to climb out of the hole. Brandi taught me to feel joy despite the regrets of the past and to not let others tear me down.

In December 2015, my company – DreamGames[122] – launched sales of MetaCheckers from a website and online store. After that, we started making sales at game conventions and in local stores around Horseheads. Through all of this, I continued to answer emails about canine distemper as we waited for news from Dr. Harkin.

In early March 2016, more news about the Kansas State study came. But it was not what I had been hoping for. A key issue was the myoclonus – or chorea – the spasmodic, jerky contraction of the muscles. Dr. Harkin wrote:

> "Just thought I'd pass on some thoughts/observations about the NDV treatment. The first few dogs that I treated has an abnormal CSF analysis with lots of inflammation. After treatment that inflammation was gone, so my initial impression was that the treatment effected that response. Having evaluated more dogs, I realize that many of them will have a normal CSF and that this is likely not an uncommon event when the virus becomes dormant. So, in that respect, I'm not sure the treatment really does anything. For those dogs with myoclonus (which has been all but one of these dogs), they do seem to improve within the first 2-3 weeks with less whining, but not really any significant reduction in their myoclonus.

"The myoclonus hasn't terminated in any of these dogs, yet, and although these dogs have a reduction in it over time and seem to have a bit better function, I'm not convinced the treatment is responsible for this change. I was able to convince one person from Florida not to come up for the treatment and that dog had similar improvement without any therapy at all (I know, n of 1, but interesting). I'm also concerned about the quality control of the vaccine. Although I've been using the same vaccine the entire time, I've recognized some of these dogs (3-4 now) that appear to have developed meningitis that is distinct from their distemper. I'm beginning to wonder if this vaccine could be intermittently contaminated with bacteria that results in a meningitis and death of the dogs. I always presumed that descriptions of meningitis was a consequence of poor technique, but now I'm wondering if it's a consequence of contaminated vaccine. I'm going to start culturing the vaccine after reconstitution, but then this study is almost done so I've arrived at that party a bit late. Ultimately, I'm not sold on this therapy. Although I had a few amazing results (2-3 dogs, one (maybe 2) prior to the study and one during the study), my general impression is that this is not the godsend as it is promoted. Oddly, the only dog that I had in this study that had been treated with the NDV serum several weeks prior to coming up here is the only dog that still had circulating distemper virus in the blood based on PCR."

The study was not over, but he was giving me a heads up. This won't be the happy ending. But at least the truth was being pursued. The possibility of a meningitis infection from contaminated NDV made a lot of sense to me because I do remember cases where dogs seemed to be dealing with an additional infection post spinal tap.

My reply:

> "First of all, I have to thank you so much for being so willing to examine this treatment so thoroughly and so fairly.
> Before you, so many experts simply rejected this treatment by saying it was impossible without even looking at it. They simply proved their point through the absence of a scientific study.
> But the absence of a study doesn't mean something doesn't work. It just meant it hadn't been put to the test. You did put it to the test. You sought the truth, and if this is where your pursuit of truth has led you, then so be it.
> I still hold to the opinion that the NDV serum used before the onset of the neuro stage can save the lives of dogs. But that was not what this study was about, and proving that would take a massive study involving a lot of dogs. Perhaps I could make that happen if I won the Powerball.
> Of course, my hope had been that if your study had a different outcome, it might have sparked further interest from other researchers to explore other possibilities including the NDV serum. I hope you do complete this study and publish your results and conclusions whatever they are. If you have done as thorough and fair a job as I believe you have, the world should know."

After responding to Dr. Harkin, I wrote a long email to my sister Jane – copied to Amy – about where I saw things. Here's some of what I had to say:

Distemper update

As Ben Carson would say, I don't see a path forward.
It took nearly 4 years to get Kansas State to this point,
and if his final conclusion is that the NDV spinal tap
doesn't have any benefit, then I am out of options.
His study is nearly finished, so I think this is just his way
of giving me a heads up ... Had they come out with a
positive conclusion that could have been the spark to
create more interest and further studies. But I don't think
that's happening.
I've put more than 7 years into this. I still believe that
what we have done has saved a lot of dogs. But my plan
has always been to get this into the hands of scientists,
doctors and vets and then let them put this discovery to
good use.
People should not be coming to me to save their dogs
from distemper. That was never my goal. They should be
going to their vets. And the vets should be going to the
best scientific research to find answers to treat their
patients.
I just felt that the system had broken down because the
vets and the scientists were so unwilling to even consider
the possibility they could save the lives of these dogs.
Imagine if humans got sick from a virus and the doctors
would just shrug and say, "Too bad. We can't do
anything. Better just euthanize you."
It was an attitude that not only killed thousands of dogs,
but also shut down an entire field of inquiry into
distemper ... the progression of the disease and finding
out what worked and what didn't work.
So many vets knew so little about the disease that they
didn't know they had a distemper case until it was too
late and then had no idea about what they could do to
help ...

I don't know if I can take any credit for the changes I have seen in the past 7 years, but it does seem to me that more vets and owners are now at least willing to try to save distemper dogs, even if they don't subscribe to the NDV treatments.

But the whole point of this social media campaign has been to open doors, to network and find at least one person in the respected, scientific world to take this seriously.

We found that person with Dr. Ken Harkin. I think he has been MORE than fair, and if his conclusion is that the NDV spinal tap does not make a difference, then I have to respect his decision. ... If that is his conclusion after actually conducting a study, then that is the truth of the matter. Let the chips fall where they may.

I think the NDV serum and NDV straight vaccine definitely saves the lives of dogs if it can happen before the onset of the neurologic stage. However, it has been explained to me that to account for all the variables needed to prove that in a scientific study you would need hundreds of dogs and A LOT of funding. ... Bottom line, I think I've played my role as well I can and it's time to step out. Between now and whenever Dr. Harkin publishes, I plan to shift away, downplay the effectiveness of the NDV spinal tap but still encourage people to get their dogs treated before the onset of the neuro stage ...

I will still maintain the Kind Hearts In Action website and I will still help with Under the Porch Dogs in any way that you want. But I never planned on fighting the distemper cause for the rest of my life. I feel that if I don't step out now, that's what I will end up doing.

Jane's reply: "It is hard but right-thinking conclusion. You accomplished what you set out to do and that is truly commendable. Makes me sad but proud of you and the good you've done in the world."

Amy's reply: "What Jane said. You fought hard and valiantly."

But I still had one card left to play. I made a poster of Tug, Selkie and Galen with the words, "We loved our distemper dogs" and the hashtag #distemperdogs. Amy and I stood out on the deck, held up the poster and Jack took our picture. I posted the photo to the Save Dogs From Distemper Facebook page, which sent it out to Twitter, and also posted to the Kind Hearts In Action website:

> "We're asking all of our followers and anyone who cares about the cause of canine distemper to make a sign like this one, using a photo of the distemper dog you've had in your life and add words like "We loved (or love) our distemper dog." Take a picture of yourself holding up the sign.
> Add a hashtag on the photo #distemperdogs and post it to the Save Dogs From Distemper Facebook page or if you are on Twitter, tweet it to @distemperdogs with the hashtags #distemperdogs and #dogs. Or you can email it to me at ed.bond.new.york@gmail.com, and I can post them for you.
> If your distemper dog is still alive, put him or her in the picture.
> The point is we know there are hundreds, probably thousands of dogs dying of distemper all over the world. But the scientists, researchers and veterinarians are not aware of what a big problem it is.
> No one tracks how many dogs die of distemper each year because it is not a reportable disease. This will be an undeniable way of showing how many people care about this disease.
> Our goals:

To end the systematic euthanasia of distemper dogs. This has shut down an interest in research into finding effective treatments.

To promote research into effective treatments and methods of saving distemper dogs.

To promote education among veterinarians to recognize distemper cases and to learn which treatments help.

We need to demonstrate this is a HUMAN issue as well as a dog problem. Not only are thousands of dogs dying of this disease, it is causing heartache and grief to the countless human companions to these animals.

One photo may not make a difference. But what about thousands?"

— Ed Bond
March 7, 2016

Over the next couple of months, we received, were shared or were Tweeted more than 200 photos just like ours. The Save Dogs From Distemper Facebook page has nearly 5,000 followers and more than 2,600 on Twitter. The website has had nearly 400,000 hits since it began in 2009. At last count, the Kind Hearts In Action YouTube channel had more than 177,000 views and more than 500 subscribers. At least I know Amy and I are not the only ones who want to stop dogs from dying of canine distemper.

In the meantime, I started work on the book again, knowing that I could not have the ending I had hoped for. But it was still a story worth telling. Dr. Sears and I pursued these possibilities honestly and in good faith. I wanted the world to understand at least that.

Even though I had begun bracing myself for an ending, the message of hope kept rippling through the Web, emails and social media, still knocking over dominoes on the other side of the world I didn't know existed.

In August, Santerpaws Bulgarian Rescue in Pleven, Bulgaria, messaged me through the Save Dogs From Distemper Facebook page and asked for help. They'd make some NDV serum and later sent me video of two dogs they saved with it. [123] They kept making serum and over the next couple of years sent me updates of saved dogs.

In September 2016, I received another email from Dr. Harkin:

> "I've wrapped up the distemper study. I haven't had time to go over all of the results, yet, but I certainly have the impression that I'll be able to provide some additional insight into CDV infections in dogs when I do. I think I told you previously that I did not appreciate improvement in dogs with myoclonus and that still stands. None of those dogs really got better. Many are still alive, and the jerking is maybe a little lessened in all of them over time, but I'm not convinced that wouldn't have happened without the treatment. Some clients suggested that they would see a marked abatement in the myoclonus right after the injection, but when I saw many of these dogs 3 months later I couldn't really tell a substantial improvement from the initial visit. Maybe the inflammation induced by the NDV suppressed the myoclonus temporarily. I don't know. I just didn't have enough dogs that didn't have myoclonus, which are the ones that I felt were the most likely to respond. So, even though a subset might do better with the NDV therapy, I don't know that those dogs wouldn't have improved with time anyhow. I also don't have any stats on the long-term survival of these dogs, yet.

"I am still happy to speak to clients about their dogs with distemper. I spoke to someone from Illinois today to whom you must have recently spoken. I think her dog is misdiagnosed and really doesn't have distemper (a surprising number of those that you've sent my way didn't have distemper, but I'm ok speaking with them, too). I will still consider doing the NDV therapy in specific cases, but in my experience it isn't the holy grail for CDV."

Through the website and the emails, I shifted the message to let people know the study had concluded, and dogs might still be treated at Kansas State so long as they did not have myoclonus, the spasmodic, jerky contraction of the muscles. Dr. Harkin sees the recovery of dogs in neurologic distemper in a different light from Dr. Sears. Instead of the NDV spinal tap killing or eliminating the distemper virus, according to Dr. Harkin these dogs were most likely recovering as the disease naturally went into remission.

Perhaps there is further knowledge to be learned from additional study.

More bad news

That night, the other shoe finally dropped. The vet under investigation in California emailed: "Hi Ed. So that investigation I told you about a couple years back finally came to head. They fined me $1500 and told me to cease and abate all 'experimental' treatment. This sucks. So to say the least I will not be treating for distemper any more. Please don't refer patients to me, as I have a tough time saying no ... Anyway thought you should know and let other vets know that they risk the same penalty as well. Until there are proven studies. Honestly I don't know if it worked, but I was just trying to save dogs that would otherwise die ... I'm getting punished for trying to do my job as a veterinarian."

Jane's reply when I told her: "Shit."

At the end of October, Elizabeth Nelson and I checked in with each other. Neither of us had heard anything more from her professor. We felt a shared disappointment that he had apparently dropped interest in the NDV serum. Elizabeth told me publication was at first expected in a few months. When she contacted him a year later to remind him she was still waiting, he replied, "you and 100 other people." He wanted to repeat the trial to "make sure." She wrote:

> "He knows better than anyone how devastating distemper is and he now knows it can be prevented. How he can withhold this information is beyond me. He knows the veterinary community would listen to him. ... But I don't know how the scientific publishing world works or what his life circumstances are so I'm no one to judge."

I can't judge either. Elizabeth is right there. It's hard to know the reasons for resistance when you can't get an answer. My best guess is that the professor doubted his results because of the earlier studies in which some dogs with distemper recovered without going into the neurologic stage. That is a claim I still can't wrap my head around, though. Over the years, I had seen dramatic recoveries in many dogs. In some cases, their health turned around in a matter of hours or days, not weeks or months.

A week later, I made one final try and wrote this professor an old-fashioned snail mail letter. In it, I reminded him it had been three years since he studied the NDV serum. Then I added:

"If you know this treatment could relieve suffering and prevent the death of distemper dogs, I do not understand why you would just sit on that. In my seven years as a volunteer on this issue for a small non-profit, I have received emails from more than 4,000 people who would be relieved to know that a respected scientist could verify an effective treatment. ...

"As for myself, I have done my best to document cases on our website – as a former journalist. But I have always known my information was only anecdotal. I did not have the means to prove this scientifically. My hope had been for scientists to study this on their own terms and see for themselves if it works. Has that happened? I guess that's up to you."

I received no reply. A draft of the manuscript for this book had also been sent to him, also with no reply.

Had all our efforts been for nothing?

"You are looking at this all wrong," Tal Shohamy at White Angel told me after reading a draft of this book. "Our mission was never to change the veterinary world. Our mission was to save dogs."

In the years since White Angel began using the NDV spinal tap in January 2009, Tal estimates they performed 200 to 300 spinal taps and saved at least half of those dogs. They also consulted with other vet clinics on hundreds of cases.

"The point is it's a 50-50 chance," he said. "I don't think we should back off on the CSF taps."

Dr. Zilkha would get sad when a dog was lost, but Tal encouraged her to keep trying. When the next dog is saved, that would be worth it, he told her. For example, one of their first cases, Hunter – who is now Sophie – is still "doing great, almost 10 years old and full of life and energy," according to Suzanna Urszuly.

Tal asked me how long my dog Galen had survived after treatment. Nine years.

"The same miracle is happening in hundreds of families," he said. "Do you know what a difference those 9 or 10 years would mean for that family? Why would you not call this a success after saving the lives of hundreds of dogs?"

Tal remained unbothered by the failure to get acceptance in the academic world. "We don't have to change their minds [in academia]," he said. "We just have to let the public know it's available … I'm very happy we were involved in this project. See what a big difference you made. We should keep giving people hope."

As I said earlier, the purpose of a journalist is to illuminate the issues for others to act on. So as it turns out, I ended up returning to journalism after all.

As Dr. Sears has always hoped, some scientist, academic, veterinarian or animal philanthropist could still pick this up and see where else it might lead. Someone reading this book may look at all of this and see the potential being missed and have the means to do something about it. On that day, we may be on the way to finding more answers. I wish that person good luck.

Here is my last report on outcomes of distemper cases treated with NDV, as posted to the Kind Hearts In Action website in 2016:

REPORTS FROM VETS

23 veterinarians treat 611 dogs with NDV

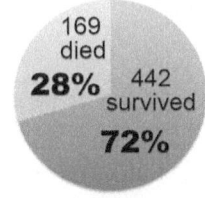

169 died
28% 442 survived
72%

305 dogs treated with NDV serum	162 dogs treated with NDV as IV	144 treated with NDV spinal taps

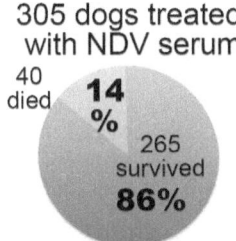

40 died **14%**
265 survived
86%

32%
51 died 111 survived
68%

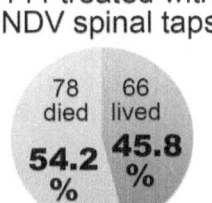

78 died 66 lived
54.2% **45.8%**

Kind Hearts In Action website
Feb.13, 2016

REPORTS FROM DOG OWNERS/CAREGIVERS

1062 dogs with distemper

768 treated with NDV

227 died
30% 541 survived
70%

294 not treated with NDV

225 died
76.5% **23.5%**
69 lived

383 dogs treated with NDV serum	160 dogs treated with NDV as IV	225 treated with NDV spinal taps

24%
67 died 316 survived
82%

23%
37 died 123 survived
77%

123 died 102 lived
55% **45%**

Kind Hearts In Action website
Feb. 13, 2016

Questions and Answers
with Dr. Harkin

In June 2017, Dr. Ken Harkin was selected as the recipient of the E.R. Frank Award by the Kansas State University College of Veterinary Medicine and Veterinary Medical Alumni Association. According to the university's website, the award is presented to a faculty member who displays meritorious service and must have at least a 15-year relationship with the college, possess a noteworthy record of service and display an unassuming and unpretentious manner throughout their careers. In my dealings with Dr. Harkin, I can see why he had been honored like this. In September 2018, Dr. Harkin sent me replies to some questions I had. Here they are:

Q: If the NDV spinal tap is not beneficial to dogs in neurologic distemper, is the conclusion that these dogs would have recovered on their own?

A: No, I do not believe the NDV spinal tap is beneficial and I do believe that the dogs that recovered would have recovered on their own. I had a few clients that wanted to come for the study that I convinced to not have the treatment done. Two of those dogs went on to recover completely with nothing othe than good supportive care at home. I know that clients report "improvement" in the symptoms after the treatment, but when they returned here for their recheck I did not appreciate significant improvement in any of them. Maybe there was fractional improvement, but nothing I wouldn't have expected with time. I do suspect that the NDV vaccine when given intrathecally does cause a transient inflammatory response in the central nervous system (spinal cord, specifically). I think that was manifested in several dogs with significant discomfort/pain that prompted the use of codeine or other analgesic therapy. It is my belief that this inflammation blunts the repetitive firing of the nerves responsible for the chorea (distemper myoclonus). I think that's why clients see an improvement but I don't. I had one dog die several days after the NDV treatment that exhibited severe pain for several days. I had a full necropsy performed on that dog and they did not identify any evidence of bacterial meningitis (the tap procedure itself did not introduce a new problem), but they also didn't find anything other than distemper encephalitis. It's possible that the inflammation induced by the NDV was just not appreciated. That dog was also NDV negative on PCR.

Q: Nilla had been scheduled to be euthanized two days after Clark first contacted me. The vet would have euthanized on that Monday. Instead, she got the spinal tap on Tuesday, and her vision began to return on Thursday. If Nilla was simply going to have a spontaneous recovery on her own, do you think it possible we are giving up on these dogs too early?

A: I had three dogs that did not have myoclonus: Nilla, Coal, and one other dog. Nilla was the most severely affected. Both dogs recovered completely. Is it possible that the NDV works in a small subset of dogs? I suppose that's possible, but I doubt it. I think both dogs would have recovered without any therapy. They showed evidence of demyelination and it's likely that remyelination was happening but that's a process that just takes time. Early on every dog I saw had a very inflammatory CSF, but then post-NDV it would be normal, so I thought the NDV was inducing remission. But, then I had a bunch of dogs that presented with CDV-encephalitis that had completely boring CSF samples, just like the dogs that were post-treatment. It's just that none of those dogs had been treated. I think the disease can and does go in remission. Interesting, Nilla developed myoclonus long after she left here and recovered. She didn't have it originally. That myoclonus also eventually subsided. I think we are giving up on some of these dogs way too soon. I have also worked with a shelter in Denver that has saved a number of these dogs with nothing other than good nursing care.

Q: I believe Nilla had originally been diagnosed via smear. Did she also show positive for distemper in the cerebrospinal fluid? Did that reading change after treatment? I believe I had it from Clark that it did, but I wanted to double check.

A: Nilla was positive on conjunctival scrape and CSF PCR. The conjunctival scrape was still positive after treatment. The CSF was negative. That's how all of the dogs went. They all stayed positive on conjunctival scrape, so long as a good scrape was performed.

Q: Do you have any new insights on diagnosing distemper? At one point, you mentioned that distemper titers in CSF are not enough to confirm distemper. Can you elaborate?

A: New insights on diagnosing? It's important to do the PCR. Titers are not the way to go. Some of these dogs have variably complete vaccination histories and some get vaccinated on entry into the shelter but then develop signs shortly after. We had dogs with positive PCR that were negative on titers. I don't think it's a reliable test. I helped a veterinarian with a dog that clearly had distemper based on my evaluation of video of the dog. She then told me the PCR was negative. I described the procedure with caveats of how to make sure the sample was good. The follow-up was positive. So long as the collection method is good, dogs with distemper will test positive.

Q: You had said that after you evaluate things you might have some further insights about canine distemper infections. Can you share anything else?

A: Additional insights? I just wonder why people get a dog and don't vaccinate it. The vaccines work wonderfully. I know a big issue are abandoned puppies that end up in shelters. We really can't do anything about that situation on the front end other than having better shelters that prevent cross-contamination of dogs. As for CDV-encephalitis, I think great nursing care is the only thing that makes a difference in these dogs. If you have a client that is dedicated to the level of care needed, many of these dogs are going to survive. But many don't and that's a viral strain issue, too. … I appreciate your efforts in educating people about Canine Distemper. Having lived in the Central Valley of California for two years and working there as a veterinarian, I saw way more canine distemper than I ever hope to see again. I guess I was lucky in that I've seen just about every manifestation of that disease one could imagine so I don't struggle with a presumptive diagnosis when a case is presented to me (and don't waste a lot of client money in the process of getting a diagnosis), but I would love to never see another case so long as I live. But, I realize it's a societal problem. I just wish more non-veterinary people cared about it at least half as much as you.

– Ken

What's Next

"The end of this story is up to you," I said into the camera for the conclusion of the DVD filmed in 2009. As I reach the end of this book, my message is the same.

Ultimately, as an ordinary guy on a computer in Horseheads, New York, I cannot prove that the NDV treatments can save dogs from canine distemper. But I still believe it could be proven by someone who had the time, money, interest and ability. If Dr. Sears had encountered such a person at the right point in his career, these treatments might have been published. But he had also been given the wrong mindset and goals that were out of reach. He didn't need a half million dollars. He didn't need to be a university professor. He just needed enough experienced, specialized help to present his case effectively.

I certainly had the interest and found the time, but lacked the money, the training and the ability. Had I talked to Jim Radke before starting Project Carré, I might have had a better outcome with that effort. I missed that chance. Had Jim Radke or some other medical writer or some of the other people of science I have met in the past few years been around Lancaster in the early 1970s, this story might have gone a different way. Then again, you can't change the past.

It is time for me to step back. Because the treatments remain unpublished, veterinarians are reluctant to publicly embrace them. Most still keep me at arms length. The list of willing vets has dwindled over the years. Owners of distemper dogs had sent me that contact information after a successful use of NDV and after getting the OK from the vet, but that is still second-hand information. Too often I end up hearing rumors about willing vets dropping the treatments and then maybe picking them up later. But this is not reliable. I've lost complete contact with some. White Angel in Austin closed its doors in 2018. However, Tal reassured me that their use of NDV did not play a role in that. Still, I think it best for clinics using NDV to reach out to the public in a way that works for them. If they would like me to help refer clients to them, they can always contact me directly and let me know their wishes. But ultimately, I've done what I needed to do. My best way to help now is offer advice and insights to anyone else who would take up this cause.

Saving Dogs: The Next Generation

You might call the anti-distemper campaign in Britain in the 1920s and 1930s as "Save Dogs From Distemper I," with a goal of identifying the cause and developing the first vaccine. They largely succeeded but also closed the book on developing treatments for dogs after they fall ill. The campaign of "Save Dogs From Distemper II" began on Facebook at the end of 2008, with a goal of demonstrating the need for a treatment and to prove NDV could save dogs from this disease. That goal had not been met, but the campaign did identify some of the issues that must be overcome. However, I would also point out that the first campaign raised more than £8 million in today's value. My campaign operated on barely a shoestring budget.

It is now time for "Save Dogs From Distemper III," a concerted effort to test the contending treatments that are now emerging to determine which offers the best benefits and chance of survival for distemper dogs. The message has to get out that distemper does not have to be a death sentence. That's a fact many are now realizing, but Dr. Alson Sears knew decades ahead of anyone else.

I've often told dog owners distemper is a nasty, terrible disease that is difficult to defeat and does not play fair. In writing this book, I have learned how true that is. Our enemy kills dogs without creating a massive outcry. Defeating that enemy requires an increase in public awareness and scientific curiosity.

Clarifying where we are:

- The NDV spinal tap MIGHT have a benefit in some cases, depending on the type of neurologic problems present. However, the main investigator on this procedure is doubtful.
- The NDV serum or NDV as IV treatment before the onset of neurologic problems MIGHT save the lives of these dogs, but it would take a very large study to establish that and eliminate all the factors. A university researcher has reportedly taken a closer look at the NDV serum but has said nothing publicly and it is unknown whether anything will come of that.
- Despite the development of a distemper vaccine in 1950, dogs continue to get sick and die of distemper. So more work remains to be done.
- Some agency needs to be tracking how many cases there are and what the survival rates are in the populations at large. In some places, like Los Angeles County, canine distemper is now locally required to be reported. But there is still no one keeping track of the overall picture. If the public knew how big a problem a canine distemper is around the world, there may be more of a push for research.
- Even if NDV does no good, then many dogs are recovering and having a decent quality of life after a distemper attack. [Nilla, Coal, Max, Icy, Kaliber, and many, many others.] Ordinarily,

those dogs would have all been euthanized. If time is all that was needed to save them, we are giving up on dogs way too early.

- Save Dogs From Distemper ran into the limitations of a social media campaign. The power of social networking can only go so far. But as I say, you don't know if something will work until you try.
- More education is needed on the diagnosis of canine distemper cases. Despite the recent shifts to giving dogs a chance to live, some clinical vets still shrug and say they can't know for sure they have a distemper case until the neurologic stage begins – or that they can't do anything for the dog except to euthanize.

Action plans

For anyone willing to pick this up and run with it, I see two possible paths. The smallest, simplest plan for an interested veterinarian, shelter or rescue group has already been explained by my friend Jim Radke:

- You'd need a budget of at least $10,000.
- A veterinarian would need to make the NDV serum and document the treatment of dogs in the pre-neurologic stage of the disease. Each case would be confirmed by a lab test, although treatment would not wait for the results of those tests. That's about half your budget.
- That veterinarian would need to hire a medical writer ahead of time to ensure that the measurements are properly made and scientific procedures followed. That's the other half of your budget.
- The medical writer would compile the information into charts and presentations that the veterinarian would take to a conference.
- The veterinarian would have to be willing to stand in front of a crowd of skeptics and explain what they did and what results they found. But they would have good records, lab reports and stats to back them up.
- Most in this crowd will not believe this, but perhaps a handful might be willing to talk about what happens next. Then, who knows?

But what if all the resources needed were available? What could be done to prove the value of these treatments beyond any doubt? To meet all the requirements of a well-designed study? To address all the questions from the skeptics? As I worked through the various drafts of this book, I received an unexpected invitation to apply for a program that funds lifesaving ideas for animals in need. Although my application was not selected, it allowed me to think about what the ideal study might be like.

While working out those ideas, I came upon the ancient story of Odysseus and Argos. After being away for 20 years – fighting in Troy and then lost in his eponymous ordeal – Odysseus returns home in disguise to defeat the suitors who were seeking to marry his wife. On his way up to his house, he encounters the dog he left behind, Argos. After two decades, Argos had become old, tired, sick and flea-infested. The dog recognizes his master and is barely able to wag his tail in recognition before dying.

Looking back, I realized my journey has been more than 20 years, and dogs with distemper still wait for an effective treatment for this disease. But as Galen did in his final days, dogs will endure much pain and suffering on behalf of their humans. It is time to repay their loyalty.

Even though my proposal was not chosen, it helped me clarify what was needed, but I welcome amendments by whoever picks this up. Here is what I wrote, with some minor revisions:

The Argos Trial

Because dogs have waited long enough

Prediction: If Dr. Alson Sears' 12-hour NDV serum treatment for dogs in the pre-neurologic stage of canine distemper could be put to the test by approved scientific methods they would dramatically out-perform the survival rates of traditional veterinary medicine. The result would be faster recoveries, fewer cases reaching the neurologic stage, a decrease in long-term symptoms and more distemper dogs surviving.

Double-blind study

Two batches of dog serum would be made, each enough to treat 20 adult dogs. One would be made following Dr. Sears' protocols for 12-hour NDV induced serum. The other would simply be dog serum with no special treatment given. The vials or bottles of serum would be labeled and coded so that no one would know which was which until after the trial was over. A sick dog would be treated from only one batch or the other. No mixing of batches.

Healthy dogs would not be given the disease. Instead, we would find distemper cases as they occur in veterinary clinics, animal shelters and among rescue groups. Ideally, investigators would find a large number of sick dogs in one location. However, this will probably require the need to travel to the site of outbreaks, ensure data is collected properly and treatments performed consistently.

The risks and possible outcomes will be explained to owners or caregivers of dogs involved in this study, and they would need to sign forms granting informed consent.

In addition to at least one veterinarian, the project would need a medical writer or a professional trained in collecting scientific data. They would either write a journal article or prepare a presentation for a conference. Other staff may be needed.

When a sick dog is identified, these would be the steps taken:

• Complete record of symptoms, overall health and description of the dog including age, breed, color, size, weight, temperature, etc.

• The owner or caregiver should be reminded of the importance of documenting the outcome throughout the treatment.

• Samples taken to test for distemper, mostly likely conjunctiva smear sent to a lab for PCR testing.

• If possible, additional samples may be taken to actually measure the number of virus particles at the onset.

• All standard protocols of supportive therapy of a distemper dog would be followed in each dog. This would include antibiotics and nebulizers for pneumonia, efforts to stimulate the appetite to keep the dog eating and addressing other symptoms as they arise.

• The dog should be within the first 6 days of the onset of symptoms and NOT be in the neurologic stage of the disease.

• The dog would be treated with serum according the to the protocol:
1 ml per dog plus 1 ml per 10 lbs, 12 hours apart for 3 treatments.   So, 20 lb dog would be 3 ml sub Q 12 hours apart 3 times. [or to say it another way, within 24 hours: At 0 hour, 12 hours and 24 hours.]

• Observation and documentation of symptoms of the dog in the following days/weeks.

• Follow-up distemper testing and checking virus particle levels as appropriate.

• Measures could be taken to permanently preserve samples of the virus and blood serum.

• Photos and videos taken at regular intervals from intake to at least the end of the first month of illness.

• Documentation of outcome, either the death of the dog or complete record of symptoms, size, weight, temperature, etc.

Any dogs who reach neurologic stage would NOT be automatically euthanized. We believe that even in this stage many dogs can eventually recover with proper nursing care. If a dog keeps eating, there is hope. If a dog no longer can eat, or if seizures become unstoppable or the dog is paralyzed to the point of complete immobility, euthanasia could be considered with the consent of, or at the direction of the owner/caregiver.

Someone should perform a mass spectrometry comparison of the NDV serum and the control serum to see whether a unique compound could be identified.

One other thought and/or question: Since humans can donate plasma without losing blood cells, could NDV-induced serum be collected from dogs in the same way? It might allow for more serum to be collected with even less of a risk of shock to the donor dog.

A few words of advice

BE SKEPTICAL
Doubt until you see verification. Don't oversell the possibilities. Don't make promises you can't keep. Don't let enthusiasm overcome the skepticism, let the facts do that. Respect the scientists. Their brains are hardwired for this. They don't want emotion to muddle up their results, which is why they keep people who are not trained scientists at arms length. But I have to believe that if you stay with the facts, you have a better chance of being listened to.

BE HOPEFUL
But you should also practice what I call "cautious optimism." There is a worthwhile goal here. This may prove to save the lives of dogs and spare their human families untold grief. If anything, we might be able to show the mortality rates in distemper cases can be significantly reduced. According to Cornell University, the death rate is now at 50 percent for adult dogs and 80 percent for puppies. The chance to save a lot more of those dogs makes this worthwhile.

BE PATIENT AND UNDERSTANDING

Know that the people who contact you are often in crisis. They need your support and compassion. Don't throw blame at people. Sometimes vaccinations fail. It doesn't matter as much how the disease happened. What is important is what they need to know and what they need to do at that time. Promote vaccination whenever possible, but without the guilt trip.

BE RESPECTFUL

Respect the veterinarians, the clinics and their staff. If they do not choose to use these treatments, they have good reason to. They have to make the best judgment for the long-term health of their patients, clients and staff. One bad decision could end the business and leave everyone without the care and services they provide, so many will not be willing to make a leap of faith on your behalf. They have a business to run and they must calculate the costs, benefits and risks in a way that works for them.

BE HONEST

Be honest to the humans desperate to save their canine friends. Make sure they understand the risks. Not every dog can be saved, but more are saved when their owners and vets are willing to give them a chance. Don't take advantage of anyone desperate to save a pet. Don't pretend to be something you are not. Don't use terms like "miracle cure" or make guarantees. Explain the realities as well as you can. But remember that unless you are a veterinarian, you are not an expert. Reading this book does not make you an expert. Writing this book does not make me an expert. These are serious medical procedures meant for veterinarians who have assessed the risks and benefits and are willing to proceed. This is not a way for people to treat their dogs at home without going to a veterinarian.

BE ACCEPTING

Don't chase people. If a dog owner or vet or scientist does not want to hear about the treatments for canine distemper, accept that. Leave them be. Instead, let the willing and interested find you on their terms.

STAY SANE

Save your sanity. Don't let the cause take over everything. Don't miss out the big moments of your life. Seek balance and other interests. Give yourself distance and a way of disconnecting when you need to. Don't hold onto the frustration, the losses and disappointments. Let them go. Be grateful for what you have and try not to despair over what you do not.

Do what you can, with what you have, where you are.

Epilogue

The first draft of this book was completed and sent to Dr. Sears in July 2017, not long before Jack and I left for the World Boardgaming Championships in Seven Springs Pa. where we ran the annual MetaCheckers tournament. After Dr. Sears and my friend Jeff Schnaufer gave it a read, I began circulating either the whole manuscript or parts of it to everyone who was involved in this story while also doing some further research into the science. The final draft was uploaded to Amazon Print On Demand in July 2020, three years later.

That sounds like a long time, and it is, but if you look back you'll see this story ranged over decades and all over the world. Some people took months to get back to me, but with good reason. Some had health scares and serious crisis in their lives. Many were professionals and academics who are extraordinarily busy. I was also one of the busy people too because I was trying to move forward with my life.

Through all of this, I strove to get some traction in my board game business. Going to conventions and demos and events. Making prototypes. Buying equipment and supplies. Taking classes on entrepreneurship. Jumping through all the legal hoops required of a small business. You get the idea.

On top of that, I ran for county legislature in 2018. As a former journalist, I was reluctant to become political, but my friends kept encouraging me. The biggest nudge into running for office came from a non-partisan organization, which had recently started in Horseheads called the Trailblazers PAC. This group aimed to create candidates who avoided big money donations and would fight for honesty, accountability and openness in government. As a former newspaper reporter, this lined up with everything I wanted to see in politics.

Campaigning turned out to be familiar territory for me. I'd been a politics major in college, and I'd spent much of my adult life writing about politics and government. No longer was I trying to make headway in a field where I had no standing. Early in the campaign, I stopped taking the anti-depression medication and never needed it again.

After knocking on hundreds of doors and making hundreds of calls, I got over my fear of rejection and anxiety about using the phone. The Trailblazers endorsed my campaign. By election night, I knew I had done everything I could and was still standing. I lost, but voter turnout reached 58 percent. So, that made it worthwhile to me. Taking action out in the real world ended the last remnants of depression.

Jumping into crowded field of candidates for local office also helped me get to know an immunology researcher at Cornell University. Christa Heyward Ph.D., a molecular biologist and immunologist, was also running for a seat on the county legislature, but in a different district. Our paths kept crossing at campaign events, so I privately broached the subject of canine distemper with her at one. After the election, Christa left Cornell to move into the private sector, but we still ran into each other at mixers for local entrepreneurs, so I could not help but pick her brains at any opportunity.

More than anything, I think she helped me to realize there are other interpretations and conclusions to be made about the NDV treatments. We exchanged journal articles about distemper and Edward Jenner. She explained neurologic retraining in which patients can recover motor functions when healthy neurons take over the work performed by ones that had been damaged. She talked about how the immune system attacks myelin in MS patients. She reminded me that viruses are not living organisms and so it is problematic to claim a treatment had killed the disease.

She raised the possibility that the timing of the blood withdrawal following the NDV injection may not be as crucial as Dr. Sears believed. She was the one who explained mass spectrometry could be used to identify the unknown materials within the NDV serum. She also gave me advice on other ways to get this into the hands of scientists.

In all, she pointed out there were a lot of questions to be answered and pure science for a researcher to explore. I am grateful for her help and insight.

Meanwhile, updates and replies kept coming in as the manuscript kept circulating around the world. This became one of the joys of writing this book. Many of the dog owners reported their dogs either were still alive or had lived for years after treatment.

When I wrote to Pippit Carlington about her dog, Carmella, who had been treated with the NDV spinal tap in Georgia in 2009, she had good news. "At the age of 5 Carmella's myoclonus in her right front leg suddenly disappeared and had never come back," she wrote, grateful to see how the neurologic system can repair itself.

Pamela Nabors, whose border collie, Mojave, had been treated with the NDV spinal tap in California, also wrote to say her dog was "doing fantastic! He can finally wag his tail after, what (seven) years? He's a trooper."

She often posts photos of Mojave and her other dogs on Facebook, as when they played on the beach in Carmel, California. "Ed, did I ever thank you for the guidance you gave during Mojave's fight against distemper?" Pam said in a post to my Facebook page. "I love my dog and thanks to you and your information he survived this horrible disease."

"As of current, Kali is doing GREAT!!!" Mia Shark replied. "At 8 years old, he is still as loving and energetic as a puppy. I am so grateful to have such a wonderful dog, and best friend. There are slight residual twitches that come about every now and then in his nose and last for about a week but go away. Other than that though, there are no other signs of distemper!!! :D"

"Sochi is healthy and happy," Amanda Bird wrote. "He's a big goofball, and you would never know he had such a horrible history. The only sign would be his size because he's small for a German shepherd, but that's it. He loves running circles in our yard, gets overly excited about walks, and begs for belly rubs."

Barbara Bias wrote with a cheerful update on Coal.

"Coal is a very happy and active dog," she wrote. "He loves to race around the living room couch playing with his toys. I love him very much. Thank you for everything you did for him. Thank you for helping my friend Debby Simms find the right place to take Coal. Dr. Harkin at Kansas State was very happy with Coal's improvement."

"Your email has put a smile on my face and joy in my heart," Joyce Burton Titular of the Philippines wrote. "Bailey is now a senior dog at 12 years old and doing fine! No more twitching the past 4 years. She would not have reached this far if it were not for you, Ed. Every time I see her so happy, I thank God I found you and Kind Hearts in Action online. I will always forever be thankful."

White Angel Animal Hospital closed its doors in 2018, but when I reconnected with Jeff Wells, it brought back some overwhelming memories of when his dog, Max, was treated there. "It was such a tumultuous, emotional, challenging time for us and it all happened so fast," he wrote. "Discovering that Max indeed had distemper, finding out about the treatment, and getting him to a vet that provides the treatment (happily, in the same state as us), all over the course of a weekend. As commonly happens, the first vet in Houston told us there was no treatment and he'd have to be euthanized. Also, his pneumonia was so bad that Dr. Zilkha told me that up to that point she hadn't successfully treated a dog that was so far gone. When I signed the paperwork to proceed, I thought I was signing his death certificate."

"My Bella and so many others I have watched recover from this disease after NDV treatments will always be in my heart," wrote Elizabeth Nelson of San Antonio. "Bella is sleeping peacefully next to me right now, 8 years after being treated. How brave these dogs have all been to have fought so hard to survive."

"Thank you so much for keeping on this path and helping others get the help that Icy got," wrote Andre Marcelo-Tanner, whose dog Icy lived for 6 years after treatment.

Tjoppie, the South African dog treated with NDV serum in a spinal tap, lived for more than 5 years. Chantel van Rensburg's husband Noel wrote me with an update: "Unfortunately Tjoppie passed away last year on the 25th of October 2016. We made the hard choice to put him to sleep as his symptoms flared up again and had just too many seizures a day and not recovering well after them. But he was almost 6 years old and if I had to do it again, I would. Thank you for everything."

"You might be aware that after the success with Muttu, several other vets in different cities in India are now aware of this treatment procedure and have been using it," wrote Kaveri Uthaiah. "Muttu is a senior girl now but doing ok. Thank you for sharing this."

After reading a later draft, Dr. Sears' wrote: "Ed, it took 2 days to read the whole book. I am impressed that you have come up with such a book. I actually learned things I did not know, which means your research was deeper than mine ever was."

When Dr. Amber Melton sent back the manuscript, she wrote:

"I am so proud to be involved in the distemper NDV treatments! I am also very happy to be a part of your book. Thank you! …We continued to use both the IV and intra-thecal (A-O taps with NDV serum) with success. Luckily (knock on wood) we have not seen a distemper case for a year at least. I speak for everyone here in saying that we are all grateful for the NDV protocols. This has saved a significant amount of animals that otherwise would have most likely died. I certainly plan to use both NDV protocols in the future if we see more distemper cases. Not everyone vaccinates their dogs for distemper, especially in rural areas with many low-income families unfortunately. … Thank you for what you have done."

Dr. Sinem Karsli Parmaksizoglu in Istanbul also emailed.

"I have read your book in two days with a lot of emotions," she wrote, expressing regret at not sending more data. She had just been overwhelmed with cases. I told her she had nothing to regret because it is the vets who do all the real work saving lives. "After starting to treat distemper dogs with Dr Sears serum the word just travelled so quickly that we were loaded with puppies from all around Turkey. I couldn't keep myself away from them because distemper was the first disease I heard about with dogs when I was little. Maybe the first reason I wanted to be a veterinarian. Dr Sears and you, Ed Bond, made my dream come true. … I believe you and Dr Sears made and will make a huge difference. Thank you for being who you are."

No … Thank you all.

My undying gratitude goes out to the countless dog owners, rescue volunteers, foster caregivers and veterinary professionals who took a leap of faith and gave these dogs a chance at life. Before 2008, I was determined to not get involved in this cause. Only because other people kept contacting me did I realize I needed to do something and to keep trying and not give up. You drew me out and made me tell a story that needed to be told. This story would have ended in Chapter 5 without your help, prodding and encouragement. We may not have achieved the acceptance we had been hoping for, but looking back I realize there are hundreds of dogs alive today because of what we did together.

In January 2019, Clark Audiss wrote with an update that they had recently been able to bring Nilla home after being away for three years. She had been boarded at a farm, and Nilla had encountered hundreds of dogs without causing any new distemper cases and without getting any phenobarbital for seizures. He respected Dr. Harkin's conclusion on NDV, but Clark said he still believes in the treatment. "I am 100% certain Nilla would not be here without the NDV treatment," he wrote, adding, "Nilla's myoclonus is completely gone. She does suffer still from stiffness in the hind quarters, diminished hearing and vision and occasional seizures."

A couple of months later, Nilla began to make a turn for the worse. Clark called me to say that her seizures had increased to 2 to 3 times a day, often taking hours to recover after each one. Her quality of life had diminished. I helped Clark reconnect with Dr. Harkin and braced for the worse. Clark wanted to at least make sure that after Nilla passed that her brain and tissues could be documented by Kansas State.

In June, Clark wrote to say that Nilla's condition had stabilized with the warmer weather. "Nilla's seizures have subsided as we moved into the spring and summer so that has been a welcome relief," he wrote in an email to Dr. Harkin and copied to me. "She is now able to be out on the lawn and she has a long leash so she can go wherever she likes. She spends most of her time just laying in the shade and then we bring her in for the night. Seizures seem to be mostly affected by atmospheric pressure, even when we're getting a thunderstorm or low-pressure system, that's when she'll get antsy and start circling and then seize. I still believe her quality of life isn't what I would like to see seizures or no, and still feel we need to put her down before the fall. I also believe strongly that the research is vital and so I want to honor the study and bring her to you for any research you feel is necessary."

The end came when Clark was out of town and Nilla was being boarded. She stopped eating and deteriorated dramatically. Clark called me July 7 to tell me he was having their local vet put her down but would be working with Dr. Harkin to ensure the brain and spinal tissue were properly preserved. As we talked, I realized it had been more than seven years since her treatment at Kansas State. Seven years since Clark's local vet recommended euthanasia. I thanked him for being so willing to give Nilla a chance, and we agreed we were grateful to have been a part of this story.

Clark's tribute on Facebook:

"Thought we lost her once then God gave her back. She's gone now and our hearts are heavy. Even so, God has been faithful and true! Job 1:21 'The LORD gave and the LORD has taken away. Blessed be the name of the LORD.' Tears are flowing but Joy is coming! Psalm 30:5 'Sorrow may last for the night but JOY comes in the morning!' Love you Nilla Bear!"

Despite the sadness over the loss of Nilla, new signs of hope soon followed. In early October 2019, I received a Facebook message from Mada Lixandru of Romania, who had now become a veterinary student. Her message in December 2008 had launched me into this campaign that has dominated nearly 12 years of my life.

She wrote:

"Hey Ed! Hope you're doing well. I am writing just a quick message to tell you that I have been thinking of you all morning. I am on a month-long research trip to Colombia with my vet school, and I am helping a friend do a presentation on canine distemper and treatments. Of course, the Sears serum will be featured in it. And of course, I had to dig up the book, and our conversations, to remember parts of the stories we shared together. And I wanted to tell you, that although I buried it for many years, and ran away as far as I could for many years (because of the trauma), I won't let the serum die in some corner of the Internet and will see if we can get it properly studied and published. My decision to start studying vet medicine was largely based on the need to help the next generation of vets to do better, and our common history was a big influence. So, I am writing to say thank you for giving me a nudge in the right direction, and that I hope some day we'll have some good data to show the world."

At the turn of the decade, I had big plans for my game business. New designs and innovations, fantasy themes, multiplayer versions, ways to change the game board every time you played. My plan for 2020 had been to get out on the board gaming circuit, test the audience interest and hopefully build a following. And then in March, the novel coronavirus crisis wiped out my whole schedule and all my plans.

As I complete this book in the midst of quarantine, the devastating power of viruses looms over us. Amy works from home. Liam does his schoolwork remotely. Jack makes deliveries for a local restaurant wearing a mask. He just had his first COVID-19 test, which was negative, thankfully. Every excursion into the world requires planning for social distancing and sanitization.

Today, the COVID-19 death toll in the U.S. has climbed above 130,000. So I had to give some thought into whether to publish a book that recommends an unconventional protocol for viruses.

But even during this pandemic, emails and messages from around the world still arrive in my computer. The Philippines, Turkey, India, Ohio, Texas, California, most recently. Dogs still get distemper, and I still hear from owners who aren't given many options beyond supportive therapy and euthanasia.

Yet even in the midst of the crisis, progress happens, even if I don't realize it at first. By the way, I sometimes miss emails, which is something I really regret when it happens. But I'm only one person and sometimes I make mistakes and I miss email. One such email came in February from a veterinary student in Britain. Fortunately, she didn't give up on us and wrote me again in April 2020. She had gone to Bulgaria to work with the Santerpaws Bulgarian Rescue in Pleven. She wrote:

> "I have recently visited Bulgaria to help with a charity that rescues and rehabilitates street dogs. It was here where I heard about the NDV serum treatment for distemper. After returning back to the UK, I was inspired to undertake a research project at my university into the treatment and its effectiveness. I was amazed by what this treatment has done for many dogs across the world, and shocked at how little was known about it. I hope to prove the treatment's effectiveness and so make it widely accepted across the world. I am extremely passionate about this cause and want to do all I can to make it known and accepted."

What happens when you send hope out into the world? It comes back.

Acknowledgments

I'd like to thank my parents and my sisters, Jane and Karen, for instilling in me a love of animals. Through that, you have taught me a valuable lesson in empathy. I'd like to thank Amy for standing by me through all my crazy schemes, causes and dreams. I would not have made progress in any of them without your support. I'd like to thank our boys, Jack and Liam, for embracing the lessons of empathy we have tried to teach through our own pets.

Many thanks to Jeff Schnaufer, who has been my solid friend for 27 years. We have been reporters, editors, teachers, science fiction writers, non-profit advocates, and founders of a newspaper. Our lives kept changing and even though I moved back to Upstate New York, we remain close friends. His advice and guidance kept me going through all of this.

I'd like to thank Dr. Alson Sears for sharing his wisdom and insights with me over the past few years. I'd also like to thank Ruth and his family for sharing him with the world during what should have been the tranquil retirement he deserved.

I owe a deep debt to the professionals and academics in the world of science and veterinary medicine who were patient enough to explain what I needed to know and advance my understanding. That includes my cousin, Dr. Kathleen Triman, now retired from Franklin and Marshall, Dr. Ken Harkin, Dr. Kim Hee Young, Dr. Amber Melton and the staff at the Mountain View Veterinary Clinic, Dr. Sinem Karsli Parmaksizoglu, Jim Radke, Ph.D., Christa Heyward, Ph.D., and Tal Shohamy. Their contributions helped improve this book. Any flaws that remain are my responsibility.

The volunteers, dog owners, rescuers and advocates who played a part in this story are too many to name here. Even in the book, I could only focus on the highlights. There are literally thousands who played a role in spreading the message of hope. I can think of many off the top of my head who might have been included in this book, but I had to go with the examples that best advanced the story. So whether I named you or not, I am grateful for your help. But the people I would especially like to thank for your support are Clark Audiss, Joyce Burton Titular, Pippit Carlington, Pamela Nabors, Elizabeth Nelson, Vickie Novak, Jamie Thomas, Adriana Robles and Kaveri Uthaiah, as well as Sherry Parker, J.D. Ward, Mike Ward, and The Rescue Ranch Animal Sanctuary.

To anyone who gave a dog a chance to live and shared your story with us, thank you. This would not have been possible without you. In no order of importance, here is a partial list of some of those people and their dogs, including some whose dogs did not survive. My apologies to anyone omitted.

Brittany R. and Mary B. with Pax; Arthur Mondejar with Simba in Miami, Florida; Sam Yen with Mr. Blue in The Philippines; Kelly Huntsinger Chasnov of Wee Waggin Rescue; Annie Mimi Savage Chaskalson with Apple; Zahra Arbelo and Scout; Lori Kalef and Bosco; Sheri Burtch with Lucky in Houston Texas; Ashley Cannon with Hachi in Houston, Texas; Cresta Rumery with Otis and Olive in Austin, Texas; Amberley Parker with Phantom in Fort Worth, Texas; Nalua Cuenca with Sumi in Florida; Sydney Adams with Adrian in Texas; Sachin Patel with Belle in Austin, Texas; Eden Smith with Basher in Florida; Charlese Uribe with Trixie in Florida; Helena Nesbitt with Mimi in Florida; Jennifer Tseng Yarbrough with Dwight in the Dallas area; James and Shari Nadal with Buddy; Dawn H. with Cookie in Riverside, California; Susan M. Kovacs with Bailey in Elberta, Alabama;

Monica and David Erlich with Bear in California; Blake
Donovan with Kasi; Gulcin Goker with Puik in Istabul; Chip
Bissell with Rosie in Del Mar, California; Ellen Parks with
Bartley in Texas; Joanna Hackney with MJ in Austin, Texas;
Bezen Kiper with Dexter in Istanbul, Turkey; Kumar Gaurav
with a Labrador in Delhi, India; Haydee Crystal Acosta
Bustamante with Tigger in El Paso, Texas; Rochelle
Puczkowskyj with Buddy, Treasure and Finnegan in Arizona;
Cortney Lea Adams with Becca of Tucson, Arizona; Nuria
Enciso with Bear in Baytown/Houston area of Texas; Anna
Alexis Bariring with Michelia in the Philippines; Amy Jaramillo
Ureste with Missy of Brownsville, Texas; Leah Keuroghlian
with T-Bone of Tucson, Arizona; Katrina Pontanar with Czar of
the Philippines; Valerie Grzesikowski with Loucca in South
Korea; Linda Hendricks with Anya and Dexter; Brian Hodgson
with Kimba in Toledo City, Cebu, in the Philippines; Mae Calle
with Cookie in the Philippines; Mhica Martinez with Keiko in
the Philippines; Nikki Brannon with Mira; Diana with Pinky of
Río Grande, Puerto Rico; Sara Matza with Feisty in Houston;
Ecem Süme with her dog in Istanbul; Rachael Marshall with
Duke in Killeen, Texas; Farrah Payumo with Lucky in Manilla,
The Philippines; Monty G. Broughton with Chopper in
Houston, Texas; Liz Bartolazo with Venus in The Philippines;
Lindsay, Joe & Boomer in Phoenix, Arizona; Craig Blackburn
with Mater; Josh Zepeda and Titan in Miami, Florida; Laurie
Lilley with Ptarmigan, Annie Oakley, & Sully in Vail, Colorado;
Jenny Cope of Give a Dog a Home; Arthur Mondejar with
Simba in Miami, Florida; Harold & Pamela Allen with Sammie
in Kendall, Fl; Kari Crist and London; Ashley Anne and Miss
Boston; Belinda Aiken and Caesar; Cris Rankin and Buster in
Arizona; Linda Badgett Forward and Winston; Tony Toby with
Anya and Dexter; Nicole Brannon and Mira; Amanda Ramirez
with Azog, Otso and Goldee; Debbie Glenn and Bailey;
Samantha Lopez and Aalto; Judy Fender with Maggie Mae,
who died from distemper; Scott Nadeau with Tucker, who did
not survive; Viji Vijimnm of India who lost his dog to
distemper; David, Abby, and Neneth with Claire-Bear in

the Philippines who did not survive; Mary Randolph with Millie in East Texas who did not survive; Amelia Rohrmoser with Darwin in Costa Rica, who did not survive; Kandy and Brian Bouquet with Nanook who did not survive in California; Dimas De Moya with Dixie who did not survive in the Dominican Republic.

For more on these and other stories, including pictures, videos and documents, go to **http://www.kindheartsinaction.com** or to the **Save Dogs From Distemper** Facebook page.

GLOSSARY

My intent here is to explain these scientific terms so the average reader will better understand them, not provide the complete, expert definitions.

Acute phase – When the symptoms of the disease last for a short period of time, as opposed to the **chronic** phase, where systems persist long-term. In distemper, the respiratory symptoms are acute. The neurologic symptoms can often be chronic.

Acyclovir – An antiviral drug.

Antibiotic – A material that can destroy or inhibit bacteria.

Antibodies – Proteins in the blood that can attach themselves to attacking foreign bodies such as bacteria, viruses and other pathogens.

Antigen – A substance that prompts an immune response within a body.

Ataxia – Loss of muscle control and balance.

Atrophic – Wasting away tissues.

B cell – A type of white blood cell not made by the thymus.

Bacterium – (bacteria is the plural form) A single-celled organism. Some bacteria are responsible for disease.

Blood-brain barrier – A semi-permeable barrier that separates the brain and spinal cord from the rest of the body. It allows some materials to pass, but blocks others.

C-peptides – A material that aids in the formation of insulin.

Canid – A mammal related to the dog.

CDV – Canine Distemper Virus

Catarrh – A buildup of mucus in the nose or throat.

CNS – Central nervous system

Cerebrospinal fluid (CSF) – A clear protective fluid found in the brain and spinal canal.

Chorea – Also called myoclonus, it is a spasmodic twitching of the muscles.

Conjunctiva – Mucous membrane of the eye and eyelids.

Conjunctivitis – Inflammation of the mucus membranes of the eye and eyelid.

Cytokine – A group of proteins that send signals between cells. Interferon is one type of this protein.

Cytoplasm – The material within a cell that is not the nucleus.

Demodex – Mange. A mite that infects the skin of animals, especially dogs. It impairs the immune system.

Diluent – A fluid used as a medium to inject or apply the vaccine particles. Newcastle's Disease Vaccine often comes with a bottle of blue diluent.

Diphasic – Two-stage

Double-blind study – When neither the researcher nor the subject knows which type of treatment has been received until after clinical trial is over.

Dystocia – A difficult birth, typically caused by the size and position of the fetus in relation to the mother's uterus, cervix or pelvis.

Encephalitis – An infection of the brain, as with Old Dog Encephalitis (ODE).

Encephalomyelitis – Inflammation of brain and spinal cord.

Epithelial – The surface layer of a body or of the esophagus, stomach and intestines.

Fauces – Part of the pharynx at the back of the mouth and nasal cavity.

Fomites – Objects or materials that are likely to carry infection, such as clothes, utensils, and furniture. Dust and fine particles in the air can also transmit pathogens.

Foramen magnum – An opening at the base of the skull, through which the spinal cord passes to connect with the brain.

Formalin – An antiseptic, which also acts as a fixative so tissue can be preserved.

Ganglia – A structure of nerve cells.

Genotype – The genetic makeup.

Humoral – Relating to body fluids.

Hyperkeratosis – Hardpad and the drying/thickening of nasal planum in distemper dogs.

In vitro – Outside a living body, usually in a test tube or petri dish. From the Latin for "in glass."

In vivo – Inside a living body.

Inclusions – Foreign granules, particles or droplets caused by infection, such as viruses in stained nuclei.

Incubation period – The time between exposure to a pathogen and the onset of symptoms.

Inducer – A microbe such as a virus or bacteria that prompts a cell to create interferon or other desired effect.

Interferon – A protein made by cells to inhibit the replication of viruses and some cancers.

Intranuclear – Within the cell nucleus.

Lymphocytes – A type of white blood cell in the lymphatic system.

Macrophages – White blood cells, which capture and destroy foreign materials, such as viruses and damaged tissues. They also prepare antigens for the B and T cells to process.

Mucopurulent – Fluid containing mucus or pus.

Multiple sclerosis – A disease that destroys the oligodentrocytes that generate the protective myelin of nervous system and causes a range of neurologic problems. Suspected causes are genetics, environment or an attack from a virus.

Myoclonus – A sudden, involuntary jerking of a muscle or group of muscles.

Myelin – Fatty white material that insulates the neuron. Loss of myelin causes a disruption in nerve function.

Nasal planum – The tip of a dog's nose.

Necropsy – An autopsy on an animal.

Necrosis – Cell death.

Neonate – Newborn.

NDV – Newcastle's Disease Vaccine.

Oculonasal – Relating to eyes and nose.

Oligodentrocyte – The cell that produces myelin in the central nervous system.

Optic neuritis – Infection of the optic nerve, which connects the eye to the brain.

Pathogen – A microorganism that causes disease.

Placebo – A material without a therapeutic benefit used to help establish controls in scientific studies.

Plasma cell – A kind of B cell that produces a specific antibody.

Plasmids – Small strands of DNA that float and replicate in the cytoplasm of the cell.

PCR or polymerase chain reaction – Another method of detecting virus first developed 35 years ago. It works by making a copy of a piece of genetic information from the virus and then making thousands to millions of copies.

Reassortment – When the genes of a virus exist as segments and the gene segments of one virus swap with the gene segments of another virus. This usually happens as both viruses infect the same host cell.

Recombinant – Created by combining other genetic material.

Recombination – The swapping of a gene within a single segment to form a new virus or a variation of the original.

RNA interference – When an RNA strand binds with another RNA strand and blocks the genetic message.

Sclerosing – Causing the overgrowth and/or hardening of tissues.

Serum – What remains when blood cells are removed from blood. The liquid usually has a yellowish tint from the fats present.

Sequelae – The results or effects of a disease.

Specific-pathogen-free (SPF) – Laboratory animals established to be free of particular pathogens to ensure they do not affect the outcome of tests.

Subcutaneous injection – An injection made just below the skin, as opposed to a vein. Frequently referred to as "sub-Q."

Taxonomy – How organisms are classified.

T-cell – A type of white blood cell produced by the thymus gland. It plays an essential role in immunity by maintaining long term memory to any antigen to which it has been sensitized through vaccination.

Thoracic – Relating to chest cavity between neck and abdomen.

Titer – The amount of antibody in the blood.

Trachea – The windpipe.

Vaccination – The administration of a dead, weakened or altered version of a microorganism (vaccine) with the intent to trigger the immune system. After a vaccination, the body's immune system should be able to recognize and destroy the full-strength version.

Variolation – Scratching material taken from a smallpox victim into the skin of a healthy person. This would result in sickness, but if the person survived they should have immunity to small pox. Used before the development of vaccination.

Virotherapy – Genetic reprogramming of viruses so they might be used to treat disease.

Virus – A small packet of genetic information, usually covered in an envelope of protein. It causes disease by invading a living host cell and using the cell's energy to replicate itself and spread.

Bibliography

Adams JM, Brown WJ, Snow HD, Lincoln SD, Sears Jr AW, Barenfus M, Holliday TA, Cremer NE, Lennette EH. 1975. Old Dog Encephalitis and Demyelinating Diseases in Man. Vet. Pathol. 12: 220-226

Adams JM, Snow HD. 1973. Viral Demyelinating Encephalitis And Old Dog Encephalitis: Possible Relationship To Distemper Measles, And Dermyelinating Disease Of Man. Calif. Vet. 27: 8-10

Adams JM, Imagawa DT, Chadwick DL, Gates EH, Siem RA. 1958. Relationship of Measles and Distemper. AMA Am J Dis Child.;95(6): 601-608

Alonso M, Jiang H, Gomez-Manzano C, Fueyo J. 2012. Targeting brain tumor stem cells with oncolytic adenoviruses. Methods Mol Biol. 2012;797:111-25. doi: 10.1007/978-1-61779-340-0_9.

AnimalResearch. Dog [Internet] [cited Jan. 25, 2018] Available from http://www.animalresearch.info/en/designing-research/research-animals/dog/

Babcock S, Jack D, Lacroix C, Pfeiffer C, Thomas J, March 2009. The American Veterinary Medical Law Association White Paper, "Vaccine Liability Issues for Veterinarians," [Internet] Edited by Settles E. Available from https://avmla.org/wp-content/uploads/2011/09/Vaccine_Liability_AVMLA.pdf

Bond E. 2000. How Galen was saved. [Internet] Available from http://www.edbond.com.

Bond E. 2009. Kind Hearts In Action. [Internet] Available from htttp://www.kindheartsinaction.com

Bresalier M, Worboys M. [Internet] 2014. 'Saving the lives of our dogs': the development of canine distemper vaccine in interwar Britain. Br J Hist Sci. Jun; 47(173 Pt 2):305-34. Available from https://www.ncbi.nlm.nih.gov/pmc/articles/PMC4014013/pdf/S0007087413000344a.pdf

Centers for Disease Control and Prevention website https://www.cdc.gov/coronavirus

Cornell University's Wildlife Health Lab website https://cwhl.vet.cornell.edu/disease/canine-distemper

Csatary L. 1971. Viruses in the treatment of cancer. Lancet; Oct 9;2(7728):825.

Csatary L, Bakács T. 1999. Use of Newcastle Disease Virus Vaccine (MTH-68/H) in a Patient With High-grade Glioblastoma. JAMA;281(17):1588-1589

Dr. Jenner's House Museum and Garden [Internet] https://jennermuseum.com/ Dr Edward Jenner 1749-1823. [cited January 2018] Available from https://drjennershouse.files.wordpress.com/2016/09/jenner-for-website2.pdf.

Faustman D, Wang L, Okubo Y, Burger D, Ban L, Man G, Zheng H, Schoenfeld D, Pompei R, Avruch J, Nathan D. August 2012. Proof-of-Concept, Randomized, Controlled Clinical Trial of Bacillus-Calmette-Guerin for Treatment of Long-Term Type 1 Diabetes. PLoS ONE, Volume 7, Issue 8, e41756

Ferry N. 1911. Etiology of canine distemper. Journal of Infectious Diseases 4, pp. 399–420.

Gonzalez G, Marshall J, Morrell J, Robb D, McCauley J, Perez D, Parrish C, Murcia P. 2014. Infection and pathogenesis of canine, equine and human influenza viruses in canine tracheas. Journal of Virology, Aug;88(16):9208-19. doi: 10.1128/JVI.00887-14. Epub 2014 Jun 4.

Gloyd J. Jan. 1987. Editorial: Protecting your practice and the food animal industry. JAVMA (Vol. 190, No. 1) p. 34.

The Guide for the Care and Use of Laboratory Animals. 8th edition. 2011. National Academies Press.

Han GZ, Liu XP, Li SS. 2008. Cross-species recombination in the haemagglutinin gene of canine distemper virus. Virus Res 2008;136(1-2):198–201.

The Humane Society of the United States. Questions and Answers About Biomedical Research [Internet] 2018. Available from http://www.humanesociety.org/issues/biomedical_research/qa/questions_answers.html

Jenner E. Observations on the Distemper in Dogs. 1809. Medico-Chirurgical Transactions. 1: 265-270.

Kapil S, Yeary T, 2011. Canine Distemper Spillover in Domestic Dogs from Urban Wildlife. Veterinary Clinics: Small Animal Practice, Volume 4 , Issue 6, pp. 1069-1086.

Kay N. 2011. Speaking for Spot: Be the Advocate Your Dog Needs to Live a Happy Healthy Longer Life. CreateSpace Independent Publishing Platform.

Kind Hearts In Action YouTube channel. 2009. [Internet] Available from **https://www.youtube.com/channel/UCUIFS3ZgmVLkrvt1w2v peAQ?**

Kirk H. 1922. Canine Distemper: It's Complications, Sequelae and Treatment. London. Bailliére, Tindall and Cox.

Ma W, Kahn R, Richt J. 2008. The pig as a mixing vessel for influenza viruses: Human and veterinary implications. J Mol Genet Med. 2008 Nov 27;3(1):158-66.

Maddie's Fund. Maddie's Story. [Internet] [cited October 2013] Available from http://www.maddiesfund.org/maddies-story.htm

Maddie's Fund Education YouTube channel. April 9, 2014. Everything Shelters Need to Know About Canine Distemper, a webinar by Dr. Cynda Crawford. [Internet] Available from https://youtu.be/LekbdFETyEw

Maddie's Fund Education YouTube channel. Oct. 2, 2012. Treating Canine Distemper Virus, a lecture by Dr. Ellen Jefferson. [Internet] Available from https://youtu.be/rq-mwDrJVE4

Malisow, Craig. May 4, 2015. Tens of Thousands of Dogs are Still Used in Laboratory Testing Every Year [Internet] Houston Press. Available from http://www.houstonpress.com/news/tens-of-thousands-of-dogs-are-still-used-in-laboratory-testing-every-year-7400834

May, K. 2018, Extralabel Drug Use and AMDUCA: FAQ, American Veterinary Medical Association, [Online]. Available: https://www.avma.org/KB/Resources/FAQs/Pages/ELDU-and-AMDUCA-FAQs.aspx

McCullough, B. 1972. Interferon Response in Cats. The Journal of Infectious Diseases, 125(2), 174-177. Available from http://www.jstor.org/stable/30111561

Mentis A, Dardiotis E, Grigoriadis N, Petinaki E, Hadjigeorgiou G. ePub May 23, 2017. Viruses and endogenous retroviruses in multiple sclerosis: From correlation to causation. Acta Neurologica Scandinavica 2017 Dec;136(6):606-616. doi: 10.1111/ane.12775.

M'Gowan JP. 1911. Some observations on a laboratory epidemic, principally among dogs and cats, in which the animals affected presented symptoms of the disease called "distemper." Journal of Pathology and Bacteriology 15, pp. 372 ff.

National Cancer Institute website November 2, 2016. [Internet] Newcastle Disease Virus (PDQ®)–Health Professional Version. Available from https://www.cancer.gov/about-cancer/treatment/cam/hp/ndv-pdq

The New England Anti-Vivisection Society (NEAVS) [Internet] [cited Jan. 25, 2018] Available from https://www.neavs.org/research/laws

Nobelprize.org. October 2, 2006. [Internet] The Nobel Prize in Physiology or Medicine 2006 Andrew Z. Fire, Craig C. Mello. Available from http://www.nobelprize.org/nobel_prizes/medicine/laureates/2006/press.html

Oldstone M. 2010. Viruses, Plagues & History: Past, Present and Future. Oxford University Press.

Paff ML, Nuismer SL, Ellington A, Molineux IJ, Bull JJ. (2016) Virus wars: using one virus to block the spread of another. PeerJ 4:e2166 https://doi.org/10.7717/peerj.2166

Pringle C. 1991. The Genetics of Paramyxoviruses. In Kingsbury D, editor. The Paramyxoviruses. Springer Science & Business Media. pp. 1-40.

Randall R, Russell W. 1991. Paramyxovirus Persistence Consequences for Host and Virus. In Kingsbury D, editor. The Paramyxoviruses. Springer Science & Business Media. pp. 299-322.

Riedel, Stefan. "Edward Jenner and the history of smallpox and vaccination." Proceedings (Baylor University. Medical Center) vol. 18,1 (2005): 21-5. doi:10.1080/08998280.2005.11928028

Samal S, editor. 2011. The Biology of Paramyxoviruses. Norfolk UK. Caister Academic Press

Sánchez, D.; Pelayo, R.; Medina, L.A.; Vadillo, E.; Sánchez, R.; Núñez, L.; Cesarman-Maus, G.; Sarmiento-Silva, R.E. Newcastle Disease Virus: Potential Therapeutic Application for Human and Canine Lymphoma. Viruses 2016, 8, 3.

Schubert T, Clemmons R, Miles S, Draper W. 2013. The use of botulinum toxin for the treatment of generalized myoclonus in a dog. J Am Anim Hosp Assoc. 2013 Mar-Apr;49(2):122-7. doi: 10.5326/JAAHA-MS-5786. Epub 2013 Jan 16.

Singer P, 1975, 2002. Animal Liberation. Harper Collins.

Soave, O. 1997. Animals, the Law and Veterinary Medicine. Lanham, New York, Oxford, Austin & Winfield Pub.

Song Q, Cao Y, Li Q, Gu M, Zhong L, Hu S, Wan H, Liu X. 2011. Artificial Recombination May Influence the Evolutionary Analysis of Newcastle Disease Virus . Journal of Virology. 2011;85(19):10409-10414. doi:10.1128/JVI.00544-11.

Summers B, Greisen H, Appel M, January 1984. Canine distemper encephalomyelitis: Variation with virus strain. Journal of Comparative Pathology, Volume 94, Issue 1, pp. 65-75

Swaminathan, Nikhil. August 8, 2008. Viruses: They're alive, and they can infect each other [Internet] Scientific American. Available from https://blogs.scientificamerican.com/news-blog/viruses-theyre-alive-and-they-can-i-2008-08-08/

Tayeb S, Zakay-Rones Z, Panet A. 2015. Therapeutic potential of oncolytic Newcastle disease virus: a critical review. Oncolytic Virother. Mar 27;4:49-62. doi: 10.2147/OV.S78600. eCollection 2015.

Tisoncik JR, Korth MJ, Simmons CP, Farrar J, Martin TR, Katze MG. 2012. Into the Eye of the Cytokine Storm. Microbiology and Molecular Biology Reviews. MMBR;76(1):16-32. doi:10.1128/MMBR.05015-11.

Tsai SC, Appel MJ. 1979. Interferon induction in dogs. Am J Vet Res. 1979 Mar;40(3):356-61.

Uhl, E. W., Kelderhouse, C., Buikstra, J., Blick, J. P., Bolon, B., and Hogan, R. J. (2019). New world origin of canine distemper: interdisciplinary insights. Int. J.Paleopathol. 24, 266–278. doi: 10.1016/j.ijpp.2018.12.007

Zamarin D, Palese P. 2012. Oncolytic Newcastle Disease Virus for Cancer Therapy Future Microbiology. Future Medicine Ltd. 2012;7(3):347-367 Available from https://www.medscape.com/viewarticle/760002_1

Mountain View Vet Clinic records

Use of 12-hour NDV-induced serum

DATE: 2/18/12
DOG NAME: Lara
OWNER: *****
Woodlawn VA Consent – N

DESCRIPTION
Staffordshire terrier
Brindle and white
F - b. 11/20/2011

DIAGNOSIS 3/27/12
PCR Canine Distemper
Result: Positive Ct= 31.10

Abaxis Veterinary
Reference Laboratories
Olathe, Kansas

TREATMENT NOTES
HBC ... *
2/29/12
O relinquished Lara to Jen Roberts
Verified by Jen Roberts and Jodie P.

Naxcel 0.15ml IV
Famotidine 4ml IV
10 a.m. NDV serum 1.5mlSQ fm Jett
10 p.m. NDV serum 1.5mlSQ fm Jett
3/15/12

3/13/12
Coughing, losing weight
BW - 7# puppy vacc.

BAR
Metacam 0.25ml PO
Naxcel 0.15ml IV
Famotidine 4ml IV

3/14/12
Bloody diarrhea - parvo test POS!
Metacam 0.25ml PO

10 a.m. NDV serum 1.5mlSQ fm Jett
...
6/2/12
Adopted by Mack and Bradi Tolbert!

OUTCOME	SURVIVED

DATE: 3/6/12
DOG NAME: Pax
OWNER: ****
Lexington KY Consent – Y

DESCRIPTION
Cocker Spaniel mix
White, F/12wks/
b. 12/31/2011

DIAGNOSIS 3/14/12
PCR Canine Distemper
Result: Positive

Abaxis Veterinary
Reference Laboratories
Olathe, Kansas

TREATMENT NOTES
NDV protocol - PE: nasal & ocular
hardened paw pads
Brd until Friday; coughing & saw
focal seizure on drive
PCR test Nasal swab in today
9 p.m. 2.5 ml NDV serum SQ
3/7/12
9 a.m. 2.5 ml NDV serum SQ
9 p.m. Very BAR
2.5 ml NDV serum SQ
3/8/12

Orbax 1 1/2ml PO QD
pm - pneumonia dev., coughing
Cough tablet 1/2 tab PO
Amoxi 250 mg PO pm
3/9/12
BAR
Orbax 1 1/2ml PO QD
Cough tablet 1/2 tab PO
Amoxi 250 mg PO BID
OK TO GO HOME
Rx Cough tablet 1/2 tab PO BIDx14d
Rx Orbax 1 1/2ml PO QDx 14d
Rx Amoxi 250 mg PO BIDx14d

OUTCOME	SURVIVED

DATE: 4/3/12
DOG NAME: Jubilee
OWNER: *****
Ballard WV Consent – Y

DESCRIPTION
Chihuahua mix Brown
Spayed female
b. 4/4/2008   4yrs

DIAGNOSIS 4/9/12
PCR Canine Distemper
Result: Positive

Abaxis Veterinary
Reference Laboratories
Olathe, Kansas

TREATMENT NOTES
Rescue group w/recent distemper
outbreak. Dog is unable to stand
Possible injury from other dog.
No coughing, sneezing, nasal D/C
or seizures
Metacam 0.17ml IV QD
Naxcel 0.18ml IV
Distemper PCR corneal swab
… CD deficits in gron and rear legs…
unable to hold head steady…
harsh lung sounds, bilaterally sm.
amt mucupurulent discharge ocular
6 p.m. NDV induced serum 2ml SQ
[from Jett]

4/4/12
6 a.m. NDV serum 2ml SQ
6 p.m. NDV serum 2ml SQ
Metacam 0.17ml IV QD
Naxcel 0.18ml IV
Hand fed 1/2 can food & 20mls H2O
4/5/12
BAR - barking, unable to stand.
Hand fed 1/4 can food. Seizuring
this p.m. …
*
Seizuring activity recorded 4/7 and 4/8
"almost comatose" …
4/9/12
Deceased in kennel
Owner will bury

OUTCOME	**DIED 4/9/2012**

DATE: 4/5/12
DOG NAME: Sadie Mae
OWNER: *****
Austinville VA– Y

DESCRIPTION
Cocker Spaniel Blonde
F/10/5/2010/18mos
BW 17.8#

DIAGNOSIS 4/19/12
PCR Canine Distemper
Result: Negative

Abaxis Veterinary
Reference Laboratories
Olathe, Kansas

TREATMENT NOTES
paralyzed in rear
can't control bladder
P.E. deep pain present; small amt
movement in both rear legs …
4/6/12
Urine in kennel. Did not eat overnight
… *
4/15/12
Ocular and nasal discharge. Cough.
Depressed anorexic
7 p.m. NDV serum 2.8 ml SQ
Cough tab - 1 tab PO BID

Simplicef 100mg PO QD …
4/16/12
7 a.m. NDV serum 2.8 ml SQ
Cough tab - 1 tab PO BID
Caught urine for distemper test
Simplicef 100mg PO QD …
Meloxicam 7.5 mg
7 p.m. NDV serum 2.8 ml SQ
…*
4/19/12
Dog depressed, not eating. Highly
recommend euth due to declining
quality of life. Owner OK'd over phone

OUTCOME	**DIED 4/19/2012**

DATE: 4/9/12 DOG NAME: Sam OWNER: ***** Elm City NC	DESCRIPTION Lab Retriever, Chocolate M 12mos, b. 4/10/2011
DIAGNOSIS 4/16/12 PCR Canine Distemper Result: Negative	Abaxis Veterinary Reference Laboratories Olathe, Kansas
TREATMENT NOTES NDV protocol BW 60# IV Catheter 1.2ml Naxcel IV pm Benadryl 50 mg PO *... unable to stand without support; unable to hold head steady; mild Rythmic tremor of rear leg ... Owner reports eats and drinks well. Head bob started about 1 wk ago ... ... no focal seizures of head and face and no generalized seizures 4/10/12 NDV spinal tap today. 11 ml Propofol IV 200 ml LRS IV 1.3ml Morphine SQ 1.2ml Naxcel IV 1.1 ml Metacam IV	Distemper PCR 0.5ml CSF Spinal tap 0.5ml serum from "HS Lab" intrathecal; Flushed w/0.5ml sterile saline ... 4/12 and 4/13 QAR, eating v well, unable to stand very ataxic ... 4/14/12 ... Phenobarb 1gr PO BID Ate well this a.m. No movement. Few tremors this a.m. Wagging tail. 4/15/12 Eating hand fed. Will not eat gravy 4/17/12 Goes home with Rx for Phenobarb, simplicef, and Meloxicam
OUTCOME	**SURVIVED**
DATE: 4/11/12 DOG NAME: Baloo OWNER: ***** Fayetteville NC	DESCRIPTION Bluetick coonhound, Blue and white Neutered male, b. 4/12/2010, 24ms
DIAGNOSIS 4/17/2012 Spoke w/ Highland Animal Hospital. Distemper test postive according to Antech	[Note on records from Highland reads: Igg: 1 – 320; Igm: 1 – 110; positi]
TREATMENT NOTES P.E. Mucopurulent ocular & nasal Dyspneic Tachypnic Depressed v. thin No neurologic signs Ciprofloxacin 1/2x500mg PO BID 6p.m.: NDV serum 6 ml SQ 4/12/12 6 a.m.: NDV serum 6 ml SQ 6 p.m.: NDV serum 6c ml SQ Ciprofloxacin 1/2x500mg PO BID Meloxicam - 1/4x7.5mg PO BID Cough tab - 1 tab BID Lungs v. harsh. Eating very well.	4/13/12 BAR eating well 1/4 meloxicam 7.5mg PO 1 Cough tab PO BID Ciprofloxacin 1/2x500mg PO BID BAR this p.m.; coughs occasionally; 4/14/12 1/4 meloxicam 7.5mg PO 1 Cough tab PO BID Ciprofloxacin 1/2x500mg PO BID Eating great. BAR 4/16/12; 4/17/12 5/30/12 BAR appears normal this a.m
OUTCOME	**SURVIVED**

NDV SPINAL TAP CASES

DATE: 4/10/12
DOG NAME: Pooka
OWNER: *****
Corolle NC

DIAGNOSIS
No record

TREATMENT NOTES
NDV protocol w/A-O tap
IV Catheter 3.8ml Propofol IV slowly
spinal tap - 0.2ml serum from HS lab
intrathecal
flushed w/0.5ml sterile saline
Distemper test on CSF
Naxcel - 0.25ml IV
Morphine - 0.3ml SQ
Metacam - 0.2ml SQ

DESCRIPTION
Toy Poodle mix
Male, neutered
Black and white
b. 8/21/03 8yrs old

Email follow-up
to owner not returned

4/11/11
QAR - can stand and walk with
assistance this a.m. but still ataxic.
Urine and feces in kennel. Offered food
and H2O no interest.
4/12/12
BAR Eating very well. Still ataxic
OK to go home today
Owner to keep confined and
quarrantined for 2 months
RX Metacam, Simplicef and
Phenobarb1.1 ml Metacam IV

OUTCOME	**SURVIVED**

DATE: 5/2/12
DOG NAME: Pistachio
OWNER: Sanchez

DIAGNOSIS ??

TREATMENT NOTES
Trembles constantly; can stand & walk
Mildly ataxic; Heart WNL
harsh lung sounds bilaterally
IV Cath 250 ml LRS IV
valium 0.3ml IV
RX Phenobarb Elixir 1.4ml PO BIDx3oz
RX Cephalexin 2ml PO BIDx40ml
5/7/12
Recheck - did well for a few days,
trembling decreased; was eating and
drinking. Now O is hand fee ding
and syringing water; Had 1st seizure
5/6; O thinks he's had several minor
ones since as well. Vocalizes almost
constantly.
Diazepam 0.4ml rectally @8:45 a.m.

DESCRIPTION
Chihuahua mix Golden Male
7mos/ b. 10/5/2011

NDV spinal tap - 1.3ml Propofol IV
.4ml Morphine SQ IV
.05ml Metacam SQ
IV Catheter 100ml LRS IV
.1ml NDV induced serum + 1ml NaCL
injected intrathecal at the Atlanto-
Axial Space; Applied pressure &
elevated head for 10 min. afterward
5/8/12
Lateral recumbancy this a.m.
0.1ml Naxcel IV
60mls LRS IV
0.09 ml Metacam IV ...
5/10/12
QAR v. ataxic. ...

OUTCOME	**UNKOWN**

DATE: 5/10/12
DOG NAME: Kitana
OWNER: *****

DESCRIPTION
Siberian Husky mix White
Spayed female b. 1/19/2012 16w

DIAGNOSIS
Referral hospital called
reported distemper pos
PCR test taken

TREATMENT NOTES
.P.E. Twitching. Fly biting seizures
started yesterday. Lungs harsh. Paw
pads severely crusted. IV cath already
placed
P. spinal tap - NDV serum
.3 Benadryl SQ
.37 morphine SQ
0.2ml NDV serum intrathecal
0.5ml Rectally diazepam
Dopram 0.5ml sublingually
Propofol 4.5ml IV
0.25ml Diazepam Rectally
5/11/12
Lateral recumbency, muscle twitching
moaning. Referal hospital called
reported distemper pos.

Phenobarb 1/2x1/4 gr PO BID
Morphine 0.3ml SQ
RX: Phenobarb 1/2 tab PO BID
Naxcel 0.25ml SQ
Standing this p.m. Uninterested in food
Does not seem very painful
5/12/12
Phenobarb 1/2x1/4 gr PO BID
Simplicef 1/2x100mg PO QD
5/13/12
[Handwriting illegible]
7 p.m. NDV serum SQ 2 ml
200ml SQ LRS
5/14/12
Deceased

OUTCOME	DIED 5/14/12

NDV SERUM

LIVED	DIED
4	2

NDV SERUM SPINAL TAP

LIVED	DIED
1	1

Unknown outcome on 1 case
Follow-ups needed on spinal tap cases

Use of NDV as IV injection *

Owner	Name/Descript.	Treatment notes	Outcome
	10/11/11		
Laurie's Rescue Dogs	Meg Boxer mix/ tri-color F/16w/7/12/2011	NDV Protocol 2mls NDV mixed w/33 mls LRS IV 0.3 ml Benadryl SQ IV cath 12/2/11 Rx Drontal 20#	**Survived**
	Aussie Mix 1 Shepherd/ Australian mix U/16w/7/8/2011	NDV Protocol 2 mls NDV mixed w/33 mls LRS IV 0.3 ml Benadryl SQ 0.15 ml Naxcel SQ IV cath 10/28/11 RX Clavamox to share w/Germ. Shep RX Clavamox 62.5mg PO BIDx7d 11/2/11 Refill Clavamox 62.5mg PO BIDx7d	**Survived**
	Aussie Mix 2 Shepherd/ Australian mix U/16w/7/8/2011	NDV Protocol 2 mls NDV mixed w/33 mls LRS IV 0.3 ml Benadryl SQ 0.15 ml Naxcel SQ IV cath 11/2/11 RX Clavamox 62.5mg PO BIDx7d	**Survived**
	Boxer Mix 1 Boxer Mix/ tri-color U/16w/7/12/2011	NDV Protocol 2 mls NDV mixed w/33 mls LRS IV 0.3 ml Benadryl SQ 0.15 ml Naxcel SQ IV cath	**Survived**

	Boxer Mix 2 Boxer Mix/ tri-color U/16w/7/12/2011	NDV Protocol **Survived** 2 mls NDV mixed w/33 mls LRS IV 0.3 ml Benadryl SQ 0.15 ml Naxcel SQ
	Germ. Shep 1 German shep. m Black and Tan M/17w/7/5/2011	NDV Protocol **Survived** 2 mls NDV mixed w/33 mls LRS IV 0.3 ml Benadryl SQ 0.15 ml Naxcel SQ
	Germ. Shep 2 German shep.mi Black and Tan F/17w/7/5/2011	NDV Protocol **Survived** 2 mls NDV mixed w/33 mls LRS IV IV Cath. 0.3 ml Benadryl SQ 0.15 ml Naxcel SQ 11/2/11 RX Clavamox 62.5mg PO BIDx7d
10/12/11		
Wythe Co. H. Society	Ashley Australian Cattle Dog red F/5m/5/15/2011	NDV vacc - 2cc + 33ml LRS **Deceased** Naxcel 0.3ml IV 10/25/11 LRS __ ml IV 8% dehydrated. Previous diarrhea Cough. Nasal discharge. Weak, depressed Eating dry food, dog gags, salivates Does not happen with canned food*
	Zeus Daschund, minature mix black and tan M/12w/7/14/2011	NDV Vaccine Protocol **Survived** Mucopurulent ocular/nasal discharge Productive cough Naxcel 0.2 ml IV NDV vaccine. 2 ml diluted in 33 ml LRS IV

10/15/11		
Wythe Co.	Trixie	NDV vac **Deceased**
H. Society	Shih Tzu	Mucopurulent ocular dischar 10/19/11
	U/12m	Very depressed
		NDV vac - 2cc IV + 35 ml LRS
		Ampicillin - 0.4ml SQ BID
		bnp - apply OU BID
		IV cath
		Corneal swab for distemper PCR
		250ml Bolus LRS
10/21/11		
Wythe Co.	Sitta Lee	NDV treatment - 35ml LRS+ **Deceased**
H. Society	Puggle	S/R from spay 10/22/11
	Spayed Female/	Benadryl 0.1 ml SQ
	5yrs	Polyflex - 0.4 ml SQ BID
		Metacam 0.15 ml
		Lasix 0.1 ml IV BID
		10/22/11
		Dead in kennel this a.m.
10/24/11		
Wythe Co.	Timmy	NDV 2ml NDV vacc in 33 ml **Survived**
H. Society	Chihuahua Mix	
	Brown	10/25/11
	M/24m/10/26/20(	.25ml Naxcel .1ml Benadryl SQ/ IV Catheter
10/24/11		
Wythe Co.	Sugar	NDV 2 ml NDV vacc given ir **Survived**
H. Society	Maltese mix	LRS IV
	white	.37 ml Naxcel SQ .1 ml Benadryl SQ
	F/24m/10/26/20(	IV Catheter
		RX Doxt 100 mg Give 1/4 tab PO BIDX14 days

10/24/11		
Wythe Co. H. Society	Baby Schnauzer mix black Spayed Female/ 5yrs/10/27/2006	NDV **Survived** 2mls NDV Vacc w/ 33 mls LRS IV IV cath 0.37 ml Naxcel SQ 0.3 ml Benadryl SQ RX Doxy 100mg Give 1/4 tab PO BIDx14days
10/24/11		
Wythe Co. H. Society	Thomas Terrier, Cairn mix Blonde M/24m/10/26/20(	NDV 2ml NDV mixed w/33 n **Survived** 10/26/11 1/2 Polyflex SQ IV Catheter Rx Doxy 100mg 1/4 tab PO BIDx14days
10/24/11		
Wythe Co. H. Society	Shelby Chihuahua mix tri-color F/12m/10/26/201	NDV 2ml NDVmixed w/ 33 n **Survived** 10/26/11 IV Catheter RX Doxy 100 mg 1/4 tab PO BIDx14dys
10/24/11		
Wythe Co. H. Society	Hairy Fox terrier mix Black M/24m/10/26/20(	NDV 2ml NDVmixed w/ 33 n **Survived** 10/26/11 IV Catheter RX Doxy 100 mg 1/4 tab PO BIDx14dys
10/24/11		
Wythe Co. H. Society	Shelly Chihuahua mix tri-color F/12m/10/26/201	NDV 2ml NDVmixed w/ 33 n **Survived** 10/26/11 IV Catheter RX Doxy 100 mg 1/4 tab PO BIDx14 days

10/24/11		
Wythe Co. H. Society	Katie Terrier, Jack Russell mix brown and white F/17wks/6/28/20	NDV 2ml NDVmixed w/ 33 n **Survived** 10/26/11 IV Catheter RX Doxy 100 mg 1/4 tab PO BIDx14dys
10/24/11		
Wythe Co. H. Society	Lacey Terrier, Jack Russell mix brown and white F/17wks/6/28/20	NDV 2ml NDVmixed w/ 33 n **Survived** 10/26/11 IV Catheter RX Doxy 100 mg 1/4 tab POBIDx14 days
10/26/11		
Wythe Co. H. Society	Oreo Shih Tzu mix black and white M/3yrs/10/26/200	NDV 2ml NDVmixed w/ 33 n **Survived** IV Catheter .2ml Benadryl SQ RX Doxy 100 mg 1/4 tab PO BIDx14dys
10/26/11		
Wythe Co. H. Society	Peanut Cairn Terrier mix - tan M/24m/10/26/200	NDV 2ml NDVmixed w/ 33 n **Survived** IV Catheter .2ml Benadryl SQ RX Doxy 100 mg 1/4 tab PO BIDx14dys
10/28/11		
Wythe Co. H. Society	Blue Toy Poodle black and tan M/8yrs/11/3/2003	NDV vacc - 2ml NDV + 35 m **Survived** Benadryl - 0.1 ml SQ Doxycycline - 50 mg PO QD q 10d Very severe dry, non-productive cough PolyFlex 0.4 ml SQ Dog received 50 ml LRS during vac.

10/28/11		
Wythe Co. H. Society	Sugar Yorkie mix N/A	NDV vac - 2ml + 35 ml LRS **Survived** Benadryl 0.1 ml SQ Doxycycline 50 mg PO QD q10days 50 ml LRS during vaccination
10/28/11		
Wythe Co. H. Society	Spike Scot terrier black N/A	NDV vac - 2ml + 35 ml LRS **Survived** Benadryl 0.1 ml SQ Doxycycline 50 mg PO QD q10days 50 ml LRS during vaccination [Sugar, Spike records on same form]
10/28/11		
Wythe Co. H. Society	Shorty Poodle mix white N/A	NDV vac - 2ml + 35 ml LRS **Survived** Benadryl 0.1 ml SQ 50 ml LRS during vaccination
10/28/11		
Wythe Co. H. Society	Happy Yorkie poo tan/black N/A	NDV vac - 2ml + 35 ml LRS **Survived** Benadryl 0.1 ml SQ 50 ml LRS during vaccination
10/28/11		
Wythe Co. H. Society	Red Pekinese red N/A	NDV vac - 2ml + 35 ml LRS **Survived** Benadryl 0.1 ml SQ 50 ml LRS during vaccination [Shorty, Happy, Red records same form]

11/28/11		
***	Buddy	NDV protocol **Deceased**
	Collie Mix	Dog is on Doxycycline, Phenobarbital
	Sable and White	Meloxicam & tramadol
	M/9yrs/11/30/200	IV catheter 2 ml NDV mixed w/35 ML LRS IV
		1 ml Benadryl SQ
		12/4/11
		RX Lixotinic 2 oz - Give 5cc PO SID until gone
12/8/11		
***	Oz	**Deceased**
	Golden Retr.	Bilat ocular discharge, severely harsh lungs
	golden	[lab test confirms distemper]
	M/5yrs/12/9/200	NDV vaccine - 3ml in 32 ml LRS IV
		…
		12/14/11
		Seizure -- euthanized
5/23/12		
***	Gizmo	Coughing, not eating, vomiti **Survived**
	Yorkshire Terr.	lethargic
	Brown and tan	Blood panel
	M/6ys/2/9/2006	Naxcel - 0.2ml IV
		Metacam - 0.06ml IV
		Cerenia 0.3ml IV
	5/24/12	Distemper test - ocular swab
		NDV vacc - 2ml diluted in 35 ml LRS IV
		Benadryl - 0.3ml IM
	5/28/12	BAR - Eating well. Urinated outside,
		Sneezing while on walk.
		Naxcel - 0.2ml IV
		Famotidine 0.2ml IV
		Metacam - 0.06ml IV
		OK TO GO HOME
		Rx for Amoxi, pepcid, metacam, doxycycline

	5/23/12		
***	Bubby	puppy vacc.	**Survived**
	Yorkshire Terr.	Deworm	
	Black and tan		5/29/12
	BW 3.2#	Possible distemper. Coughing, watery	
	M/9wks/3/21/201	eyes, sneezing.	
		NDV protocol	
		RX Amoxi 0.75ml PO BIDx14days	
		Rx Metacam 0.1ml PO QDx5days	
		Rx Cough tabs 1/2 tab PO BID DRN	
		6/14/12	
		RX Amoxi 0.75ml PO BIDx14days - out of stock	
		Rx Cough tabs 1/2 tab PO BID	
		Rx Clavamox 1/2 ml PO BID	

32 dogs treated with NDV as IV

27 survived

5 died

NDV: Newcastle Disease Vaccine
LRS: Lactated Ringer's solution
SQ: subcutaneous
Drontal: dewormer
PO: by mouth
BID: Twice a day
P.E.: Physical exam
BNP: ointment
Bolus: Form of sub-Q injection
(sometimes a tablet in other animals)
S/R: suture removal
QD: 4 times a day
BAR: Bright and alert
HBC: Hit by car

FHO: Femoral head osteotomy
CD Deficits: Neurol unable to make
paw upright
CRT: Capillary refill time
PE - WNL: within normal limits
No SIR: No suture removal
Rx: prescription
O: Owner
BW: Body weight
WNL: within normal limits
Bolus: Form of sub-Q injection
(sometimes a tablet in other animals)
H. Society: Humane Society

* These are the initial outcomes of
these distemper cases after
treatment with NDV as IV. One of the
first group of 7 puppies died weeks
later of a respiratory infection.

THE NDV PROTOCOLS
by DR. ALSON SEARS

**Making the 12-Hour NDV-Induced Serum
(Anti-Morbillivirus Serum)**

for distemper dogs in pre-neurologic stage

1. DOG: Use a 10- to 12-month-old, mixed-breed dog, 60-90 lbs, 27.27kg to 40.91kg, young and healthy.

2. Do full lab work-up to eliminate all possible health problems, especially blood-born diseases.

3. Must be previously vaccinated against all local diseases.

4. Do not use breeds or individuals known to have immune deficiency problems.

5. Make up Newcastle Disease Vaccine 1000 dose vial. (Use only the 6 cc of diluent vial that comes with the NDV or Saline if Diluent is not available). Inject 6.0cc of Diluent or Saline into the NDV vial. Discard the balance remaining from the Diluent vial. The La Sota strain or B-1 are most common. Other strains of this virus should work as well but do not use Killed Virus NDV Vaccine. Use Modified Live NDV. This virus is your cell immunity inducer.

6. Place IV Catheter in dog.

7. Inject 2.0 or 3.0cc of Newcastle virus I.V. from your vaccine bottle depending on the official weight of the dog. (Treat dog with I.V fluids accordingly) (Do Not use Corticosteroids)

8. Induction of Newcastle's disease virus for cellular immune serum may only be done once on any dog. The second time around, antibodies to Newcastle's disease are present. These are of no use and can cause an adverse reaction.

9. Timing is absolutely essential for taking serum against distemper. Take blood 11-12 hours post injection (11-12 hrs post injection= Anti-viral factors=Very effective against Distemper Virus in VIVO.) Timing is important. (Interferon, antiviral, regulatory, anti-inflammatory cytokines all have different times of production).

10. All procedures must be sterile. Just prior to the 11-12 hours post- injection, anesthetize donor dog (approx. 5-10 minutes before).

11. Place Jugular catheter.

12. Start I.V. fluids.

13. Withdraw blood between the 11th and 12th hour and inject into 10cc blood vials [sterile no additive vials] and allow the blood to clot. All VETS please take out only up to maximum amount from donor dog. Remove blood just short of putting the dog into shock. That can be determined by the color of the gums and respiratory rate. What is amazing is the speed with which a healthy dog recovers. Fluids of course help recovery. We could take about 250 cc whole blood from a 90 lb dog and get about 100 cc of usable serum (A.W. Sears DVM 6/8/09)

14. Centrifuge immediately after clotting for clear serum. Do not allow RBC's to lyse.

15. Remove serum and place into sterile bottles.

16. Place serum bottles in baggies and store in refrigerator. Bottles of serum can be stored for up to five years in a refrigerator; longer if frozen.

17. Cryo-precipitates may form after refrigeration. Mixing causes clouding. This is not harmful.

18. May be filtered out with a .02 micron filter. Keep sterile.

19. All my donor dogs have survived. I have not lost any.

Dosage

From Dr. Sears: Dose of the serum depends on age of the dog. If for herpes, single shot 1 cc to each pup at birth. If for distemper of any age the dose is 1 cc per dog plus 1 cc per 10 lbs 12 hours apart for 3 treatments. So, 20 lb dog would be 3 cc sub Q 12 hours apart 3 times. for a 30 lb dog would be 1 cc plus 3 cc for a total of 4 cc given 3 times. Not NDV as some dogs cannot or do not respond. UPDATE: Give the injection sub Q on the rear legs--left or right--anterior to the great muscle, NOT between the shoulders or neck area.

Screening Tests/Criteria for Donor Dogs

1) Most important is parasites; must not have any ascarids; (roundworms), as these severely change the ability to create the NDV reaction and also interfere with the ability to make antibodies against distemper and interferes with vaccines.

2) Look for skin parasites such as demodex. (All these things cause a change in the way the inducer works).

3) Full blood count

4) Full urine test

5) Thyroid test

Unfortunately, not all large dogs are eligible to be donor dogs. Mixed breeds are usually best, and some pure breeds do not create a serum that can save other dogs. Those that can't be donor dogs include German shepherds, poodles, Irish setters, Gordon setters, English bulldogs and shar peis. There are other mixed-breed dogs that are not good donors, but fewer than the purebred dogs.

Treatment Of Neurologic Distemper
With The NDV-Induction Tap

This medical protocol covers neurologic forms of distemper, which include chorea, seizures, progressive paralysis, blindness. This medical protocol pertains to dogs of all ages who ARE infected with the neurologic forms of distemper.

Medical procedure protocol for NDV-induction tap
1. Place an IV catheter.

2. Anesthetize the dog as for surgery.

3. Prep for surgery at the foramen magnum.

4. Spinal tap at the Foramen Magnum.

5. Remove 0.1 cc to 1.0 cc of spinal fluid based on the size of the dog.

6. Send the spinal fluid to a lab for testing for anti-distemper antibodies. Antech Labs.

7. Inject using the same placed needle from 0.1 to 0.5 cc of NDV depending on size of the dog directly into the spinal canal and flush the needle with ½ to 1 cc of saline.

8. Treat the dog for shock with fluids after giving this injection.

Send saved spinal fluid to Lab for Anti-Distemper Antibodies in the CSF. Any distemper antibody found is totally diagnostic for Neurologic Distemper. Must verify the CSF antidistemper antibodies.

Other tests to be deemed necessary by the attending veterinarian. Toxoplasmosis, immune cells, Infection, other causes of neuropathology, cancer.

Regenerative ability of the brain stem cells (Schwann cells or oligodendrocytes, and the replacement of myelin, stem cells) will allow for healing over a period of time and it will vary depending on the genetics of the dog and its ability to recover.

Control of the seizure activity at this time can be controlled with Phenobarb and other seizure medications until all symptoms come under control and disappear. The time involved here depends on the severity of the damage and the ability and genetics of the animal to recover. This can be a long-term recovery.

Life long immunity to distemper is conferred with infection from distemper virus.

NDV once given to any dog establishes NDV antibody for which there is no need. It precludes the use of NDV in any particular dog in the future as the antibody will neutralize this virus and prevent its activity on the immune system.

Recommended Treatment After Spinal Tap

Drug therapy can help limit the pain dogs experience after a spinal tap treatment. The pain control and extra rest and sleep in the first week after the treatment is key. Otherwise a dog who had seemed to be rebounding will have sudden difficulties, as they crash from buildup of pain.

UPDATE, APRIL 7, 2010: "I talked to an old friend vet in Calif today who treated a case neurologically and had pain. He treated with Buprenorphine and said the dog was much more comfortable. And did well. I would suggest this as a post brain tap treatment to see if it helps with the pain. Buprenophine 0.005 - 0.03 mg/kg IV or IM or SQ . 2 to 4 times daily. Also comes under the names of Buprenex, Buprenor, or Tumgesic. Vets have access to this drug. Worth a try.

"I'm hearing of a large group of dogs that are having problems with lock jaw after being treated intrathecally. Do not know the cause. But, most of these cases go on to die or be euthanized. I think this needs to be put into the protocol as an exception. I know of no way to help this situation at this time."

Additional information, endorsed by Dr. Sears: "Also use valium orally or rectally. Between pain control and keeping them relaxed/sleeping for the first week, this helps them recover from the tap and seizures. For a 4 lb dog, we used 0.7ml up to three times a day of liquid valium--per treating vets tried both the cherry kid's oral and the IV valium in her rectum. I was given pre-filled syringes of buprenorpnine for a week--in a big jar, and several days of pre-filled syringes of valium plus a prescription was called into my local pharmacy."

The Brush Border Smear

Because distemper must be treated quickly, a fast diagnosis is essential. Often waiting for the results of a blood test may push the dog past the sixth day of treatment, after which the odds of saving the dog drop dramatically.

The best test for rapidly diagnosing acute, systemic distemper is to do what is called a brush border smear of the cells of the lining of the bladder. These cells always have inclusions if distemper is present. So, easy to collect, easy to stain (quick dip) and instantly diagnosed inclusions in these cells are carmine red and paranuclear. These inclusions will NOT be present in long term distemper cases.

Any medical person can tell you how to get cells from the bladder. Urinary catheter. Empty bladder, flush with saline and collect some of the last saline. Spin down the saline and remove the cells. Place on slide and dry stain with diff-quick. Very common stain used by most medics or lab people who use medical microscopy. Everyone? I should hope so. Very fast, very cheap, very accurate for diagnosis of distemper. If present, then distemper. If negative, then either kennel cough or respiratory herpes or toxoplasmosis.

Treatment Of Acute Upper Respiratory Disease

Tamiflu–Turns out some of these other viruses are extremely sensitive to this medication. I would recommend that 1 mg/lb be given twice daily for at lease 7 days. Should block most of the viruses we are discussing.

Antibiotics.–All these viruses cause inflammation in the lungs. (flu causes hemorrhagic pneumonia) All leave a BACTERIAL SECONDARY PNEUMONIA. My recommendation is

Penicillin -G and Baytril inj three times daily in older dogs 9 Mos or older for at least 10 days.

Penicillin -G and Chloromycetin (25 mg/lb) three times daily for 10 days in younger dogs. (Baytril causes joint problems in younger dogs)

Supportive fluids and feeding as necessary.

INDEX

END NOTES

[1] His complete protocols are in the appendix before the Index at the back of the book.

[2] He used Diff-Quik.

[3] When I do use a year in this book, it is because I am able to confirm it from another source.

[4] Adams JM, Snow HD. 1973. Viral Demyelinating Encephalitis And Old Dog Encephalitis: Possible Relationship To Distemper Measles, And Dermyelinating Disease Of Man. Calif. Vet. 27: 8-10

[5] Uhl, E. W., Kelderhouse, C., Buikstra, J., Blick, J. P., Bolon, B., and Hogan, R. J. (2019). New world origin of canine distemper: interdisciplinary insights. Int. J.Paleopathol. 24, 266–278. doi: 10.1016/j.ijpp.2018.12.007

[6] "Dog" AnimalResearch.info [Online]. Available: http://www.animalresearch.info/en/designing-research/research-animals/dog/. [January 2018].

[7] New England Anti-Vivisection Society. (2018). Laws and Regulations. [Online]. Available: http://www.neavs.org/research/laws. [Jan. 24, 2018]

[8] Singer, P. 2002. Animal Liberation. New York. Harper Collins pp. 25-94.

[9] Singer. p. 77.

[10] Singer p. 86.

[11] Malisow, C. (May 4, 2015) "Tens of Thousands of Dogs are Still Used in Laboratory Testing Every Year," Houston Press [Online] Available: http://www.houstonpress.com/news/tens-of-thousands-of-dogs-are-still-used-in-laboratory-testing-every-year-7400834. Jan. 24, 2018.

[12] http://www.humanesociety.org/issues/biomedical_research/qa/questions_answers.html

[13] Adams JM, Brown WJ, Snow HD, Lincoln SD, Sears Jr AW, Barenfus M, Holliday TA, Cremer NE, Lennette EH. 1975. Old Dog Encephalitis and Demyelinating Diseases in Man. Vet. Pathol. 12: 220-226

[14] Kapil S, Yeary T, 2011. Canine Distemper Spillover in Domestic Dogs from Urban Wildlife. Veterinary Clinics: Small Animal Practice, Volume 4 , Issue 6, pp. 1069-1086

[15] Riedel, Stefan. "Edward Jenner and the history of smallpox and vaccination." Proceedings (Baylor University. Medical Center) vol. 18,1 (2005): 21-5. doi:10.1080/08998280.2005.11928028

[16] "Dr Edward Jenner 1749 – 1823" Dr. Jenner's House Museum and Garden https://jennermuseum.com/ [Online] Available: https://drjennershouse.files.wordpress.com/2016/09/jenner-for-website2.pdf (Jan. 2018)

[17] Oldstone, Michael B.A., 2010, <u>Viruses, Plagues & History: Past, Present and Future.</u> Oxford University Press, p. 78.

[18] Jenner E. Observations on the Distemper in Dogs. 1809. Medico-Chirurgical Transactions. 1: 265-270.

[19] Oldstone. p. 16.

[20] Kirk, H. 1922, <u>Canine Distemper: It's Complications, Sequelae and Treatment.</u> London. Bailliére, Tindall and Cox, pp. 29-34.

[21] Ferry N. 1911. Etiology of canine distemper. Journal of Infectious Diseases 4, pp. 399–420.

M'Gowan JP. 1911. Some observations on a laboratory epidemic, principally among dogs and cats, in which the animals affected presented symptoms of the disease called "distemper." Journal of Pathology and Bacteriology 15, pp. 372 ff.

[22] Kirk, p. 66.

[23] Kirk, p. 61.

[24] Kirk, p. 156

[25] You can read the series here: http://www.museumofquackery.com/ephemera/oct7-01.htm

[26] Bresalier M, Worboys M. <u>'Saving the lives of our dogs': the development of canine distemper vaccine in interwar Britain.</u> Br J Hist Sci. 2014 Jun; 47(173 Pt 2):305-34. [Online]. Available: https://www.ncbi.nlm.nih.gov/pmc/articles/PMC4014013/pdf/S0007087413000344a.pdf

[27] By the 1970s, canine distemper had been classified as a morbillivirus, which grouped it with measles. Morbilliviruses are a genera of Paramyxoviridae, which also include Newcastle Disease, mumps and human parainfluenza. The group of paramyxoviruses also include Hendra virus, which attacks horses as well as their owners, and Nipah, which originates in flying foxes and can attack pigs and humans. In 1971, David Baltimore of MIT proposed a classification system which placed paramyxoviruses as a Class V virus with a single-stranded RNA.

[28] Kapil S, Yeary T, 2011. Canine Distemper Spillover in Domestic Dogs from Urban Wildlife. Veterinary Clinics: Small Animal Practice, Volume 4 , Issue 6, pp. 1069-1086.

[29] Kapil S, Yeary T, 2011. Canine Distemper Spillover in Domestic Dogs from Urban Wildlife. Veterinary Clinics: Small Animal Practice, Volume 4 , Issue 6, pp. 1069-1086.

[30] Kapil S, Yeary T, 2011. Canine Distemper Spillover in Domestic Dogs from Urban Wildlife. Veterinary Clinics: Small Animal Practice, Volume 4 , Issue 6, pp. 1069-1086.

[31] Babcock, S., Jack, D., Lacroix, C. , Pfeiffer, C., Thomas, J., The American Veterinary Medical Law Association White Paper, "Vaccine Liability Issues for Veterinarians," Editor: Elizabeth Settles, [Online]. Available: https://avmla.org/wp-content/uploads/2011/09/Vaccine_Liability_AVMLA.pdf. March 2009, p. 10.

[32] Babcock et al., p. 10.

[33] Bacock et al. p. 11

[34] Babcock et al. p. 10.

[35] Babcock et al. p. 13.

[36] Gloyd, J. Protecting your practice and the food animal industry JAVMA (Vol. 190, No. 1) p. 34, Jan. 1987

[37] May, K. 2018, Extralabel Drug Use and AMDUCA: FAQ, American Veterinary Medical Association, [Online]. Available: https://www.avma.org/KB/Resources/FAQs/Pages/ELDU-and-AMDUCA-FAQs.aspx

[38] Gloyd, J. p. 32.

[39] Oldstone, p. 79.

[40] You can still read the original story, starting here: https://edbond.com/distemper_first.html

[41] http://www.edbond.com

[42] We now have nearly 5,000 Facebook followers.

[43] Hunter's name was later changed to Sophie, and as of November 2017 was reported to be "doing great, almost 10 years old and full of life and energy."

[44] "Icy, a distemper dog in Philippines, successfully treated" KindHeartsInAction YouTube channel, https://youtu.be/2Vjkm3nGV_s

[45] She later told me Kaliber had a positive distemper test.

[46] "Kaliber treated for neurologic distemper," Kind Hearts In Action, [Online]. Available: http://www.kindheartsinaction.com

[47] Kapil S, Yeary T, 2011. Canine Distemper Spillover in Domestic Dogs from Urban Wildlife. Veterinary Clinics: Small Animal Practice, Volume 4 , Issue 6, pp. 1069-1086.

[48] Kapil S, Yeary T, 2011. Canine Distemper Spillover in Domestic Dogs from Urban Wildlife. Veterinary Clinics: Small Animal Practice, Volume 4 , Issue 6, pp. 1069-1086.

[49] Bresalier and Worboys, p. 318

[50] Summers B, Greisen H, Appel M, January 1984. Canine distemper encephalomyelitis: Variation with virus strain. Journal of Comparative Pathology, Volume 94, Issue 1, pp. 65-75

[51] Randall R, Russell W. 1991. Paramyxovirus Persistence Consequences for Host and Virus. In Kingsbury D, editor. The Paramyxoviruses. Springer Science & Business Media. pp. 299-322.

[52] Kapil S, Yeary T, 2011. Canine Distemper Spillover in Domestic Dogs from Urban Wildlife. Veterinary Clinics: Small Animal Practice, Volume 4 , Issue 6, pp. 1069-1086.

[53] Kapil S, Yeary T, 2011. Canine Distemper Spillover in Domestic Dogs from Urban Wildlife. Veterinary Clinics: Small Animal Practice, Volume 4 , Issue 6, pp. 1069-1086.

[54] https://cwhl.vet cited in May 2020.

[55] The appearance of the slides has been adjusted for publication in a book.

[56] 1 CC is equal to a milliliter.

[57] Tisoncik JR, Korth MJ, Simmons CP, Farrar J, Martin TR, Katze MG. 2012. Into the Eye of the Cytokine Storm. Microbiology and Molecular Biology Reviews. MMBR;76(1):16-32. doi:10.1128/MMBR.05015-11.

[58] Dr. Sears' notes on treating parvovirus: http://www.kindheartsinaction.com

[59] Kapil S, Yeary T, 2011. Canine Distemper Spillover in Domestic Dogs from Urban Wildlife. Veterinary Clinics: Small Animal Practice, Volume 4 , Issue 6, pp. 1069-1086.

[60] Kapil S, Yeary T, 2011. Canine Distemper Spillover in Domestic Dogs from Urban Wildlife. Veterinary Clinics: Small Animal Practice, Volume 4 , Issue 6, pp. 1069-1086.

[61] Kapil S, Yeary T, 2011. Canine Distemper Spillover in Domestic Dogs from Urban Wildlife. Veterinary Clinics: Small Animal Practice, Volume 4 , Issue 6, pp. 1069-1086.

[62] Kapil S, Yeary T, 2011. Canine Distemper Spillover in Domestic Dogs from Urban Wildlife. Veterinary Clinics: Small Animal Practice, Volume 4 , Issue 6, pp. 1069-1086.

[63] Adams JM, Brown WJ, Snow HD, Lincoln SD, Sears Jr AW, Barenfus M, Holliday TA, Cremer NE, Lennette EH. 1975. Old Dog Encephalitis and Demyelinating Diseases in Man. Vet. Pathol. 12: 220-226

[64] Randall R, Russell W. 1991. Paramyxovirus Persistence Consequences for Host and Virus. In Kingsbury D, editor. The Paramyxoviruses. Springer Science & Business Media. pp. 299-322.

[65] Mentis A, Dardiotis E, Grigoriadis N, Petinaki E, Hadjigeorgiou G. ePub May 23, 2017. Viruses and endogenous retroviruses in multiple sclerosis: From correlation to causation. Acta Neurologica Scandinavica 2017 Dec;136(6):606-616. doi: 10.1111/ane.12775.

[66] Csatary L. 1971. Viruses in the treatment of cancer. Lancet; Oct 9;2(7728):825.

[67] Csatary L, Bakács T. 1999. Use of Newcastle Disease Virus Vaccine (MTH-68/H) in a Patient With High-grade Glioblastoma. JAMA;281(17):1588-1589

[68] Newcastle Disease Virus (PDQ®)–Health Professional Version, National Cancer Institute at the National Institutes of Health, Updated: August 22, 2018 [Online]. Available: https://www.cancer

[69] Tayeb S, Zakay-Rones Z, Panet A. 2015. Therapeutic potential of oncolytic Newcastle disease virus: a critical review. Oncolytic Virother. Mar 27;4:49-62. doi: 10.2147/OV.S78600. eCollection 2015.

[70] Sánchez, D.; Pelayo, R.; Medina, L.A.; Vadillo, E.; Sánchez, R.; Núñez, L.; Cesarman-Maus, G.; Sarmiento-Silva, R.E. Newcastle Disease Virus: Potential Therapeutic Application for Human and Canine Lymphoma. Viruses 2016, 8, 3.

[71] Alonso M, Jiang H, Gomez-Manzano C, Fueyo J. 2012. Targeting brain tumor stem cells with oncolytic adenoviruses. Methods Mol Biol. 2012;797:111-25. doi: 10.1007/978-1-61779-340-0_9.

[72] Notes and photos from Dr. Sears on diagnosing and treating respiratory herpes and other diseases can be found here: http://www.kindheartsinaction.com

[73] For full description of both treatments, go to: http://www.kindheartsinaction.com/archives/2963

[74] Soave, Orlando Animals, the Law and Veterinary Medicine Lanham, New York, Oxford, Austin & Winfield Pub p. 18.

[75] "HOUSTON: Max fights distemper" KindHeartsInAction YouTube channel [Online]. Available: https://youtu.be/DO-GaEvZYbY

[76] http://skeptivet.blogspot.com/2010/01/canine-distemper

[77] "Muttu Made It!!" Jan. 28, 2010, Kind Hearts In Action [Online]. Available: http://www.kindheartsinaction.com

[78] You can now watch the lecture for free here: http://www.kindheartsinaction.com

[79] "Distemper dogs saved in Hungary" Dec. 17, 2010, Kind Hearts In Action, [Online]. Available: http://www.kindheartsinaction.com

[80] Enzyme-linked immunosorbent assay

[81] "Hector gets NDV spinal tap" February 20, 2011 http://www.kindheartsinaction.com

[82] Kay, N., Speaking for Spot: Be the Advocate Your Dog Needs to Live a Happy Healthy Longer Life CreateSpace Independent Publishing Platform, 2011, P. 15.

[83] "Distemper dog saved in South Africa" Dec. 5, 2011, Kind Hearts In Action, [Online]. Available: http://www.kindheartsinaction.com

[84] "Story failed to note vaccine for distemper" Ithaca Journal, Ithaca N.Y. Jan. 31, 2012. p6.

[85] Their last names omitted because I was unable to reconnect with them before publication.

[86] It remained available until October 2016 when I was no longer able to keep up with the updates required for the iOS systems. My game has now been renamed MetaCheckers and is available as a real-world board game through Amazon. www.metacheckers.com

[87] #stealthhistory, later it became #mockhistory

[88] Yes, this book! Look at the appendix in the back for the data on Project Carré.

[89] Name omitted at her request.

[90] You can watch them all here: https://www.youtube.com/user/25swagger/videos

[91] Zamarin D, Palese P. 2012. Oncolytic Newcastle Disease Virus for Cancer Therapy Future Microbiology. Future Medicine Ltd. 2012;7(3):347-367 Available from https://www.medscape.com/viewarticle/760002_1

[92] Zamarin D, Palese P. 2012. Oncolytic Newcastle Disease Virus for Cancer Therapy Future Microbiology. Future Medicine Ltd. 2012;7(3):347-367 Available from https://www.medscape.com/viewarticle/760002_1

[93] Swaminathan, N. Aug. 8, 2008, "Viruses: They're alive, and they can infect each other" Scientific American [Online]. Available: https://blogs.scientificamerican.com/news-blog/viruses-theyre-alive-and-they-can-i-2008-08-08/

[94] Paff ML, Nuismer SL, Ellington A, Molineux IJ, Bull JJ. (2016) Virus wars: using one virus to block the spread of another. PeerJ 4:e2166 https://doi.org/10.7717/peerj.2166

[95] "The Nobel Prize in Physiology or Medicine 2006, Andrew Z. Fire, Craig C. Mello" Nobelprize.org. [Online]. Available: https://www.nobelprize.org/nobel_prizes/medicine/laureates/2006/press.html

[96] In 2018, a drug using RNAi gene-silencing to fight disease won regulatory approval. https://vis.sciencemag.org/breakthrough2018/finalists/#rna-drug

[97] http://www.imdb.com/title/tt1598778/

[98] https://www.cdc.gov/coronavirus/2019-ncov/cases-updates/summary.html

[99] Oldstone, pp. 202-3.

[100] Ma W, Kahn R, Richt J. 2008. The pig as a mixing vessel for influenza viruses: Human and veterinary implications. J Mol Genet Med. 2008 Nov 27;3(1):158-66.

[101] Pringle C. 1991. The Genetics of Paramyxoviruses. In Kingsbury D, editor. The Paramyxoviruses. Springer Science & Business Media. pp. 1-40.

[102] Samal S, editor. 2011. The Biology of Paramyxoviruses. Norfolk UK. Caister Academic Press

[103] Pringle C. 1991. The Genetics of Paramyxoviruses. In Kingsbury D, editor. The Paramyxoviruses. Springer Science & Business Media. pp. 1-40.

[104] Song Q, Cao Y, Li Q, Gu M, Zhong L, Hu S, Wan H, Liu X. 2011. Artificial Recombination May Influence the Evolutionary Analysis of Newcastle Disease Virus . Journal of Virology. 2011;85(19):10409-10414. doi:10.1128/JVI.00544-11.

[105] Han GZ, Liu XP, Li SS. 2008. Cross-species recombination in the haemagglutinin gene of canine distemper virus. Virus Res 2008;136(1-2):198–201.

[106] But a study did come out in 2014 proposing the possibility for dogs to mix influenza virus. "Infection and pathogenesis of canine, equine and human influenza viruses in canine tracheas." Gaelle Gonzalez, John F. Marshall, Joanna Morrell, David Robb, John W. McCauley, Daniel R. Perez, Colin R. Parrish and Pablo R. Murcia, Journal of Virology, June 2014

[107] McCullough, B. 1972. Interferon Response in Cats. The Journal of Infectious Diseases, 125(2), 174-177. Available from http://www.jstor.org/stable/30111561

[108] Tsai SC, Appel MJ. 1979. Interferon induction in dogs. Am J Vet Res. 1979 Mar;40(3):356-61.

[109] Faustman D, Wang L, Okubo Y, Burger D, Ban L, Man G, Zheng H, Schoenfeld D, Pompei R, Avruch J, Nathan D. August 2012. Proof-of-Concept, Randomized, Controlled Clinical Trial of Bacillus-Calmette-Guerin for Treatment of Long-Term Type 1 Diabetes. PLoS ONE, Volume 7, Issue 8, e41756

[110] Name and university omitted because this professor did not respond to later phone calls or emails.

[111] http://www.maddiesfund.org/maddies-story.htm

[112] She asked that her real name not be used. Lizzy is the English name she goes by.

[113] Schubert T, Clemmons R, Miles S, Draper W. 2013. The use of botulinum toxin for the treatment of generalized myoclonus in a dog. J Am Anim Hosp Assoc. 2013 Mar-Apr;49(2):122-7. doi: 10.5326/JAAHA-MS-5786. Epub 2013 Jan 16.

[114] "Everything Shelters Need to Know About Canine Distemper" Maddie's Fund Education YouTube channel https://youtu.be/LekbdFETyEw

[115] http://www.maddiesfund.org/topic-shelter-medicine.htm

[116] I made repeated attempts to contact Dr. Crawford without success. I understand why she would not want to respond because I have no standing in the veterinary community. I decided to go ahead and post these excerpts as fair use of public comments about the campaign to save dogs from distemper.

[117] "Treating Canine Distemper Virus" Oct 2, 2012, Maddie's Fund Education YouTube channel [Online]. Available: https://youtu.be/rq-mwDrJVE4

[118] http://www.kindheartsinaction.com

[119] http://www.herald-dispatch.com/features_entertainment/kansas-treatment-has-dog-celebrating-second-new-year/article_53cd1d4e-33fd-5af2-9a91-459991ebf4d7.html

[120] http://www.kindheartsinaction.com

[121] http://www.kindheartsinaction.com

[122] It reorganized as MetaDreams LLC in 2019.

[123] "First Use of NDV serum in Bulgaria"
https://www.kindheartsinaction.com